# Drug Use in Respiratory Disease

# Drug Use in Respiratory Disease

Edited by
*J. D. Wilson*

WILLIAMS & WILKINS and ASSOCIATES PTY LIMITED
Sydney • Baltimore • London

# Drug Use in Respiratory Disease

Drug Use in Respiratory Disease

Includes index.
ISBN 0 86433 029 4.

1. Respiratory agents. 2. Respiratory organs — Diseases — Chemotherapy. I. Wilson, J.D. (J. Douglas).

615'.72

WILLIAMS & WILKINS and ASSOCIATES PTY LIMITED
43 Herbert Street, Artarmon, N.S.W. 2064, Australia

Printed in Australia by Hogbin, Poole (Printers) Pty. Ltd., Redfern

# Preface

In recent years so many new drugs have been developed to treat respiratory diseases, and so many clinical studies of various drug combinations have been published that now is an appropriate time to present an overview of this important area.

The text of *Drug Use in Respiratory Disease* assembles a group of international authorities who give their views and concepts of the current state of the basic pharmacology of drugs used in respiratory disease and a series of reviews of their role in treatment. The book's aim is to be topical and practical. Space constraints have required some limitation of the subjects covered (for example, upper respiratory tract diseases are not included), while details of the investigations, natural history and non-drug aspects of treatment are kept brief. But drug treatment is the prime role of this text so discussion is extensive and well annotated to serve as a permanent reference.

The first eight chapters address the pharmacology of common respiratory drugs, and include principles of pharmacokinetics in lung disease and modes of drug delivery. The second section examines various major respiratory problems including pneumonia, bronchial asthma, acute respiratory distress syndrome, non-infective parenchymal diseases, chronic bronchitis and emphysema and respiratory failure. As adverse effects of drugs are not uncommonly directed towards the lungs this topic is extensively reviewed by Allen Cooper and Richard Matthay at Yale to complete the book.

One central purpose of this book was to invite writers from a number of different countries to provide a more international perspective. A consequence of this policy has been a little duplication, which has been left to enable individual chapters to be read alone; in addition, some differences of emphasis emerge. With optimal practices of many aspects of drug therapy in respiratory disease still in the process of being established, these differences serve accurately to demonstrate the current state of treatment.

J. D. Wilson
Riyadh, Saudi Arabia
June 1986

# Preface

# Contributors

*Asher, M. Innes* *BSc, MB, ChB, FRACP*
Senior Lecturer, Department of Paediatrics, University of Auckland, Auckland, New Zealand; and Consultant Paediatrician, Auckland Hospital, Auckland, New Zealand.

*Baker, G.J.* *BSc(Med), MB, BS, FRACP*
Fellow in Thoracic Medicine, Royal North Shore Hospital, Sydney Australia.

*Berend, N.* *MD, BS, FRACP, FCCP*
Associate Professor of Medicine, University of Sydney; Head, Department of Thoracic Medicine, Royal North Shore Hospital, Sydney, Australia.

*Clarke, Stewart W.* *MD, FRCP*
Department of Thoracic Medicine, The Royal Free Hospital, Hampstead, London NW3 2QG, England.

*Cochrane, G.M.* *BSc(Physiology), MB, BS, FRCP*
Consultant Physician, Guy's Hospital, St Thomas' Street, London SE1 9RT, England.

*Cooper J. Allen D. Jr* *MD*
Assistant Professor of Medicine, Pulmonary Section, West Haven VAMC and Yale University School of Medicine, West Haven, Connecticut 06516, USA.

*Crompton, G.K.* *MB, FRCPE*
Consultant Physician, Northern General Hospital; and Part-time Senior Lecturer, Departments of Medicine (Western General Hospital) and Respiratory Diseases, University of Edinburgh, Scotland.

*Davidson, Bruce* *MD, MPH*
Assistant Professor of Medicine; and Director, Pulmonary Procedures Unit, Jefferson Medical College, Thomas Jefferson University, Philadelphia, Pennsylvania, USA.

*Glanville, Allan R.* *MB, BS, FRACP*
Fellow in Heart Lung Transplantation, Stanford University Medical Center, California, USA.

*Greening, Andrew P.* *BSc, MB, FRCPE*
Consultant Physician, Northern General Hospital; and Part-time Senior Lecturer, Departments of Medicine (Western General Hospital) and Respiratory Diseases, University of Edinburgh, Scotland.

*Hodson, Margaret E.* *MD, MSc, FRCP, DA*
Reader in Respiratory Medicine and Honorary Consultant Physician, Sub-Dean, Teaching, The Cardiothoracic Institute, British Postgraduate Medical Federation, The University of London, SW3 6HP, England.

*Horne, N.W.* *MB, FRCPE*
Formerly Senior Lecturer in Respiratory Medicine, University of Edinburgh; and Consultant Physician, Chest Unit, City Hospital, Edinburgh Scotland.

*Kolbe, John*
Department of Medicine, The University of Auckland, Auckland, New Zealand.

*Löfdahl, Claes-Göran MD, FCCP, PhD*
Associate Professor, Department of Pulmonary Medicine, Renstromska Hospital, S-402 64 Goteborg, Sweden.

*McLean, A.J. MB, BS(Hons 1), BSc(Med), PhD, FRACP*
Consultant Physician, Clinical Research Unit and Monash University Department of Medicine; Director, Department of Clinical Pharmacology, Alfred Hospital, Prahran, Victoria 3181, Australia.

*McDonnell, Timothy J. MB, MRCPI*
Cardiovascular Pulmonary Research Laboratory and Webb-Waring Lung Institute, University of Colorado Health Sciences Center, Denver, Colorado 80262, USA.

*Marlin, Graham E. MD, BS, FRACP*
Senior Specialist, Respiratory Unit, Concord Hospital, Sydney, Australia.

*Matthay, Richard A. MD*
Professor of Medicine and Associate Director, Pulmonary Section, Department of Internal Medicine, Yale University School of Medicine, New Haven, Connecticut 06519, USA.

*Newman, Stephen P.*
Department of Thoracic Medicine, The Royal Free Hospital, Hampstead, London NW3 2QG, England.

*Petty, Thomas L. MD*
Professor of Medicine and Director, Webb-Waring Lung Institute, University of Colorado Health Sciences Center, Denver, Colorado 80262, USA.

*Rothwell, Richard P.G. MB, ChB, FRCP, FRACP, FCCP*
Respiratory Physician, Waikato Hospital, Hamilton, New Zealand; and Clinical Lecturer, University of Auckland School of Medicine, New Zealand.

*Ruffin, R.E. MB, BS(Hons II), BSc(Hons), MD, FRACP*
Senior Lecturer, Flinders University, Senior Staff Specialist in Respiratory Medicine, Flinders Medical Centre, Adelaide, South Australia, Australia.

*Rutland, Jonathan BSc, MB, BS, FRACP*
Visiting Thoracic Physician, Concord Hospital and Lidcombe Hospital, Sydney, Australia.

*Seale, J. Paul MB, BS, PhD, FRACP*
Associate Professor in Clinical Pharmacology, Department of Pharmacology, University of Sydney; and Honorary Physician, Department of Thoracic Medicine, Royal Prince Alfred Hospital, Sydney, Australia.

*Sharpe, D.N.* *MD, FRACP, FACC*
Associate Professor of Medicine, Department of Medicine, University of Auckland School of Medicine; and Cardiologist, Auckland Hospital, New Zealand.

*Svedmyr, Nils* *MD, PhD*
Professor, Department of Clinical Pharmacology, Sahlgrenska University Hospital, S-413 45 Goteborg, Sweden.

*Voelkel, Norbert F.* *MD*
Cardiovascular Pulmonary Research Laboratory and Webb-Waring Lung Institute, University of Colorado Health Sciences Center, Denver, Colorado 80262, USA.

*Ward, Helen E.* *MB, BS, PhD, FRACP*
NHMRC Australian Post-doctoral Fellow, University of Sydney; and Clinical Assistant, Royal North Shore Hospital, Sydney, Australia

*Watt, S.J.*
Department of Medicine, University of Aberdeen, Foresterhill, Aberdeen AB9 22B, Scotland.

*Whelan, Anthony J.* *MB, BS*
Thoracic Registrar, Concord Hospital, Sydney, Australia.

*Wilson, J. Douglas* *MB, ChB, PhD, FRACP, FRCPA*
Professor, Department of Pathology, College of Medicine, King Saud University, Riyadh 11472, Saudi Arabia.

# Contents

# Chapter 1

# Pulmonary Pharmacology

*R.E. Ruffin and A.J. McLean*

In the past decade there has been increasing awareness of the need to study drug usage in patients with specific organ dysfunction other than hepatic and renal disorders. Respiratory disease was one of the earliest examples considered with a number of mechanisms recognised as potentially contributing to altered systemic drug requirements.[1]

In this review we update the evidence for alteration in requirement of systemically administered drugs in patients with respiratory disease and the mechanisms which may be involved. However, the major element of the review deals with inhaled therapies and the evidence that there is altered requirement for aerosol medications in respiratory disease as a result of altered handling and response.

## Respiratory Disease and Systemic Medications

### General Therapeutic Considerations

Prominent among the determinants of therapeutic outcome are drug compliance, bioavailability and drug interactions, issues not normally considered of particular importance in patients with respiratory disease. A recent computer-based study in our hospital[2,3] indicated that patients with chronic respiratory disease were heavily over-represented among patients receiving extreme 'polypharmacy' (more than 10 different medications), comprising 100% of examples of polypharmacy in the age-group below 30 years and more than 20% of all other age-groups up to 70 years of age. Accordingly, polypharmacy with consequent non-compliance and adverse effects might be considered a practical therapeutic problem with particular application to patients with respiratory disease.

Issues of bioavailability are not recognised as particular problems in patients with respiratory disease; however, multiple drug therapy adds an unknown element to this consideration.

### Drugs with Altered Systemic Effects and Handling in Respiratory Disease

The drugs involved include agents of therapeutic importance commonly used in patients with respiratory disease. Because of prior review[1,4] and little change in the data base, drugs whose handling is known to be altered in respiratory disease (or whose handling can be predicted to be changed) are listed in Table 1.1.

Theophylline remains the drug whose clearance is most commonly affected to a major degree with important clinical consequences.[5-9]

*Table 1.1* Drugs and respiratory disease

| |
|---|
| *Systemic Handling Known to be Influenced by Respiratory Disease* |
| Aminoglycoside antibiotics |
| Digoxin |
| Ephedrine |
| Procainamide |
| Theophylline |
| Tolbutamide |
| *Systemic Handling Expected to be Influenced by Respiratory Disease* (representative examples only) |
| Ampicillin |
| Baclofen |
| Carbenicillin |
| Cefamandole |
| Chlormethiazole |
| Cimetidine |
| Clonidine |
| Frusemide |
| Hydrochlorothiazide |
| Labetalol |
| Lignocaine (lidocaine) |
| Morphine |
| Pethidine (meperidine) |
| Phenacetin |
| Verapamil |

## Mechanisms Underlying Altered Drug Handling

Our understanding of the pathological changes and physiological deficits in chronic respiratory disease is somewhat changed from previous reviews of altered drug handling.[1,4] Hepatic and renal perfusion are considered to be linked directly and indirectly to the physical or physiological changes resulting from pulmonary disease.[1] The single instance where there has been a major advance in knowledge of mechanism is in the area of alteration in plasma protein binding.

Conventionally, plasma protein binding of substrate has been considered to constrain the clearance of only those substrates with a relatively low intrinsic clearance ($Cl_I$). Recently this area of clearance theory has been re-evaluated,[10] and it is now clear that drugs with intermediate to high values of $Cl_I$ can show proportionately higher changes in clearance when protein binding is changed (Figure 1.1).

The examples shown in Figure 1.1 include a model compound with a $Cl_I$ near that of propranolol (1a) and model-dependent simulations together with in-vitro experimental data for diazepam (1b). These examples illustrate the dramatic changes in extraction fraction (E) and hence clearance which are possible with both high and low clearance drugs when there is alteration in protein binding.

Despite the importance of the topic, most studies reporting changes in clearance in subjects with respiratory disease have not estimated plasma protein binding of drugs. Studies of this type are needed to resolve issues of mechanism related to important drugs such as theophylline.[1]

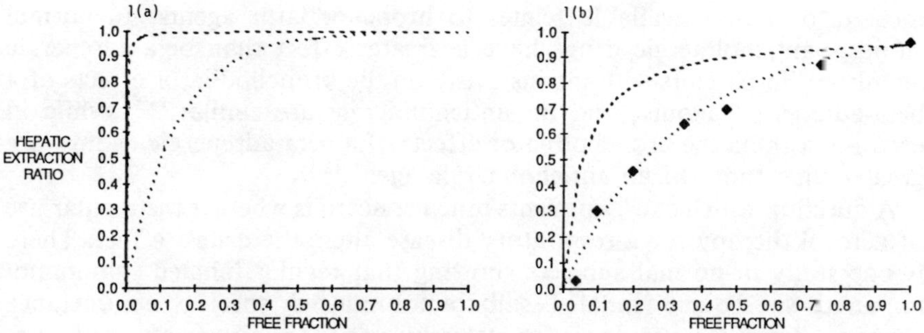


*Figure 1.1* Changes in extraction fraction and hence clearance in (1a) a model compound with a clearance near that of propranolol, and (1b) model-dependent simulations and in-vitro experimental data for diazepam. The continuous lines indicate relationships associated with the sinusoidal perfusion model, while the discontinuous lines indicate the venous equilibrium model.

Tissue binding of drugs has received little attention; however, this may be of special significance in respiratory disease. Mendelman and co-workers,[11] have shown that the sputum of patients with cystic fibrosis binds significant quantities of tobramycin so that bioassay of drug effectiveness does not parallel apparent accumulation in sputum after systemic dosing.

## Respiratory Disease and Medications Administered by Aerosol Inhalation

### General Therapeutic Considerations

Respiratory disease, dermal disease and some elements of gastrointestinal disease respond to topical therapies which remain substantially external to the systemic circulation. In respiratory disease, application of this principle represents one of the major recent advances in the field.

In order for inhaled drug therapy to be effective in respiratory diseases, drugs must reach the site(s) of action: bacteria in the airway lumen, airway mucosa or alveolar spaces; receptors on cilia; receptors on effector cells such as mast cells in either the airway lumen or airway mucosa; or receptors on airway smooth muscle. Therefore inhaled drugs must be able to enter the lower respiratory tract and penetrate to the appropriate level. The drugs must be deposited on the mucous blanket, then penetrate the mucous blanket, enter the periciliary fluid, pass through the respiratory epithelium to enter the mucosa and ultimately reach either mucosal effector cells or airway smooth muscle. It is possible that some of the inhaled drugs may have an action on effector cells within alveolar spaces and the interstitium, but this will not be considered further.

### Altered Aerosol Drug Effect in Respiratory Disease

Changes have been observed in inhaled drug effect in patients with respiratory disease. These appear to be a function of both the drug and the disease state;

most information available relates to bronchodilator agents. In normal subjects anticholinergic drugs have a greater effect than beta-adrenergic agonists;[12] in patients with intrinsic asthma the bronchodilator effects of a beta-adrenergic agonist and an anticholinergic are similar,[13,14] while in extrinsic asthma the bronchodilator effects of a beta-adrenergic agonist are greater than those of an anticholinergic agent.[13,14]

A question which causes patients much concern is whether the regular use of aerosol therapy for a respiratory disease alters the drug's effect. There is one study in normal subjects showing that regular inhaled salbutamol impaired subsequent inhaled salbutamol-induced specific conductance change.[15] There is no evidence for tachyphylaxis to the airway effect of beta-agonist aerosols in asthmatics,[16] although tachyphylaxis is observed in the skeletal muscle response to regular beta-agonist aerosols (reduced tremor). It has been suggested that oral beta-agonists can cause airway tachyphylaxis,[17] presumably by down-regulation of beta-receptors with chronic exposure to high doses of a beta-agonist. It has recently been reported that patients chronically inhaling an anticholinergic bronchodilator had rebound hyper-responsiveness to muscarinic stimulation for two to three days after ceasing therapy.[18] Despite this finding, there was no evidence of tolerance developing to the bronchodilator effect or to the protective effect against methacholine-induced bronchoconstriction.

Disease severity may also alter drug responsiveness. It has been recognised for many years that response to a bronchodilator aerosol is dependent on the initial degree of airflow obstruction[19] — the greater the obstruction the less the response. Moderate obstruction results in a larger response, and maximal obstruction obviously allows only a small response.

Clearly alterations in the biological basis of drug response could be involved in these changes; however, altered disposition must be considered in parallel.

## Administration and Disposition of Aerosol Medications

### *Aerosol Versus Systemic Administration*

Despite some observations interpreted to the contrary,[20] it is generally accepted that inhaled medications used in asthma, chronic bronchitis, chronic obstructive airways disease and cystic fibrosis act directly on lung elements. This assumption is strongly supported in part by data from animal studies.

A study in rats and mice compared the distribution of tritiated terbutaline given intravenously or via the respiratory tract.[21] Intravenous terbutaline yielded lung concentrations paralleling those found in the blood, whereas when terbutaline was administered by intratracheal instillation, the radioactivity in the lung exceeded that in the blood and was still present in the lung eight hours later. Almost all the radioactivity in the lung after intratracheal instillation was shown to be unchanged terbutaline; the lung/serum concentration ratio of unchanged terbutaline two minutes after intratracheal instillation was 54, rising to 160 at 2.25 hours after administration. The comparable study cannot be performed in man; however, drug distribution in human lungs has been studied in limited situations following administration of drugs via the respiratory tract. Laros et al[22] examined the lung tissue and blood of two patients undergoing lung resection for carcinoma some 45 minutes after the administration of tritiated fenoterol by metered dose inhaler. They found a slightly greater amount in the lung tissue as compared to plasma (wet weight of tissue compared to volume of plasma), but the site of distribution in lung tissue was not examined.

*Required Distribution of Inhaled Drug Within the Airways*

The required site(s) of deposition of inhaled agents to generate optimal effects depends on the nature of the agent and the distribution of receptor sites. Physiological responses in asthmatics to aerosols preferentially depositing beta-adrenergic agents,[23] or conventional aerosols[12,24,25] suggested uniform distribution of beta-adrenoreceptors throughout the airway, but concentration of muscarinic receptors in larger airways; a pattern of receptor distribution confirmed using autoradiographic techniques in animals.[26,27] These findings indicate that aerosols should deliver beta-agonists widely throughout the airways, while requirements for anticholinergic delivery are not so stringent. Sodium cromoglycate needs to enter the lower respiratory tract to interact with mast cells in the airway lumen and mucosa (see discussion in Chapter 7).

*Determinants of Aerosol Handling*

The principles of aerosol handling will be more fully examined in Chapter 2, but a brief review is needed here. The entry of aerosolised drugs into the lower respiratory tract of patients is dependent on factors which are aerosol-related (aerosol particle size, aerosol particle hygroscopicity, and aerosol particle velocity) and factors which are patient-related (inspiratory flow rate, degree of airflow obstruction, period of breath holding, and the patient's general technique for inhaling drugs).

Aerosol particle size needs to be in the range of 0.5 to 5μm to deposit in the lower respiratory tract.[28] Particles smaller than this tend to behave as gases and move with respiratory tidal flow; particles larger than this do not penetrate into the lower respiratory tract.[29] Particles which do not enter the lower respiratory tract do not have any therapeutic affect in asthma as instanced below.

1.Gargling and swallowing a dose of 500μg of fenoterol did not have any therapeutic effect in asthmatics, whereas 200μg of inhaled fenoterol caused a large degree of bronchodilatation.[30]

2. In a comparison of the effects of two sizes of sodium cromoglycate aerosols in protecting against exercise-induced asthma, larger particles of 10 to 12μm diameter gave little protective effect compared to a large protective effect of 2μm diameter particles.[31]

Modern metered dose inhalers (MDIs) contain solid particles of drug (milled to 5μm range) in suspension in the freon propellant with a dispersal agent to minimise clumping. In these devices the particle size is relatively fixed. However, these devices do discharge large droplets of propellant containing one or more particles of drug and the propellant must evaporate to leave the solid particles only, which may take up to several seconds. In jet nebulisers the size of the aerosols produced is widely variable and there is an inverse relationship to air or oxygen flow rate through the nebuliser.[32] There is a need to optimise the flow rates for these nebulisers to enable production of aerosols in the therapeutic size range.

Aerosol particle hygroscopicity will determine the rate of change of aerosol size in the humid environment of the respiratory tract. Particles which are small enough to penetrate into the lower respiratory tract may absorb water, increase in size and therefore deposit more proximally in the respiratory tract. This problem occurs more frequently with the powder aerosols than with nebulised liquid aerosols. Kim et al[33] showed that the size of sodium cromoglycate particles increased by 1.8 to 2.8 times when measured in air of 90% relative humidity compared to dry air.

Increase in aerosol particle velocity causes more proximal deposition of aerosol particles. The high velocity of aerosols from MDIs (more than 30m/s) causes impaction of much of the dose in the oropharynx and upper airways. In any respiratory disease it is therefore appropriate to use MDIs by a technique away from the mouth, or to introduce a spacer device to slow the particles and allow the propellant to evaporate. In the case of inhaled beclomethasone a spacer device diminishes the risk of developing oral candidiasis.[34] Positive pressure devices increase aerosol particle velocity and also promote upper airway and proximal deposition of aerosol with high losses in the delivery tubing.[35]

### *Drug Diffusion through Lung*

Drugs pass from the lumen through the mucous blanket, periciliary fluid and the mucosa to reach airway smooth muscle or mucosal mast cells. Drugs must solubilise otherwise they would be trapped in the mucous blanket and swept proximally by the ciliary clearance mechanism. The process of passage through the mucous blanket and mucosa may occur as a result of passive diffusion or there may be active mechanisms for some agents involving carrier protein. A saturable carrier-type transport has been proposed for some of the absorption of sodium cromoglycate.[36]

The process of transfer of drugs is rapid. Following inhalation of 800μg of inhaled salbutamol from an MDI, tachycardia occurs within five minutes.[37] Instillation of tritiated salbutamol into airways[38] or inhalation of tritiated terbutaline aerosol[39] leads to detectable levels of the labelled drug in plasma within a few minutes.

Accordingly it can be concluded that the transfer of drug by diffusion from lumen to tissue occurs rapidly in normal subjects and in patients with stable asthma.

### *Pulmonary Drug Clearance*

The lung contains a variety of enzyme systems which could be involved in the metabolism of drugs or agents arriving in the lung by the airways or the circulation.[40] Catechol-orthomethyl transferase is present in the lung and can methylate natural catecholamines and isoprenaline, but has no effect on the newer synthetic beta2-adrenergic agonists such as salbutamol, fenoterol, and terbutaline. This lack of metabolism accounts for the observed longer duration of effect of the newer agents compared to isoprenaline (isoproterenol). Other commonly used inhaled agents, such as sodium cromoglycate[41] and budesonide,[42] also seem not to be metabolised directly in the lung, but beclomethasone dipropionate is hydrolysed rapidly by human lung homogenate to beclomethasone 17-alphapropionate.[43]

The lung has the capacity to actively take up some substances from the blood flowing through the pulmonary circulation.[44] These substances include catecholamines such as noradrenaline (norepinephrine).[44] Animal studies have shown that lung extraction/uptake of terbutaline in single-pass perfusion experiments is low.[45]

### *Changes in Aerosol Drug Handling in Pulmonary Disease*

A variety of changes in disease can limit the effectiveness and use of aerosols so that optimal delivery cannot be achieved. Thus oral or systemic administration is required.[46]

The presence of disease does not appear to alter the distribution of receptors. In asthmatics the beta-adrenoreceptor agonists have an effect on all airways[23,25] and anticholinergic agents appear to have their main effects on central airways.[25] Respiratory diseases do have the potential for altering receptor numbers or modulating receptor enzyme systems. Evidence for this comes from in-vitro animal studies in which endogenous proteinases may inhibit the function of the beta2-adrenoreceptor-adenylate cyclase system in the rat lung,[47] and that histamine reduces the number of beta2-adrenoreceptors in guinea pig lung membranes.[48] Inflammation in the lung from any cause has the ability to increase the local level of inflammatory mediators and possibly bring the above mechanisms into play, altering expected responses of drugs such as the beta-adrenergic agonists.

The patient's overall technique for inhaling drugs will determine to a large extent what percentage of the available aerosol dose reaches the lower airway and the amount of drug deposited. Rapid inspiration by patients has the effect of increasing aerosol particle velocity and therefore promotes proximal deposition. Similarly, increasing degrees of airflow obstruction should theoretically decrease the penetration of aerosol and promote proximal deposition. Whilst this occurs with aerosols produced by nebulisers[49] it appears to be less important for MDIs where there is little difference in the amount deposited in the airways in normal subjects and in patients with moderately severe airflow obstruction from chronic bronchitis.[50,51] The amount of aerosol deposited in the airways is partly dependent on the duration of the breath-holding period after inspiration, known to be required for sedimentation of the aerosol particles. This applies to aerosols from MDIs[52,53] and nebulisers[54]

Asthma, bronchitis, emphysema, combinations of the previous three diseases, and cystic fibrosis tend to promote proximal airway deposition because of the narrowed airways from bronchoconstriction, mucosal oedema and airway secretions and the increased inspiratory flow rates as a result of the narrowed airways. As mentioned above, aerosols from MDIs appear to be less affected by increased obstruction than do aerosols from nebulisers.

The shortened duration of effect of inhaled beta-adrenergic agonists in acute asthma could result from a number of mechanisms. Diffusional processes would be altered by increased thickness of the mucous blanket caused by mucus hypersecretion. The effects of a given amount of drug may be less pronounced because of the increased time the drug takes to reach its site of effect and the smaller amount of drug which reaches the site. Such effects could be reduced if the process of transfer of drugs through the respiratory epithelium were altered by disease. It has been shown that mucosal or epithelial permeability to technetium-labelled diethylenetriamine pentacetic acid is increased in smokers,[55] but not in stable asthmatics.[56] Additive mechanisms could include increased blood flow in an area of airway inflammation with increased clearance of drug from the mucosa. Clearance of inhaled drugs can be altered by increased blood flow to the respiratory mucosa, which can occur in the common respiratory diseases such as bronchitis and asthma, but is likely to have a larger effect in cystic fibrosis and bronchiectasis. The relevance of altered mucosal blood flow is uncertain and its effect on inhaled drugs sequestered in the lung is unexplored.

## Conclusions

Alterations in requirements for systemic and aerosol drugs have been demonstrated in patients with respiratory disease. A variety of mechanisms is involved; however, it is apparent that the effectiveness of aerosol medications can be very limited in severely ill patients, requiring substitution of systemic therapy.

The use of drugs in patients with respiratory disease requires careful titration of dose against effect. Reduced effect is the general rule with aerosol modes of administration, and enhanced effect and toxicity the general rule with systemically administered drugs.

## References


1. du Souich P, McLean AJ, Lalka D, Erril S, Gibaldi M. Pulmonary disease and drug kinetics. *Clin Pharmacokinet* 1978; 3: 257-266.
2. McLean AJ, Barned J, Ionnides-Demos L, Nel D, Tong N, Mercer W, Wood TJ. Computer based prescription audit as a research, education and management tool. *Aust Health Rev* 1984; 7: 260-268.
3. McMillan DA, Harrison PM, Rogers LJ, Tong N, McLean AJ. Polypharmacy in an Australian teaching hospital. *Med J Aust* 1986; 145: 339-342.
4. du Souich P, McLean AJ, Lalka D, Erril S, Gibaldi M. Pulmonary disease and drug kinetics. In: Avery GS (ed). *Topics in clinical pharmacology*. Sydney: Adis Press Australasia, 1981.
5. Jacobs MH, Senior RM. Theophylline toxicity due to impaired theophylline degradation. *Am Rev Respir Dis* 1974; 110: 342-345.
6. Jacobs MH, Senior RM, Kessler G. Clinical experience with theophylline. Relationships between dosage, serum concentration and toxicity. *JAMA* 1976; 235: 1983-1986.
7. Weinberger MW, Matthay RA, Ginchansky EJ, Chidsey CA, Petty TL. Intravenous aminophylline dosage. Use of serum theophylline measurement for guidance. *JAMA* 1976; 235: 2110-2113.
8. Hendeles L, Bighley L, Richardson RH, Hepler CD, Carmichael J. Frequent toxicity from IV aminophylline infusions in critically ill patients. *Drug Intelligence Clin Pharm* 1977; 11: 12-18.
9. Vicuna N, Ludden TM, Schwertner H, Vicuna AV, McNay JL. Effect of heart failure upon theophylline (T) clearance in chronic airway obstruction (CAO) patients. *Clin Res* 1977; 25 (abstr): 277.
10. Byrne AJ, Morgan DJ, Harrison PM, McLean AJ. Variation in hepatic extraction ratio with unbound drug fraction: discrimination between models of hepatic drug elimination. *J Pharm Sci* 1985; 74: 205-207.
11. Mendelman PM, Smith AL, Levy J, Weber A, Ramsay B, Davis RL. Aminoglycoside penetration, inactivation, and efficacy in cystic fibrosis sputum. *Am Rev Respir Dis* 1985; 132: 761-765.
12. McIntyre EM, Alpers JH, Ruffin RE. Bronchial smooth muscle tone in normal subjects. *Chest* 1982; 81: 396.

13. Ruffin RE, Fitzgerald JD, Rebuck AS. A comparison of the bronchodilator activity of Sch1000 and salbutamol. *J Allergy Clin Immunol* 1977; 59: 136-141.

14. Ruffin RE, McIntyre E, Crockett AJ, Zielonka K, Alpers JH. Combination bronchodilator therapy in asthma. *J Allergy Clin Immunol* 1982; 69: 60-65.

15. Holgate ST, Baldwin CJ, Tattersfield AE. β-adrenergic agonist resistance in normal human airways. *Lancet* 1977; 2: 375-377.

16. Gibson GJ, Greenacre JK, Konig P, Conolly ME, Pride NB. Use of exercise challenge to investigate possible tolerance to beta-adrenoreceptor stimulation in asthma. *Br J Dis Chest* 1978; 72: 199-206.

17. Jenne JW, Chick TW, Strickland RD, Wall FJ. Subsensitivity of beta responses during therapy with a long-acting beta-2 preparation. *J Allergy Clin Immunol* 1977; 59: 383-390.

18. Newcomb R, Tashkin DP, Hui KK, Conolly ME, Lee E, Dauphinee B. Rebound hyper-responsiveness to muscarinic stimulation after chronic therapy with an inhaled muscarinic antagonist. *Am Rev Respir Dis* 1985; 132: 12-15.

19. Hume KM, Gandevia B. Forced expiratory volume before and after isoprenaline. *Thorax* 1957; 12: 276-278.

20. Symon DNK, Miller G, Russell G. Buccal administration of fenoterol aerosol in childhood asthma. *Eur J Respir Dis* 1985; 67: 37-40.

21. Ryrfeldt A, Ramsay CH. Distribution of terbutaline. *Eur J Resp Dis* 1984; 65 (suppl 134): 63-72.

22. Laros CD, van Urk P, Rominger KL. Absorption, distribution and excretion of the tritium-labelled $\beta_2$ stimulator fenoterol hydrobromide following aerosol administration and instillation into the bronchial tree. *Respiration* 1977; 34: 131-140.

23. Ruffin RE, Dolovich MB, Oldenburg FA, Newhouse MT. The preferential deposition of isoproterenol and propranolol in asthmatic patients. *Chest* 1981; 80 (suppl): 904-907.

24. Hensley MJ, O'Cain CF, McFadden ER Jr, Ingram RH Jr. Distribution of bronchodilatation in normal subjects: beta agonist versus atropine. *J Appl Physiol* 1978; 45: 778-782.

25. McFadden ER Jr, Ingram RH Jr, Haynes RL, Wellman JJ. Predominant site of flow limitation and mechanisms of postexertional asthma. *J Appl Physiol* 1977; 42: 746-752.

26. Barnes PJ, Basbaum CB, Nadel JA. Autoradiographic localization of autonomic receptors in airway smooth muscle. Marked differences between large and small airways. *Am Rev Respir Dis* 1983; 127: 758-762.

27. Carstairs JR, Nimmo AJ, Barnes PJ. Autoradiographic localisation of beta adrenoreceptors in human lung. *Eur J Pharmacol* 1984; 103: 189-190.

28. Newman SP. Aerosol deposition considerations in inhalation therapy. *Chest* 1985; 88: (suppl): 152S-160S.

29. Swift DL. Aerosols and humidity therapy. Generation and respiratory deposition of therapeutic aerosols. *Am Rev Respir Dis* 1980; 122(conf): 71-77.

30. Ruffin RE, Montgomery JM, Newhouse MT. Site of beta-adrenergic receptors in the respiratory tract. Use of fenoterol administered by two methods. *Chest* 1978; 74: 256-260.

31. Godfrey S, Zeidifard E, Brown K, Bell JH. The possible site of action of sodium cromoglycate assessed by exercise challenge. *Clin Sci* 1974; 46: 265-272.

32. Clay MM, Pavia D, Newman SP, Clarke SW. Factors influencing the size distribution of aerosols from jet nebulisers. *Thorax* 1983; 38: 755-759.

33. Kim CS, Trujillo D, Sackner MA. Size aspects of metered-dose inhaler aerosols. *Am Rev Respir Dis* 1985; 132: 137-142.

34. Toogood JH, Baskerville J, Jennings B, Lefcoe NM, Johansson SA. Use of spacers to facilitate inhaled corticosteroid treatment of asthma. *Am Rev Respir Dis* 1984; 129: 723-729.

35. Dolovich MB, Killian D, Wolff RK, Obminski G. Newhouse MT. Pulmonary aerosol deposition in chronic bronchitis: intermittent positive pressure breathing versus quiet breathing. *Am Rev Respir Dis* 1977; 115: 397-402.

36. Gardiner TH, Schanker LS. Absorption of disodium cromoglycate from the rat lung: evidence of carrier transport. *Xenobiotica* 1974; 4: 725-731.

37. Collier JG, Dobbs RJ, Williams I. Salbutamol aerosol causes a tachycardia due to the inhaled rather than the swallowed fraction. *Br J Clin Pharmacol* 1980; 9: 273-274.

38. Evans ME, Paterson JW, Shenfield GM. A technique for studying drug absorption from the lung in man. *Br J Pharmacol* 1973; 49: 153P.

39. Nilsson HT, Simonsson BG, Strom B. The fate of $^3$H-terbutaline sulphate administered to man as an aerosol. *Eur J Clin Pharmacol* 1976; 10: 1-7.
40. Philpot RM, Anderson MW, Eling TE. Uptake, accumulation, and metabolism of chemicals by the lung. In: Bakhle YS, Vane JR, eds. *Metabolic functions of the lung.* Vol 4, *Lung biology in health and disease.* New York: Marcel Dekker, 1977: 123-171.
41. Walker SR, Evans ME, Richards AJ, Paterson JW. The fate of [$^{14}$C] disodium cromoglycate in man. *J Pharm Pharmacol* 1972; 24: 525-531.
42. Ryrfeldt A, Andersson P, Edsbacker S, Tonnesson M, Davies D, Pauwels R. Pharmacokinetics and metabolism of budesonide, a selective glucocorticoid. *Eur J Respir Dis* 1982; 63: (suppl 122): 86-95.
43. Andersson P, Ryrfeldt A. Biotransformation of the topical glucocorticoids budesonide and beclomethasone 17-alpha, 21-diproprionate in human liver and lung homogenate. *J Pharm Pharmacol* 1984; 36: 763-765.
44. Gillis CN, Green NM. Possible clinical implications of metabolism of blood borne substrates by the human lung. In: *Metabolic functions of the lung.* Bakhle YS, Vane JR eds. Vol 4, *Lung biology in health and disease.* New York: Marcel Dekker 1977: 173-193.
45. Ryrfeldt A, Nilsson E. Uptake and biotransformation of ibuterol and terbutaline in isolated perfused rat and guinea pig lungs. *Biochem Pharmacol* 1978; 27: 301-305.
46. Larsson S, Svedmyr N. Bronchodilating effect and side effects of $beta_2$ adrenoreceptor stimulants by different modes of administration (tablets, metered aerosol, and combinations thereof). A study with salbutamol in asthmatics. *Am Rev Respir Dis* 1977; 116: 861-869.
47. Stiles GL, Strasser RH, Kilpatrick BF, Taylor SR, Lefkowitz RJ. Endogenous proteinases modulate the function of the beta-adrenergic receptor-adenylate cyclase system. *Biochim Biophys Acta* 1984; 802: 390-398.
48. Mita H, Yui Y, Shida T. Changes of beta-adrenergic receptor number and catecholamine-sensitive adenylate cyclase in guinea pig lung after inhalation of histamine aerosol. *Int Arch Allergy Appl Immunol* 1983; 72: 373-376.
49. Dolovich MB, Sanchis J, Rossman C, Newhouse MT. Aerosol penetrance: a sensitive index of peripheral airways obstruction. *J Appl Physiol* 1976; 40: 468-471.
50. Spiro SG, Singh CA, Tolfree SEJ, Partridge MR, Short MD. Direct labelling of ipratropium bromide aerosol and its deposition pattern in normal subjects and patients with chronic bronchitis. *Thorax* 1984; 39: 432-435.
51. Dolovich M, Ruffin R, Corr D, Newhouse MT. Clinical evaluation of a simple demand-inhalation MDI aerosol delivery device. *Chest* 1983; 84: 36-41.
52. Dolovich M, Ruffin RE, Roberts R, Newhouse MT. Optimal delivery of aerosols from metered dose inhalers. *Chest* 1981; 80 (suppl): 911-915.
53. Newman SP, Pavia D, Garland N. Clarke SW. Effects of various inhalation modes on the deposition of radioactive pressurized aerosols. *Eur J Respir Dis* 1982; 63 (suppl 119): 57-65.
54. Gottschalk B, Leupold W, Woller P. Deponierung von Aerosoler in den Atemwegen. *Z Erkr Atmungsorgane* 1978; 150: 139-146.
55. Kennedy SM, Elwood RK, Wiggs, BJR, Pare PD. Hogg JC. Increased airway mucosal permeability of smokers. Relationship to airway reactivity. *Am Rev Respir Dis* 1984; 129: 143-148.
56. Elwood RK, Kennedy S, Belzberg A, Hogg JC, Pare PD. Respiratory mucosal permeability in asthma. *Am Rev Respir Dis* 1983; 128: 523-527.

# Chapter 2

# Drug Delivery to the Lungs

*Stewart W. Clarke and Stephen P. Newman*

Inhalation therapy can be traced back to the earliest records of Hebrew, Chinese, Indian, Greek, Arabic and Roman cultures.[1] Primitive remedies usually involved aromatic fumes and incenses derived from natural plant essences or from burning organic materials. Hippocrates even described a type of inhaler incorporating a clay pot and reed pipe.[2] In Europe, interest in inhalation therapy was increased by the introduction of tobacco smoking in the 17th century, which resulted eventually in the development of herbal cigarettes containing powerful bronchodilators such as stramonium. These cigarettes are still available, but are not now recommended for treating asthmatic symptoms.

The modern era of inhalation therapy probably began with the introduction of inhaled adrenaline (epinephrine) in the first half of this century.[3] Subsequently, a range of sophisticated delivery devices has been developed, not only for chest therapy, but also for inhalation challenge testing and for delivery of radioaerosols to the lungs for ventilation scanning and for measurement of mucociliary or pulmonary clearance.[4] There is also a potential role for inhalation devices as a means of delivering drugs to the lungs for systemic rather than topical treatment.[5] This chapter will review the devices currently available for aerosol inhalation (nebulisers, metered dose inhalers (MDIs) and dry powder inhalers) with special reference to drug delivery.

## Advantages and Disadvantages of Inhalation Therapy

*Table 2.1* Inhalation therapy: advantages and proposed disadvantages

| |
|---|
| *Advantages* |
| Rapid onset of drug action |
| Small drug dose |
| Low incidence of systemic side effects |
| *Proposed Disadvantages* |
| Ineffective in presence of airway obstruction? |
| Ineffective in presence of hypersecretion of mucus? |
| Tolerance (resistance, tachyphylaxis)? |
| Safety problems? |

### Advantages

The inhaled route is used primarily to deliver bronchodilators, corticosteroids or sodium cromoglycate to the lungs, but may also be used for delivery of mucolytics, antibiotics and other drugs. As such this route has several well-recognised advantages, often exemplified by reference to bronchodilators, but probably equally applicable to many other drugs.

1. There is a rapid onset of drug action. Inhaled bronchodilators produce a significant effect within five minutes and a peak effect after 15 to 30 minutes, whereas the peak effect does not occur until two to three hours after an oral dose. This rapid onset of action is particularly useful in the treatment of acute asthmatic symptoms. The duration of action of inhaled bronchodilators is similar to that of oral therapy.

2. A small drug dose can be used. Doses of only a few hundred micrograms of inhaled bronchodilators or corticosteroids can replace oral doses of 5 to 10mg. The drugs are delivered directly to the required site of action in the lungs, rather than risking being metabolised in the liver or undergoing dilution in the bloodstream prior to arrival at the target organ via the systemic circulation; hence they are highly potent.

3. There is a low incidence of systemic side effects. The small doses of bronchodilators required to treat asthmatic symptoms give rise to insignificant tachycardia. The likelihood of systemic side effects has been further reduced by the development of selective beta2-agonists such as salbutamol (albuterol), terbutaline, rimiterol, reproterol and fenoterol. The lack of systemic side effects with modern glucocorticoids such as beclomethasone dipropionate, betamethasone valerate, triamcinolone acetonide, flunisolide and budesonide may be attributed not only to the very small doses that are effective topically, but also to low systemic absorption and rapid metabolism in the gastrointestinal tract or liver into relatively inactive compounds.

**Proposed Disadvantages**

Several potential disadvantages have been proposed for the inhaled route, although it is probable that none is of major importance. Larsson and Svedmyr[6] suggested that aerosol might not reach the area to be treated in the presence of airway obstruction or mucus hypersecretion, although there seems to be no good evidence that this is the case,[7] unless the airways are actually plugged with mucus, when intravenous therapy may be more effective.[8]

The possibility of 'tolerance', 'resistance' or 'tachyphylaxis' to the acute effects of beta-agonists resulting from long-term use has been raised. Tattersfield[9] reviewed studies in which the airway response to salbutamol was measured before and after regular therapy over periods of 2 to 15 months. Although tolerance was noted in normal subjects, the majority of studies in subjects with asthma or bronchitis showed no evidence of this problem. There is no evidence that tolerance develops in asthmatic subjects as a result of relatively large doses of bronchodilator delivered regularly by nebuliser.[10]

The safety of inhaled therapeutic agents has also given cause for concern. In the mid 1960s, there was an epidemic of asthma deaths in England and Wales, which correlated statistically with the sales of isoprenaline (isoproterenol) MDIs. However, it is more likely that this epidemic resulted from an over-reliance on MDIs and failure to give other forms of treatment necessary in severe asthmatic attacks.[11]

Chlorofluorocarbon propellants can cause palpitations, but Dollery et al[12] showed that the arterial blood concentrations of propellants attained only a fraction of the levels required to produce arrhythmias in animals, provided that inhalers were used in recommended doses. However, some patients may abuse their inhalers, and may take excessively large doses especially during acute asthmatic attacks, and some 'sniffers' who inhale propellants for kicks may also be at risk.[13]

A more recent rise in asthma deaths has occurred in New Zealand, perhaps related to over-reliance upon home nebuliser therapy, late self-referral and inadequate use of corticosteroids.[14] Because of these concerns, the desirability of home nebuliser therapy has been the subject of recent debate.[15] A survey of the use of home nebulisers in a district of West London showed confusion about their use and lack of adequate supervision of some patients using this form of therapy.[16] Several patients taking part in the survey, who had moderate to severe asthma, were not attending a hospital clinic on a regular basis, and several said that they would take further doses of bronchodilator in the event of an acute asthmatic attack, rather than seek medical advice. Tattersfield[17] has advocated that each nebuliser should carry a warning that it is dangerous to exceed the prescribed dose. Perhaps the true 'dangers' lie not in the inhalation devices or drugs themselves, but in patients' lack of awareness of the limitations of aerosol therapy, and of the measures to take if inhaled bronchodilators cease to be effective.

## Principles of Aerosol Penetration and Deposition

As a general rule, therapeutic aerosols must enter the lungs to be effective (Table 2.2). For the doses normally used, drug deposited in the oropharynx and subsequently swallowed contributes little or nothing to the overall effect.[18] The required site of deposition within the lungs themselves is, however, poorly defined at present.

*Table* 2.2 Aerosol deposition in man

| |
|---|
| *Mechanisms of Deposition* |
| Inertial impaction |
| Gravitational sedimentation |
| (Brownian diffusion) |
| (Electrostatic forces) |
| *Factors Determining Deposition* |
| Aerosol characteristics |
| Size |
| Density |
| Shape |
| Mode of inhalation |
| Flow rate |
| Inhaled volume |
| Breathing frequency |
| Breath-holding |
| Patient factors |
| Random anatomical variations |
| Degree of airway obstruction |

Two mechanisms of deposition are of major importance for therapeutic aerosols (typical size range 1 to 10μm), namely inertial impaction and gravitational sedimentation.[19] Deposition by Brownian diffusion is important only for submicronic particles. Electrical charges on aerosols may increase their deposition, especially for dry powders, but this aspect awaits clarification.

Inertial impaction occurs in the oropharynx and large conducting airways, primarily for large particles in rapid airstreams, while gravitational sedimentation is confined largely to the small conducting airways and alveoli where the airstream moves slowly and where, given time, particles may settle on to the airway surfaces under gravity.

Deposition has been calculated as a function of airway 'generation' by Gerrity et al.[20] The deposition pattern depends critically upon aerosol size: for particles less than 5μm in diameter the major deposition is by sedimentation in the peripheral airways, whereas for particles more than 5μm in diameter the major deposition occurs by impaction in the large conducting airways. Oropharyngeal deposition rises with increasing aerosol size.[21] At an inhaled flow rate of 30L/min, approximately 50% of 8μm diameter particles, and approximately 100% of 16μm diameter particles, is deposited in the oropharynx and cannot reach the lungs at all. Hence there is a practical limit on how large the particles of a therapeutic aerosol should be if they are to enter the lungs in sufficient quantity: the 'respirable range' may be defined for practical purposes as particles or droplets of 5μm diameter or less. In practice, therapeutic aerosols are heterodisperse; that is, the particles or droplets in any spray comprise a range of sizes, and the mass median diameter (MMD) or mass median aerodynamic diameter (MMAD) (the latter quantity taking particle or droplet density into account) are used to describe such aerosols.[19]

The mode of inhalation also determines the site of deposition. Inhaled flow rate is probably the most important factor, since rapid inhalation increases impaction in the oropharynx and large conducting airways, while slow inhalation allows aerosol to penetrate more readily to the peripheral parts of the lungs. A period of breath-holding on completion of inhalation allows particles entering the lungs to deposit by gravitational sedimentation. During tidal breathing, the breathing frequency may also be important. As the breathing rate decreases below 15 to 20 breaths per minute, particles spend a longer time in the respiratory tract and are more susceptible to deposition by sedimentation; conversely, as the breathing rate increases above 15 to 20 breaths per minute, the inhaled flow rate increases, and hence the probability of impaction also rises.[22]

A more 'central' deposition pattern within the lungs may occur in obstructive airways disease, when the airways are narrowed by bronchospasm, oedema and mucus hypersecretion.[23] Theoretically, slower inhalation and/or smaller particles should be used in patients with severe airways obstruction, but to date there is no evidence to prove that this is necessary in practice.

## Nebulisers

Nebulisers are available in two basic types: jet and ultrasonic.[24] The jet nebuliser (Figure 2.1) is operated by an electric compressor, an air or

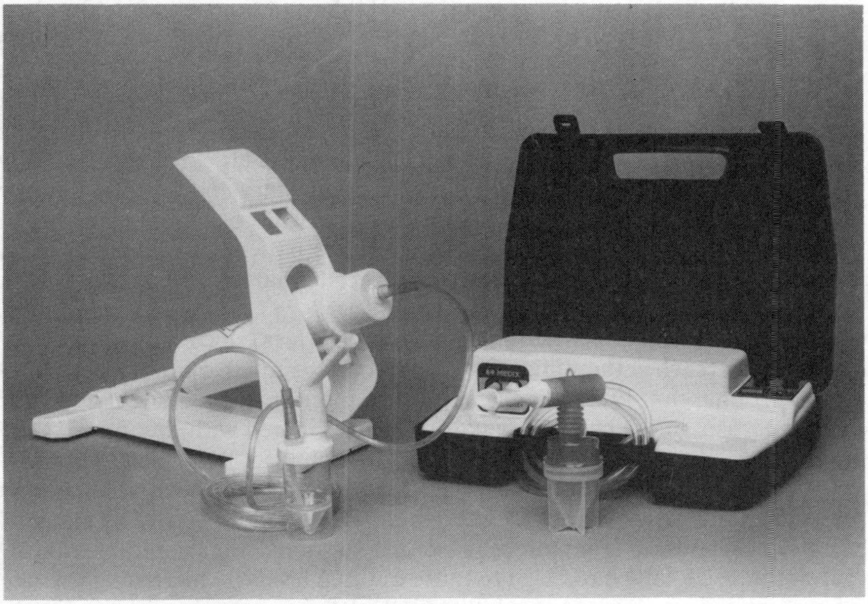

*Figure 2.1* Jet nebulisers, which may be operated by an electric compressor or even by a foot-pump.

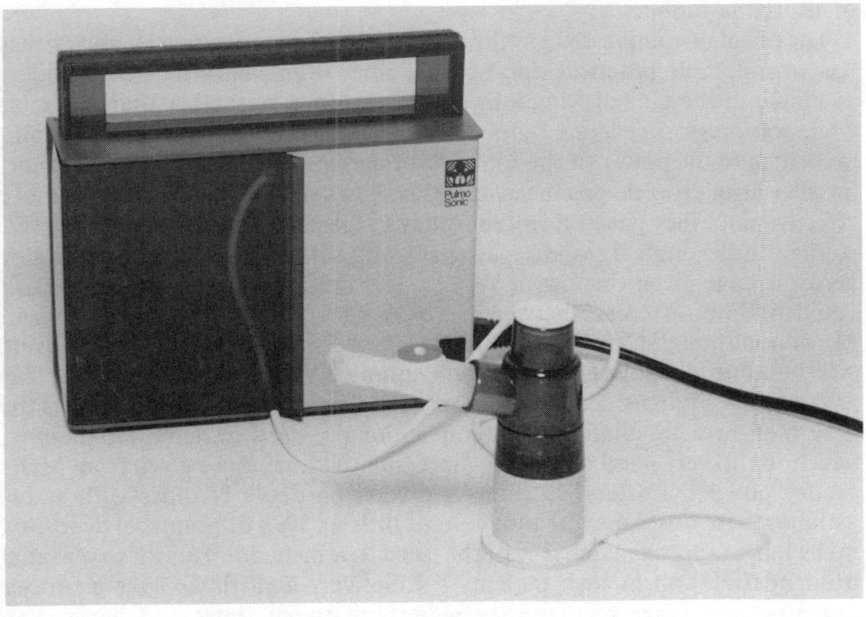


*Figure 2.2* Ultrasonic nebuliser.

oxygen cylinder, a hospital airline or even a foot-pump, although foot-pumps require considerable expenditure of effort over a lengthy treatment period.[25] In the jet nebuliser, liquid is drawn up a feed tube and fragments into droplets: large droplets impact on baffles surrounding the orifice, while small droplets are carried away in the inhaled airstream. In the ultrasonic nebuliser (Figure 2.2), high frequency (1 to 2 megaHz) vibrations in a piezoelectric crystal produce a fountain of droplets in a drug solution, and the smaller droplets are inhaled by the patient. In the United Kingdom, use of jet nebulisers greatly outweighs that of ultrasonic nebulisers for domiciliary and hospital therapy with bronchodilators: for this reason this text will concentrate on the jet nebuliser. Nebulisers are easy to use, since the patient can inhale by tidal breathing and does not need to develop a special inhalation technique as with an MDI.

Jet nebulisers are inefficient drug delivery devices, since only about 10% of the dose reaches the lungs,[26] with a broadly similar quantity deposited in the oropharynx. Either a face mask or a mouthpiece may be used,[27] but loss of aerosol in the nasopharynx is to be anticipated with the former. The majority of the dose is retained within the nebuliser as a 'dead volume', trapped on baffles and internal walls; furthermore, this dead volume may be much more concentrated than the original solution. The size of many of the droplets released from the nebuliser may be above the 'respirable range', but droplet size can be reduced to more optimal levels by increasing the rate of compressed gas flow to the nebuliser.[28] A high flow rate also reduces nebulisation time.[29] Droplet size may be reduced in the ultrasonic nebuliser by raising the frequency of the ultrasonic signal,[30] but this can only be varied in certain models. Output, droplet size and nebulisation time vary considerably among nebuliser brands, and even among individual nebulisers of the same brand.

The effect of compressed gas flow rate on nebuliser operating characteristics has considerable practical significance, since domiciliary oxygen cylinders available in the United Kingdom operate at flows no higher than 4L/min, while compressors generate flows through nebulisers between 6 and 12L/min, according to the power of the compressor and the resistance of the nebuliser. Smaller drug droplets produced at higher flows should theoretically be more effective since they penetrate more readily to the peripheral airways. However, studies on the clinical response attained with different sized bronchodilator aerosols have given conflicting results. Hadfield et al[31] and Douglas et al[32] could find no difference between aerosols generated at flow rates of 4 and 8L/min, although Clay et al[33] found improved small airways function using a terbutaline aerosol of MMD 1.8$\mu$m compared with two larger sizes. This relative lack of dependence of response on droplet size probably reflects the very high bronchodilator doses conventionally used in nebuliser therapy, which for no very good reason are more than 10 times those given from MDIs or dry powder inhalers. In many patients, particularly those with stable asthma, these doses may be too high: as little as 30$\mu$g of fenoterol deposited in the lungs (approximately 1% of the usual treatment dose) may give maximal bronchodilatation in such patients.[34] Relatively high flows have a further potential advantage in that they reduce treatment times and hence may improve patient compliance.

*Table 2.3* Factors determining output characteristics of jet nebulisers

| |
|---|
| Nebuliser design |
| Mouthpiece or face mask |
| Compressed gas flow rate |
| Volume fill |
| Physical characteristics of solution |
| Continuous or intermittent nebulisation |
| Use of trigger to synchronise inhalation with aerosol release |
| Inhalation mode |
| Ambient temperature |

Several other practical steps can be taken to improve output from nebulisers (Table 2.3). Although a volume fill of 2ml is often recommended by pharmaceutical companies, 4ml is better, because a greater proportion of the drug dose is released as aerosol.[35] In practice, many physicians prescribe therapy with low flows and small volume fills, and the output of respirable aerosol may often be inadequate.[36] Standardisation of aerosol output and droplet size is potentially important not only for therapy, but also for bronchial challenge testing.[37] Aerosol output can also be increased by tapping the walls of the nebuliser or nebulising intermittently to encourage droplets trapped on baffles to run back to the reservoir, and by use of a triggering device to synchronise aerosol generation with the patient's inhalation.

Intermittent positive pressure breathing (IPPB), intended to 'force' aerosol into peripheral airways, is not now considered to have any advantage over standard nebuliser therapy,[38] and does not in fact alter the pattern of aerosol deposition within the lungs.[39] There seems little if any indication for using this modality now.

Although nebulisers are used primarily for bronchodilators, virtually any drug suspension or solution can be nebulised. Antibiotic aerosols have been used in several centres for some years with only moderate success,[40] but recently a combination of gentamicin and carbenicillin given as aerosols to a group of patients with cystic fibrosis with *Pseudomonas* chest infection produced marked clinical improvement.[41] Mucolytic and hypertonic saline aerosols may also be useful in the management of patients with tenacious secretions.[42] For nebulising these substances, it may be important to use nebuliser systems which are as efficient as possible, delivering the maximum amount of respirable aerosol in the minimum possible time. The amount of 'respirable' (particle size less than 5$\mu$m diameter) antibiotic aerosol available to the patient, and the nebulisation time, vary widely according to the type of nebuliser, the volume fill and the compressed gas flow rate.[35] Powerful compressors may be particularly valuable for nebulising viscous antibiotic solutions since droplet size and nebulisation time are otherwise relatively high for these solutions.

Nebulisers are prone to bacterial contamination, and regular cleaning and sterilisation are essential. An individual nebuliser should not be used by more than one person in order to avoid the risk of cross-infection.

## Metered Dose Inhalers

Metered dose inhalers (MDIs) were introduced in the mid 1950s and have become very popular for their convenience, compactness and portability. More than five million MDIs are prescribed annually in the United Kingdom. MDIs (Figure 2.3) are powered by various mixtures of chlorofluorocarbon propellants at vapour pressures of approximately three to four atmospheres, and contain the drug either as a suspension of drug crystals (prevalent in European formulations) or as a solution (more usual in the USA). Surfactants are added to suspension formulations to reduce particle agglomeration, while co-solvents such as ethanol are used in solution formulations to enhance mixing of drug and propellants. The addition of co-solvents may decrease the vapour pressure, delay evaporation and generate larger droplets.[43] Since MDIs are hermetically sealed, the contents remain sterile throughout the life of the canister.

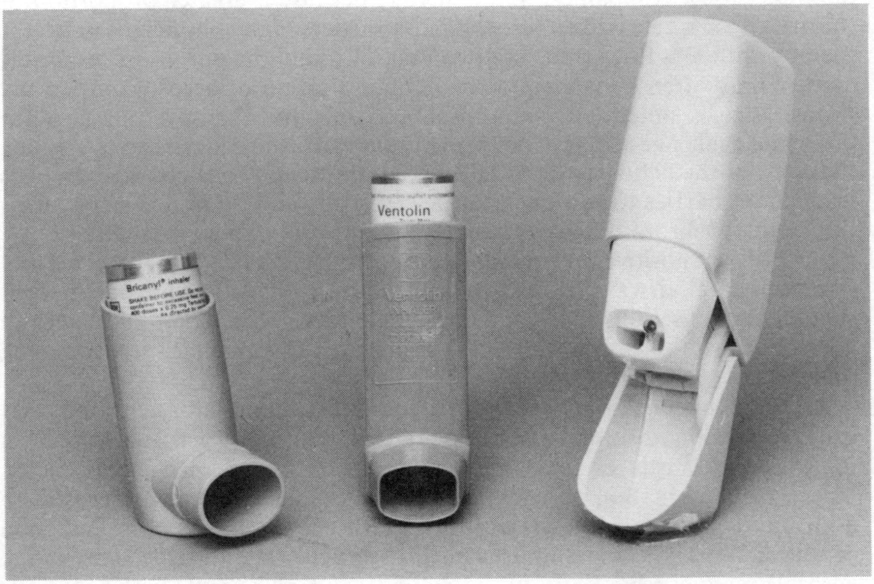


*Figure 2.3* Metered dose inhalers (MDIs). The model on the right-hand side is a breath-actuated inhaler.

Upon actuation, the contents of a small metering chamber (25 to 100μl, containing 100 to 670μg of bronchodilator, 50 to 250μg of corticosteroid or 1 to 5mg of sodium cromoglycate) are released as a spray of large, rapidly moving propellant droplets, most of which impact in the oropharynx.[44,45] Consequently only about 10% of the dose enters the lungs directly.[45-47] Typically 80% of a bronchodilator or corticosteroid dose is deposited in the oropharynx, is subsequently swallowed, and is largely metabolised and inactivated.[44]

Despite being apparently easy to use, MDIs are in fact misused by many patients.[48-52] The conflicting instructions provided with different brands of MDI may not help in this respect, although hopefully these will soon be standardised. Failure to coordinate actuation of the MDI with inhalation has long been recognised as a major form of MDI misuse (Table 2.4). Response to an inhaled bronchodilator may be reduced if the dose is fired before inhalation begins,[53] and will probably be absent if fired after inhalation ends.[54] Other forms of error may, however, be just as important, notably the 'cold freon' effect (stopping inhalation or inhaling through the nose when the spray enters the mouth)[11,51] or inhaling too rapidly and/or failing to breath-hold adequately.[53,55]

In recent years, many studies have been performed to assess the 'correct' MDI technique (Table 2.4), most of which have measured bronchodilator response following inhalation from an MDI under various systematically controlled conditions.[53,56-58] These studies have been supplemented by studies using radiotracers to measure quantities of aerosol reaching the lungs,[46,59] and by studies in which bronchodilator responses following self-administration by the patient and administration by a physician have been compared.[49,60] Broadly speaking, these studies have reached a common conclusion: namely that the MDI should be actuated during the course of a slow deep inhalation (over a period of five to six seconds), followed by 10 seconds' breath-holding. Controversy remains over the placement of the MDI (between closed lips or with the mouthpiece several centimetres from the open mouth). The 'open mouth' technique is supported by some groups,[46,61] but disputed by others.[55,62]

For patients who have difficulty using MDIs correctly, auxiliary devices may be valuable. Perhaps the earliest such device was the breath-actuated MDI (Figure 2.3) which consists of the inhaler fitted into a plastic holder incorporating a spring. As the patient breathes in through the device, the

*Table 2.4* Metered dose inhalers

| |
|---|
| *Correct Inhalation Technique* |
| 1. Shake the inhaler |
| 2. Hold the inhaler upright |
| 3. Place the mouthpiece between the lips |
| 4. Fire the inhaler while breathing in deeply and slowly |
| 5. Hold the breath for 10 seconds or for as long as possible |
| *Errors in Technique* |
| Cap not removed from mouthpiece |
| Inhaler upside-down |
| Failure to coordinate inhalation and actuation |
| 'Cold freon' effect |
| Small inhaled volume |
| Inhaling too rapidly |
| Inadequate breath-holding |
| *Alternatives for Patients with Poor Technique* |
| Breath-actuated MDI |
| Tube spacer |
| Holding chamber |
| Dry powder inhaler |
| Nebuliser |

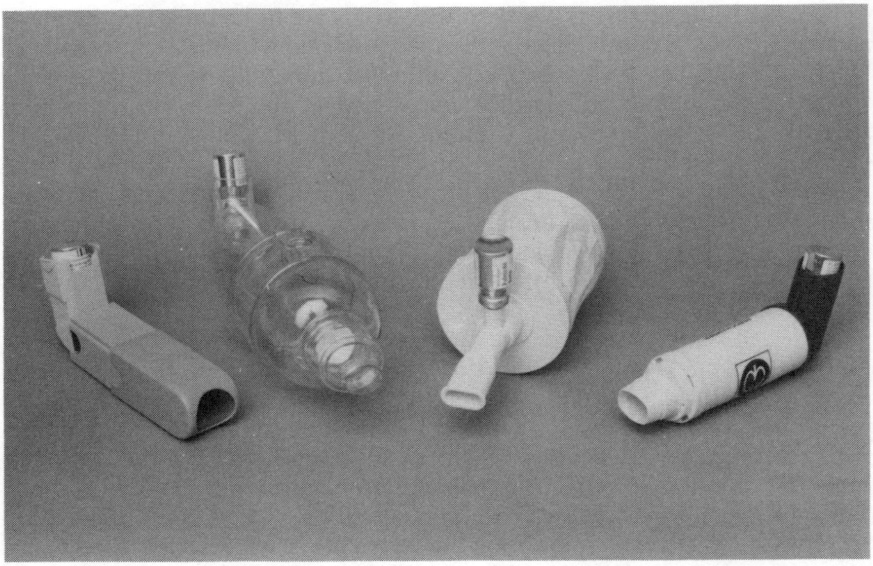

*Figure 2.4* Spacers and holding chambers for use with MDIs.

spring is triggered and thus the MDI is actuated automatically in synchrony with the inhalation.[63] Unfortunately, these devices have never been widely used, perhaps because they tend to release the dose rather noisily and violently.

A variety of extension devices has been introduced (Figure 2.4), following essentially two designs: (i) simple tube extensions to the inhaler mouthpiece, and (ii) holding chambers into which the spray is actuated and from which the subject then inhales. Tube spacers allow the propellant droplets to slow down and evaporate, so that they are less likely to deposit in the oropharynx and more likely to penetrate to the lungs.[64] In clinical trials, they generally confer greater clinical advantage than an MDI alone.[65-67] Tube spacers improve response in poor coordinators, perhaps because the spacer and mouth act as a holding chamber to contain the spray momentarily before inhalation.[65]

Several designs of purpose-built holding chambers, ranging in volume from 100 to 2000ml have been described (Figure 2.4). A 750ml pear-shaped chamber with a valve in the mouthpiece (Nebuhaler) has been tested extensively. This device can double the amount of aerosol reaching the lungs, thus giving adequate drug delivery even in patients with poor inhaler technique, while at the same time reducing oropharyngeal deposition by a factor of five.[68] In clinical trials with the Nebuhaler, the therapeutic effect was enhanced for bronchodilators[69] and corticosteroids.[70] This device is obviously large and relatively cumbersome, but it may be possible to use it as an alternative to a nebuliser for large doses of bronchodilators, either for treatment of acute severe asthma[71] or stable asthma especially in children.[72] It is acceptable to fire four doses in quick succession into the Nebuhaler and inhale all four doses simultaneously,[68] and it may also be possible to inhale from the device by tidal breathing, although this has yet to be demonstrated formally.

Several other large holding chambers perform similar functions, including the InspirEase,[73] which is collapsible for easy portability, the Aidac[74] and the InhalAid.[75] The Aerochamber[76] is a small holding chamber (volume approximately 150ml) which, although highly portable, has not been quite as successful in clinical trials as the larger chambers. Since all holding chambers markedly reduce oropharyngeal deposition, they reduce the incidence of candidiasis and dysphonia which can be troublesome side effects of corticosteroid metered dose therapy.[70,77]

Although extension devices can 'correct' for poor inhaler technique, it would be wrong to assume that there are no limitations upon the manner in which they can be used. The inhaled flow rate, breath-holding pause and the delay between actuation and inhalation will all determine the amount of aerosol reaching the lungs from an extension device, and hence the therapeutic effect produced. Poor control over the mode of inhalation may explain the relatively poor clinical response obtained in some trials with extension devices. Further work is required to determine which modes of inhalation are acceptable for each type of extension device. Additionally, some holding chambers are fitted with adaptors to accommodate any brand of MDI. It is questionable whether this is sound practice, since the vapour pressure and hence the spray characteristics vary widely between brands. It is possible that an unacceptably large amount of the dose will be impacted within the apparatus with some MDI/extension combinations.

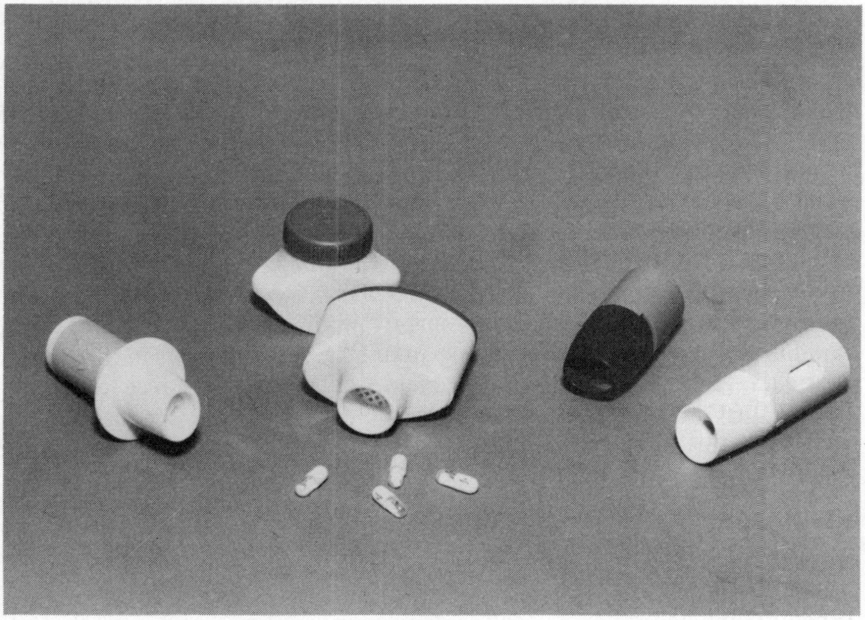

*Figure 2.5* Dry powder inhalers.

## Dry Powder Inhalers

Dry powder inhalers (Figure 2.5) are an alternative drug delivery system to MDIs for bronchodilators, corticosteroids and sodium cromoglycate which avoid the use of chlorofluorocarbon propellants. The drug is formulated as a dry powder in a gelatin capsule. As the patient inhales through the device, the powder is dispersed into the airstream. Hence these devices are 'breath-actuated', and can be used by patients who cannot successfully coordinate MDI actuation with inhalation.

The earliest dry powder inhaler (Spinhaler) was developed for the prophylactic agent sodium cromoglycate and was formulated as 20mg of sodium cromoglycate with 20mg of lactose powder in each capsule.[78] The sodium cromoglycate powder had an MMD of less than 5$\mu$m, while the lactose powder had an MMD greater than 50$\mu$m. Lactose was required because the drug material is cohesive and would not empty from the capsule on its own. Mixtures of fine and coarse particles resulted in agglomerates, and only 5% of the sodium cromoglycate was present as respirable particles in the inhaled airstream.[79] As with the MDI, the majority of the dose was deposited in the oropharynx.[44] Sodium cromoglycate has now been formulated in a new 'pelletised' lactose-free presentation, and in a new design of inhaler (Halermatic),[80] as well as in an MDI.

Other types of dry powder inhaler, such as the Rotahaler are available for powder formulations of bronchodilators and corticosteroids.[81,82] Compared to the Spinhaler, the Rotahaler has a simpler design in which the capsule is broken in half by a twisting mechanism. The resistance of the Rotahaler is lower than that of the Spinhaler and the contents of each capsule are more easily emptied. The drug dose in each capsule is approximately double the corresponding MDI dose. Lactose powder is needed as a diluent, however, in order to fill the capsules with the drug substance.

Dry powder inhalers suffer from a major drawback in that a capsule must be loaded into the device each time it is used. Hence it is less convenient than an MDI, especially in acute situations. The development of multidose systems would considerably improve the convenience and simplicity of these inhalers. Even so, some patients cannot tolerate the irritant effect of the powder.

There has been little work to date on evaluating the correct inhalation technique for dry powders. In a study on an inhaler not currently available in the UK, inhaling rapidly conferred greater response to fenoterol powder than inhaling slowly.[83] This is not surprising on theoretical grounds, since rapid inhalation promotes the break-up of large agglomerates in the inhaled airstream. However, the inhaler tested had a rather high resistance to air flow, so that 'fast' and 'slow' flow rates were only 0.5 and 0.2L/sec respectively, and it remains to be seen whether these data can be extrapolated to other types of dry powder inhaler.

## Summary

When the inhaled route is used for drug delivery, there is often a relatively rapid onset of drug action, a small quantity of drug is frequently effective, and there are few systemic side effects. Several potential disadvantages of aerosol therapy have been suggested, but it is probable that none is of major importance. Aerosol deposition in the respiratory tract takes place chiefly by the processes of inertial impaction and gravitational sedimentation; deposition depends in turn upon particle size, mode of inhalation and the degree of airway obstruction. Drugs are delivered by three types of device: the nebuliser, the MDI and the dry powder inhaler. Only about 10% of the dose reaches the lungs from each device. Nebulisers can be used to deliver virtually any drug solution or suspension, although their most common use is for the delivery of relatively large doses of bronchodilators. The output of respirable aerosol from nebulisers varies considerably upon their mode of operation, particularly the volume fill and the compressed gas flow rate. MDIs are compact and portable, but many patients use them incorrectly; spacers and holding chambers may improve drug delivery in patients with poor technique. Compared to the other two types of device, relatively little work has been done to evaluate the optimal technique for using dry powder inhalers.

## References


1. Ziment I. *Respiratory pharmacology and therapeutics.* Philadelphia: WB Saunders, 1978: 1-7.
2. Miller WF. Aerosol therapy in acute and chronic respiratory disease. *Arch Intern Med* 1973; 131: 148-155.
3. Graeser JB, Rowe AH. Inhalation of epinephrine for relief of asthmatic symptoms. *J Allergy* 1935; 6: 415-420,
4. Clarke SW, Pavia D. *Aerosols and the lung.* London: Butterworths, 1984.
5. Clarke SW, Newman SP. Therapeutic aerosols II. Drugs available by the inhaled route. *Thorax* 1984; 39: 1-7.
6. Larsson S, Svedmyr N. Bronchodilating effect and side effects of beta-2 adrenoceptor stimulants by different modes of administration. *Am Rev Respir Dis* 1977; 116: 861-869.
7. Clark TJH. Factors influencing the route of administration of airway therapy. In: Sadoul P, Milic-Emili J, Simonsson BG, Clark TJH, eds. *Small airways in health and disease.* Amsterdam: Excerpta Medica, 1979: 170-178.
8. Williams S, Seaton A. Intravenous or inhaled salbutamol in severe acute asthma. *Thorax* 1977; 32: 555-558.
9. Tattersfield AE. Albuterol in the long-term treatment of airways disease. In: McFadden ER, ed. *New concepts in the topical treatment of asthma and related disorders.* Greenwich: Cliggott Publishing Co, 1982: 33-37.
10. McGivern DV, Ward M, Revill S, Sechiari A, MacFarlane J, Davies D. Home nebulisers in severe chronic asthma. *Br J Dis Chest* 1984; 78: 376-382.
11. Crompton GK. Use and abuse of aerosol inhalers. In: McFadden ER, ed. *New concepts in the topical treatment of asthma and related disorders.* Greenwich: Cliggott Publishing Co, 1982: 10-12.
12. Dollery CT, Williams FM, Draffan GH, Wise G, Sahyoun H, Paterson JW, Walker SR. Arterial blood levels of fluorocarbons in asthmatic patients following use of pressurized aerosols. *Clin Pharmacol Ther* 1974; 15: 59-66.
13. Anonymous. Fluorocarbon aerosol propellants (Editorial). *Lancet* 1975; 1: 1073-1074.
14. Anonymous. The nebuliser epidemic (Editorial). *Lancet* 1984; 2: 789-790.
15. Cochrane GM, Prior JG, Rees PJ. Home nebulisers for airflow limitations. *Br Med J* 1985; 290: 1608-1609.
16. Laroche CM, Harries AVK, Newton RCF, Britton MG. Domiciliary nebulisers in asthma: a district survey. *Br Med J* 1985; 290: 1611-1613.

17. Tattersfield AE. Nebulisers in domiciliary practice. *Lancet* 1985; 1: 48-49.
18. Ruffin RE, Montgomery JM, Newhouse MT. Site of beta-adrenergic receptors in the respiratory tract. *Chest* 1978; 74: 256-260.
19. Agnew JE. Physical properties and mechanisms of deposition of aerosols. In: Clarke SW, Pavia D, eds. *Aerosols and the lung.* London: Butterworths, 1984: 49-70.
20. Gerrity TR, Lee PS, Hass FJ, Marinelli A, Werner P, Lourenco RV. Calculated deposition of inhaled particles in the airway generations of normal subjects. *J Appl Physiol* 1979; 47: 867-873.
21. Swift DL. Generation and respiratory deposition of therapeutic aerosols. *Am Rev Respir Dis* 1980; 122: 1-7.
22. Dennis WL. Discussion. In: Davies CN, ed. *Inhaled particles and vapours.* Oxford: Pergamon Press, 1961: 88-89.
23. Pavia D, Thomson ML, Clarke SW, Shannon HS. Effect of lung function and mode of inhalation on penetration of aerosol into the human lung. *Thorax* 1977; 32: 194-197.
24. Newman SP. Therapeutic aerosols. In: Clarke SW, Pavia D, eds. *Aerosols and the lung.* London: Butterworths, 1984: 197-224.
25. Dunn AM, Darvell F, Wilson RSE. An evaluation of the footpump as a driving source for nebuliser solutions. *Br J Dis Chest* 1985; 79: 172-176.
26. Lewis RA, Fleming JS, Balachandran W, Tattersfield A. Particle size distributions and deposition from a jet nebuliser: influence of humidity and temperature. *Clin Sci* 1981; 62: 5P.
27. Steventon RD, Wilson RSE. Facemask or mouthpiece for delivery of nebulized bronchodilator aerosols. *Br J Dis Chest* 1981; 75: 88-90.
28. Clay MM, Pavia D, Newman SP, Clarke SW. Factors influencing the size distribution of aerosols from jet nebulisers. *Thorax* 1983; 38: 755-759.
29. Clay MM, Pavia D, Newman SP, Lennard-Jones T, Clarke SW. Assessment of jet nebulisers for lung aerosol therapy. *Lancet* 1983; 2: 592-594.
30. Sterk PJ, Plomp A, Van der Vate JF, Quanjer PH. Physical properties of aerosols produced by several jet and ultrasonic nebulisers. *Bull Eur Physiopathol Respir* 1984; 20: 65-72.
31. Hadfield JW, Lowe G, Windebank WJ, Bateman JRM. Is the flow rate clinically important for nebuliser therapy? *Thorax* 1984; 39: 240.
32. Douglas JG, Leslie MJ, Crompton GK, Grant IWB. Is the flow rate used to drive a jet nebuliser clinically important? *Br Med J* 1985; 290: 29.
33. Clay MM, Pavia D, Clarke SW. Does nebulised bronchodilator aerosol droplet size matter? *Thorax* 1985; 40: 222.
34. Ruffin RE, Kenworthy MC, Newhouse MT. Response of asthmatic patients to fenoterol inhalation: a method of quantifying the airway bronchodilator dose. *Clin Pharmacol Ther* 1978; 23: 338-345.
35. Newman SP, Pellow PGD, Clay MM, Clarke SW. Evaluation of jet nebulisers for use with gentamicin solution. *Thorax* 1985; 40: 671-676.
36. Stainforth JN, Lewis RA, Tattersfield AE. Dosage and delivery of nebulised beta-agonists in hospital. *Thorax* 1983; 38: 751-754.
37. Ryan G, Dolovich MB, Obminski G, Cockcroft DW, Juniper E, Hargreave FE, Newhouse MT. Standardisation of inhalation provocation tests: influence of nebuliser output, particle size and method of inhalation. *J Allergy Clin Immunol* 1981; 67: 156-161.
38. IPPB Trial Group. IPPB in COPD. *Chest* 1984; 86: 341-342.
39. Dolovich MB, Killian D, Wolff RK, Obminski G, Newhouse MT. Pulmonary aerosol deposition in chronic bronchitis: intermittent positive pressure breathing versus quiet breathing. *Am Rev Respir Dis* 1977; 115: 397-402.
40. Williams MH. Steroid and antibiotic aerosols. *Am Rev Respir Dis* 1974; 110: 122-127.
41. Hodson ME, Penketh ARL, Batten JC. Aerosol carbenicillin and gentamicin treatment of *Pseudomonas aeruginosa* infection in patients with cystic fibrosis. *Lancet* 1981; 2: 1137-1139.
42. Hodson ME, Gaskell DV. Physiotherapy. In: Hodson ME, Norman AP, Batten JC, eds. *Cystic fibrosis.* London: Ballière Tindall, 1983: 219-241.
43. Bell JH, Brown K, Glasby J. Variation in delivery of isoprenaline from various pressurized inhalers. *J Pharm Pharmacol* 1973; 25 (suppl): 32-36P.
44. Davies DS. Pharmacokinetics of inhaled substances. *Postgrad Med J* 1975; 51 (suppl 7): 69-75.

45. Newman SP, Pavia D, Morén F, Sheahan NF, Clarke SW. Deposition of pressurized aerosols in the human respiratory tract. *Thorax* 1981; 36: 52-55.
46. Dolovich M, Ruffin RE, Roberts R, Newhouse MT. Optimal delivery of aerosols from metered dose inhalers. *Chest* 1981; 80 (suppl): 911-915.
47. Short MD, Singh CA, Few JD, Studdy PT, Heaf JD, Spiro SG. The labelling and monitoring of lung deposition of an inhaled synthetic anticholinergic bronchodilating agent. *Chest* 1981; 80 (suppl): 918-921.
48. Coady TJ, Stewart CJ, Davies HJ. Synchronization of bronchodilator release. *Practitioner* 1976; 217: 273-275.
49. Orehek J, Gayrard P, Grimaud C, Charpin J. Patient error in the use of bronchodilator metered aerosols. *Br Med J* 1976; 1: 76.
50. Epstein SW, Manning CPR, Ashley MJ, Corey PN. Survey of the clinical use of pressurized aerosol inhalers. *Can Med Assoc J* 1979; 120: 813-816.
51. Crompton GK. Problems patients have using pressurised aerosol inhalers. *Eur J Respir Dis* 1982; 62 (suppl 119): 101-104.
52. Morén F, Andersson J, Stiksa G. Mode of inhalation for trained and untrained asthmatics using a pressurised aerosol. *Respiration* 1984; 45: 56-60.
53. Newman SP, Pavia D, Clarke SW. How should a pressurised beta-adrenergic bronchodilator be inhaled? *Eur J Respir Dis* 1981; 62: 3-20.
54. Rivlin J, Mindorff C, Levison H, Kazim F, Reilly P, Worsley G. Effect of administration technique on bronchodilator response to fenoterol in a metered-dose inhaler. *J Pediatr* 1983; 102: 470-472.
55. Newman SP. The correct use of inhalers. In: Clark TJH, ed. *Steroids in asthma.* Auckland: ADIS Press, 1983: 210-226.
56. Riley DJ, Liu RT, Edelman NH. Enhanced responses to aerosolized bronchodilator therapy in asthma using respiratory maneuvers. *Chest* 1979; 76: 501-507.
57. Lawford P, McKenzie D. Pressurized aerosol inhaler technique: how important are inhalation from residual volume, inspiratory flow rate and the time interval between puffs? *Br J Dis Chest* 1983; 77: 276-281.
58. Thomas P, Williams T, Reilly PA, Bradley D. Modifying delivery technique of fenoterol from a metered dose inhaler. *Ann Allergy* 1984; 52: 279-281.
59. Newman SP, Pavia D, Garland N, Clarke SW. Effects of various modes on the deposition of radioactive pressurised aerosols. *Eur J Respir Dis* 1982; 63 (suppl 119): 57-65.
60. Epstein SW, Parsons JE, Corey PN, Worsley GH, Reilly PA. Comparison of three means of pressurised aerosol inhaler use. *Am Rev Respir Dis* 1983; 128: 253-255.
61. Connolly CK. Methods of using pressurized aerosols. *Br Med J* 1975; 3: 21.
62. Lawford P, McKenzie D. Pressurized bronchodilator aerosol technique: influence of breath-holding time and relationship of inhaler to mouth. *Br J Dis Chest* 1982; 76: 229-233.
63. D'Arcy PF, Kirk WF. Development of a new device for inhalation therapy. *Pharm J* 1971; 206: 306-307.
64. Newman SP, Morén F, Pavia D, Little F, Clarke SW. Deposition of pressurised suspension aerosols inhaled through extension devices. *Am Rev Respir Dis* 1981; 124: 317-320.
65. Bloomfield P, Crompton GK, Winsey NJP. A tube spacer to improve inhalation of drugs from pressurised aerosols. *Br Med J* 1979; 2: 1479.
66. Lindgren SB, Formgren H, Morén F. Improved aerosol therapy of asthma: effect of actuator tube size on drug availability. *Eur J Respir Dis* 1980; 61: 56-61.
67. Spicer JE, Cayton RM, Frame M, Winsey NJP. Influence of tube-spacer on aerosol efficacy. *Lancet* 1980; 2: 1248.
68. Newman SP, Millar AB, Lennard-Jones TR, Morén F, Clarke SW. Improvement of pressurised aerosol deposition with Nebuhaler spacer device. *Thorax* 1984; 39: 935-941.
69. Dorow P, Hidinger K-G. Terbutaline aerosol from a metered dose inhaler via a 750 ml spacer. Effect on large and small airways. *Eur J Clin Pharmacol* 1982; 22: 511-514.
70. Toogood JH, Baskerville J, Jennings B, Lefcoe NM, Johansson S-A. Use of spacers to facilitate inhaled corticosteroid treatment in asthma. *Am Rev Respir Dis* 1984; 129: 723-729.
71. Morgan MDL, Singh BV, Frame MF, Williams SJ. Terbutaline aerosol given through pear spacer in acute severe asthma. *Br Med J* 1982; 285: 849-850.

72. Rivlin J, Mindorff C, Reilly P, Levison H. Pulmonary response to a bronchodilator delivered from three inhalation devices. *J Pediatr* 1984; 104: 470-473.
73. Tobin MJ, Jenouri G, Danta I, Kim C, Watson H, Sackner MA. Responses to bronchodilator drug administration by a new reservoir aerosol delivery system, and a review of other auxiliary delivery systems. *Am Rev Respir Dis* 1982; 126: 670-675.
74. Freigang B. A new method of beclomethasone aerosol administration to children under 4 years of age. *Can Med Assoc J* 1977; 117: 1308-1309.
75. Huntley W, Weinberger M. Evaluation of bronchodilatation from aerosol $beta_2$ agonists delivered by the Inhal-Aid device to young children. *J Asthma* 1984; 21: 265-270.
76. Corr D, Dolovich M, McCormack D, Ruffin R, Obminski G, Newhouse M. Design and characteristics of a portable breath-actuated, particle size selective medical aerosol inhaler. *J Aerosol Sci* 1982; 13: 1-7.
77. Toogood J, Jennings B, Baskerville J, Lefcoe N, Newhouse M. Assessment of a device for reducing oropharyngeal complications during beclomethasone treatment of asthma. *Am Rev Respir Dis* 1981; 123: 113.
78. Bell JH, Hartley PS, Cox JSG. Dry powder aerosols I: a new powder inhalation device. *J Pharm Sci* 1971; 10: 1559-1564.
79. Smith G, Hiller C, Mazumder M, Bone R. Aerodynamic size distribution of cromolyn sodium at ambient and airway humidity. *Am Rev Respir Dis* 1980; 121: 513-517.
80. Berg T. Clinical evaluation of a new breath-activated turboinhaler for delivering sodium cromoglycate powder. *Eur J Respir Dis* 1983; 64 (suppl 126): 569.
81. Hallworth GW. An improved design of powder inhaler. *Br J Clin Pharmacol* 1977; 4: 689-690.
82. Pover GM, Browning AK, Mullinger BM, Butler AG, Dash CH. A new dry powder inhaler. *Practitioner* 1982; 226: 565-567.
83. Groth S, Dirksen H. Optimal inhalation procedure for the fenoterol powder inhaler. *Eur J Respir Dis* 1983; 64 (suppl 130): 17-24.

# Chapter 3

# Oxygen Therapy and Toxicity

*Helen E. Ward, G.J. Baker and N. Berend*

## Oxygen Therapy

The administration of oxygen is almost universal in acute, severe respiratory disease; oxygen saves more lives than any other drug used in respiratory medicine. Oxygen is also being used more frequently in the management of chronic respiratory disorders. It is beyond the scope of this chapter to discuss in detail the indications and therapeutic guidelines in each particular disease entity. However, the rational use of oxygen requires an understanding of the pathophysiology of respiratory disease, and the factors affecting oxygen transport. It is also important to recognise that oxygen administration is not without hazard. The aim of this chapter is to familiarise the reader, at least in broad principle, with these issues so that oxygen may be given with maximum benefit and least risk.

### Oxygen Transport

The $PO_2$ of blood returning to the heart (mixed venous $PO_2$) is determined by the balance between oxygen delivery to the peripheral circulation and oxygen requirements of the tissues. While it is not possible to alter oxygen demand under normal circumstances, oxygen transport can be markedly influenced by changes in both arterial oxygen content and cardiac output.

Oxygen is carried in the blood in two forms: physically dissolved in the plasma and chemically combined with haemoglobin. The amount of oxygen dissolved is proportional to its partial pressure (Henry's law): for each mmHg of $PO_2$ there is 0.003ml oxygen per 100ml blood. Normal arterial blood with a $PO_2$ of 100mmHg (13.3kPa) therefore contains only 0.3ml oxygen per 100ml, a small proportion of the normal oxygen content of the blood (Figure 3.1). However, the amount of dissolved oxygen can be markedly increased if the arterial $PO_2$ is increased by breathing high inspired concentrations of oxygen, particularly hyperbaric oxygen.

Oxygen combines readily and reversibly with haemoglobin to form oxyhaemoglobin. As one gram of haemoglobin can combine with 1.39ml of oxygen,[1] normal blood containing 15g of haemoglobin per 100ml can carry 20.8ml of oxygen per 100ml blood when haemoglobin is fully saturated. As the oxygen dissociation curve (Figure 3.1) is not linear, the oxygen saturation of arterial blood with a $PO_2$ of 100mmHg (13.3kPa) is about 97.5%, and the saturation remains above 90% with $PO_2$ values greater than about 60mmHg (8kPa). This flat upper portion of the oxygen dissociation curve means that loading of oxygen on to haemoglobin from alveolar gas will not be substantially reduced until the arterial $PO_2$ falls below 60mmHg (8kPa). Hence this $PO_2$ is generally accepted as 'safe' to ensure adequate oxygen

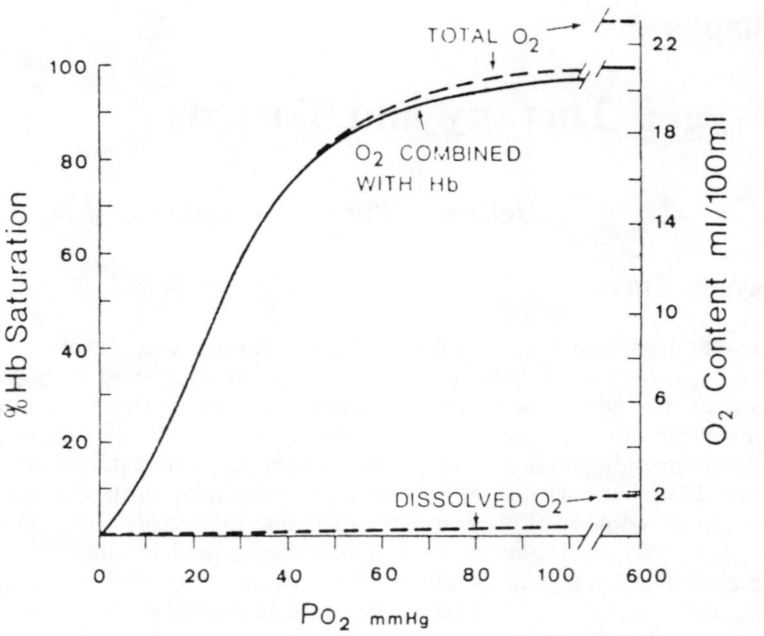


*Figure 3.1* Oxygen dissociation curve (solid line) for pH 7.4, $PCO_2$ 40mmHg and 37°C. The total blood oxygen content is also shown for a haemoglobin concentration of 15g/100ml of blood (from West JB. *Respiratory physiology — the essentials.* 2nd ed. Baltimore: Williams and Wilkins, 1979: 71).

delivery to the tissues. By contrast, due to the steep slope of the lower portion of the oxygen dissociation curve, a small fall in capillary $PO_2$ results in the release of a large amount of oxygen which can diffuse into the tissues.

Alterations in pH, $PCO_2$ and temperature affect the position of the oxygen dissociation curve. A fall in pH, a rise in $PCO_2$ and a rise in temperature all shift the curve to the right, which means that at a given capillary $PO_2$ more oxygen is released from oxyhaemoglobin. Opposite changes in pH, $PCO_2$ and temperature result in a shift of the curve to the left and impaired oxygen release from oxyhaemoglobin. Carboxyhaemoglobin and methaemoglobin also have increased affinity for oxygen.[1]

2,3-Diphosphoglycerate (DPG) is a by-product of erythrocyte glycolysis. Its concentration increases during chronic hypoxia and leads to a shift of the oxygen dissociation curve to the right, which assists the unloading of oxygen to peripheral tissues. In patients transfused with large amounts of stored blood, the 2,3-DPG levels are low and the curve shifts to the left. The position of the oxygen dissociation curve can be assessed by measuring the $P_{50}$ which is the $PO_2$ at which 50% of the haemoglobin is saturated. The normal value for human blood is about 26mmHg (3.5kPa).[1]

The oxygen content of arterial blood is therefore reduced by conditions resulting in a reduced oxygen-carrying capacity of the blood (anaemia, carbon monoxide poisoning) or reduced arterial oxygen tension (arterial hypoxaemia). However, the total amount of oxygen per unit time (oxygen flux) going to the tissues is a product of oxygen content and cardiac output. An increase in cardiac output can therefore at least partially compensate for a reduction in oxygen content; this occurs in patients with anaemia. In patients with chronic hypoxaemia, compensatory polycythaemia occurs and increases the oxygen-carrying capacity of the blood. However, when the haematocrit exceeds 65%, the blood viscosity increases markedly, countering this advantage.[2]

## Hypoxaemia

Hypoxaemia results through one or more of four mechanisms: hypoventilation, ventilation-perfusion inequality, shunt, and impairment of diffusion.[3]

### *Hypoventilation*

This occurs when the volume of fresh gas entering the alveoli per unit time (alveolar ventilation) is insufficient to replenish the oxygen removed from the blood by the metabolic demands of the body. In addition, the flow of gas leaving the alveoli is insufficient to remove the carbon dioxide entering the alveoli from the blood. Therefore, hypoventilation is always associated with an increased alveolar and arterial $PCO_2$. The relationship between arterial $PCO_2$ and alveolar ventilation in the normal lung is:

$$\text{arterial } PCO_2 = \dot{V}CO_2/\dot{V}_A.K$$

where $\dot{V}CO_2$ is the carbon dioxide production, $\dot{V}_A$ is the alveolar ventilation, and K is a constant. Thus, if the alveolar ventilation is halved the arterial $PCO_2$ is doubled once a steady state has been established. However, the hypoxaemia caused by hypoventilation can be readily abolished by administering oxygen without correcting the hypercapnia. This can be predicted from the alveolar gas equation:

$$P_AO_2 = P_IO_2 - \text{arterial } PCO_2/R + F$$

where $P_AO_2$ is the alveolar $PO_2$, $P_IO_2$ is the inspired $PO_2$, R is the respiratory exchange ratio, and F is a small correction factor. The arterial $PCO_2$ is used for the alveolar value. Assuming that alveolar ventilation and metabolic rate remain constant, it can be seen that the alveolar $PO_2$ (and therefore the arterial $PO_2$) rises approximately parallel with the inspired $PO_2$. Thus hypoxaemia due to hypoventilation is very easily reversed by a modest oxygen enrichment of the inspired gas using a simple mask. The alveolar gas equation also predicts that, even with severe hypoventilation, arterial $PO_2$ cannot fall to very low levels.[3]

The causes of hypoventilation include:

1. Depression of the respiratory centre by drugs including barbiturates, opiates or anaesthetics.
2. Disease of the medulla including encephalitis, trauma, haemorrhage or neoplasia (rare).
3. Abnormalities of the spinal cord: conducting pathways such as high cervical dislocation; anterior horn cell diseases such as poliomyelitis.
4. Disease of the motor axons to the respiratory muscles including the Guillain-Barré syndrome.

5. Diseases of the myoneural junction such as myasthenia gravis and anticholinesterase poisoning.
6. Respiratory muscle disease such as progressive muscular dystrophy.
7. Abnormalities of the thoracic cage such as flail chest and severe kyphoscoliosis.
8. Upper airway obstruction such as extrinsic tracheal compression by a thymoma, thyroid tumour or aortic aneurysm; or tracheal stenosis caused by a congenital abnormality or scarring following injury.
9. The Pickwickian syndrome. Some extremely obese patients hypoventilate and the association of obesity, daytime somnolence, polycythaemia and excessive appetite has been called the Pickwickian syndrome. Increased work of breathing associated with obesity is probably an aetiological factor, as weight loss often results in dramatic symptomatic improvement. However, the association of marked somnolence and excessive appetite suggest that an abnormality of the central nervous system may be present, at least in some patients.
10. Idiopathic hypoventilation is a rare disease characterised by impaired ventilatory response to carbon dioxide in patients whose lungs and chest wall are normal.
11. Sleep apnoea. Apnoeic periods which occur during sleep can be divided into central apnoeas, in which respiratory efforts are absent, and obstructive apnoeas, where there is no airflow in spite of respiratory muscle activity. Mixed central and obstructive apnoeas also occur. Backward movement of the tongue, or enlarged tonsils or adenoids, can cause airway obstruction. Recent studies in patients with obstructive sleep apnoea reveal a reduced pharyngeal cross-sectional area which is further reduced by recumbency.[4] However, application of continuous positive airway pressure returns the calibre to that found in normal subjects[4] and is associated with reduction or abolition of apnoeas.[5]

### *Ventilation-perfusion Inequality*

This means that ventilation and blood flow are mismatched in various regions of the lung, resulting in inefficiency of gas transfer. This mechanism of hypoxia is extremely common and is responsible for most, if not all, of the hypoxaemia of chronic obstructive lung disease, interstitial lung disease and vascular disorders such as pulmonary embolism.[3,6]

Some ventilation-perfusion inequality exists even in the normal upright lung where the ventilation-perfusion ratio decreases from apex to base. However, as pulmonary disease occurs and progresses, there is a disorganisation of the relationship between ventilation and blood flow in the alveoli. A convenient way of depicting the effect of the ventilation-perfusion ratio is to use the oxygen/carbon dioxide diagram (Figure 3.2) which shows the gas tensions in a lung which is supplied with an inspired gas composition (I), and a mixed venous blood composition ($\tilde{v}$). All alveolar gas compositions in this lung are represented and the alveolar $PO_2$ and $PCO_2$ move along the line from $\tilde{v}$ to I, as the ventilation-perfusion ratio is increased. If the ventilation-perfusion ratio in a lung unit decreases below one, hypoxaemia and mild hypercapnia occur resulting in so-called venous admixture. The extreme of this situation is a ventilation-perfusion ratio of O; that is, no

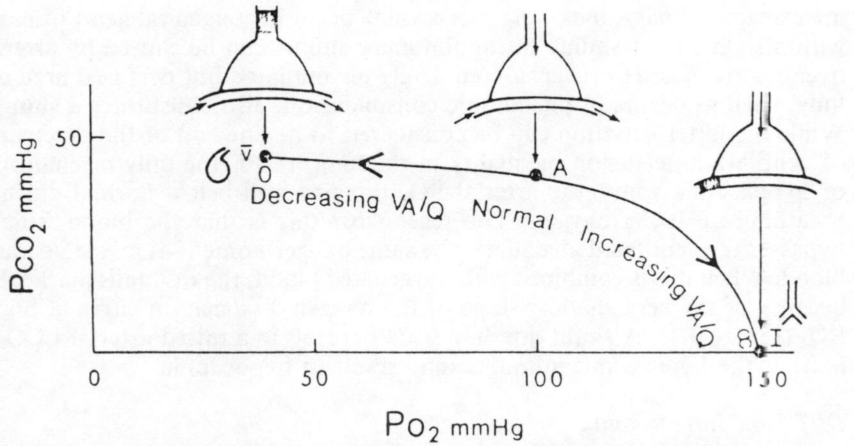


*Figure 3.2* Oxygen-carbon dioxide diagram showing a ventilation-perfusion ratio line. The $PO_2$ and $PCO_2$ of a lung unit move along this line from the mixed venous point, v̄, to the inspired gas point, I, as the ventilation-perfusion ratio is increased. Point A represents the normal alveolar gas composition (from West JB. *Ventilation/blood flow and gas exchange.* 3rd ed. Oxford: Blackwell, 1977: 37).

ventilation but persisting perfusion. This constitutes a shunt (see below). In lung units having high ventilation-perfusion ratios, the $PO_2$ can be seen to increase to a maximum determined by the inspired $PO_2$. Such an increase in arterial $PO_2$ does not significantly alter the oxygen content of arterial blood due to the almost flat upper portion of the oxygen dissociation curve (Figure 3.1). However, the $PCO_2$ in such high ventilation-perfusion lung units does fall appreciably, as does the carbon dioxide content of the blood. This is because the carbon dioxide dissociation curve is almost straight in the physiological range,[1] so that an increase in ventilation will increase the carbon dioxide clearance from lung units with both high and low ventilation-perfusion ratios.

An indication of the amount of ventilation-perfusion inequality can be obtained by measuring the overall impairment of gas exchange:

1. The alveolar-arterial oxygen difference. This is obtained by subtracting the arterial $PO_2$ from the 'ideal' alveolar $PO_2$ which can be calculated from the alveolar gas equation (see above). An increased alveolar-arterial oxygen difference reflects mainly those alveoli with abnormally low, rather than abnormally high, ventilation-perfusion ratios within the lung. In the normal upright lung this difference is about 4mmHg (0.5kPa)[1] and values over about 10mmHg (1.3kPa) are considered abnormal, although the upper limit of normal increases with age.
2. Physiologic shunt. The effect of the units with low ventilation-perfusion ratios can be assessed by measuring the physiologic shunt.[3]
3. The physiologic dead space. The effect of lung units with abnormally high ventilation-perfusion ratios is assessed by calculating the physiologic dead space.[3]

### *Shunt*

When mixed venous blood reaches the arterial system without passing through ventilated regions of the lung, this constitutes a shunt. The most common are extrapulmonary, including those which occur in congenital heart disease with a right-to-left shunt. Intrapulmonary shunts can be caused by arteriovenous fistulas. However, a completely unventilated but perfused area of lung, such as occurs in pneumonic consolidation, also constitutes a shunt. While the latter situation can be considered to be one end of the spectrum of ventilation-perfusion inequality in the lung, this is the only mechanism of hypoxaemia where the arterial $PO_2$ remains well below normal during breathing of 100% oxygen. The reason for this is that the blood which bypasses the ventilated alveoli has the same oxygen content as mixed venous blood. When this is combined with oxygenated blood, the $PO_2$ falls markedly because of the very shallow slope of the oxygen-dissociation curve at high $PO_2$ (Figure 3.1). A shunt does not usually result in a raised arterial $PCO_2$; indeed, the hypoxaemic stimulus may result in hypocapnia.

### *Diffusion Impairment*

In conditions such as interstitial lung disease, Goodpasture's syndrome and alveolar cell carcinoma, the blood-gas barrier is thickened, at least in some regions of the lung. Gaseous diffusion in these areas would be expected to be slowed, so that the $PO_2$ may not equilibrate between alveolar gas and pulmonary capillary blood. However, recent studies have shown that the hypoxaemia at rest in such diseases can be almost entirely explained by ventilation-perfusion mismatching, with only some of the hypoxaemia seen on exercise caused by diffusion impairment.[3,6]

## Methods of Oxygen Administration

### *Nasal Cannulas*

These are well accepted by patients when used at flow rates up to 3 to 4L/min. At higher flow rates, nasal crusting and bleeding may occur, although this is reduced by humidification. The inspired oxygen concentration is not predictable and varies with the inspiratory flow rate and the type of breathing. However, it is usually in the range 25 to 30%[3] and in most cases this is not critical for its effect, particularly when it is used for long-term low-dose therapy.

### *Masks*

Simple masks are well tolerated by most patients, although some patients find them hot and uncomfortable. The inspired oxygen concentration varies markedly with the flow rate and pattern of breathing, but can reach up to 60% at flow rates up to 6L/min.[3] They are therefore unsuitable for patients at risk of carbon dioxide retention due to the risk of suppression of the hypoxic drive as well as carbon dioxide accummulation in the mask.

With fixed percentage masks using the Venturi principle, a jet of oxygen at a set flow rate enters the mask and entrains air to produce a fixed oxygen concentration, usually 24, 28 or 35%. Total flow rates are high so that rebreathing of expired gas is minimal. The masks are bulky and uncomfortable, particularly with prolonged use, but they are the method of choice for administering oxygen to patients at risk of developing carbon dioxide retention.

All masks suffer from the disadvantage that they can be easily displaced by a confused or obtunded patient.

### Tents

Due to problems in keeping masks or nasal cannulas in place, oxygen tents are still used for children. Humidification can be applied to the child's environment and oxygen concentrations of up to 50% can be achieved.

### Ventilators

Mechanical ventilation through an endotracheal or tracheostomy tube allows precise control of inspired oxygen concentration. To minimise the risk of oxygen toxicity (see below), the lowest inspired oxygen concentration which provides an acceptable arterial $PO_2$ should be used. As previously discussed, in most patients, an arterial $PO_2$ of 60mmHg (8kPa) appears appropriate on physiological grounds.

### Hyperbaric Oxygen

By increasing the amount of dissolved oxygen in the blood, hyperbaric oxygen can be used to improve oxygen delivery to the tissues in conditions in which the oxygen-carrying capacity of the blood has been acutely decreased, as in carbon monoxide poisoning.

### Domiciliary Oxygen

In patients with severe hypoxaemia due to chronic lung disease, domiciliary oxygen can greatly increase exercise capacity. Oxygen is usually delivered by nasal cannulas, but masks are also appropriate. Flow rates of oxygen should be individually tailored and are generally in the range 1 to 3L/min.[7,8] The oxygen source can be compressed gas or liquid oxygen (which have a low initial but high maintenance cost) or an oxygen concentrator (which has a high initial cost but low maintenance). The latter is preferred in isolated areas where delivery of cylinders is difficult, although small portable cylinders are usually required in addition to the concentrators for mobility outside the home.

## Indications for Oxygen Treatment

Oxygen is a drug which is given to relieve hypoxaemia, but it does not replace the definitive treatment of the underlying disease.

### Hypoxaemia Without Carbon Dioxide Retention

An arterial $PO_2$ below 60mmHg (8kPa) is generally an indication for oxygen therapy. Most patients will have hypocapnia in response to the hypoxic stimulus, and the risk of carbon dioxide retention with high concentrations of oxygen is low. However, blood gas tensions should be monitored to ensure adequate oxygenation is achieved (see below).

*Hypoxaemia With Carbon Dioxide Retention*

In patients with acute-on-chronic obstructive lung disease, administration of high concentrations of oxygen may result in a dramatic increase in arterial $PCO_2$ due to supression of hypoxic drive (see later). Controlled oxygen by Venturi-type mask or graded low-flow oxygen via nasal cannulas is indicated for these patients, with careful monitoring of blood gas tensions and mental state prior to step-wise increases in oxygen concentration. In severely hypoxaemic patients, it may not be possible to achieve an arterial $PO_2$ of 60mmHg (8kPa) without significant hypercapnia, and lower values of $PO_2$ may have to be accepted. However, these patients are operating on the steep part of the oxygen dissociation curve (Figure 3.1) where a small increase in $PO_2$ results in a marked increase in haemoglobin saturation. It is essential in these patients that oxygen therapy is continuous, as intermittent therapy may result in profound hypoxaemia.[3]

*Long-term Therapy for Chronic Obstructive Lung Disease*

Two controlled trials of long-term oxygen therapy[7,8] have shown that this treatment can prolong life in patients with stable chronic obstructive lung disease with hypoxaemia. Oxygen therapy (15 hours/day) reduced long-term mortality compared to control patients receiving no oxygen,[7] while continuous oxygen therapy (average, 18 hours/day) further improved survival over that observed in patients receiving nocturnal oxygen only (average, 12 hours/day).[8] Long-term oxygen also prevents nocturnal desaturation in these patients[8,9] and may result in sustained reduction of pulmonary artery pressure.[9]

The indications for such therapy are: (i) clinical and laboratory diagnosis of chronic obstructive lung disease which is stable over approximately one month of outpatient observation; and (ii) hypoxaemia, with an arterial $PO_2$ equal to or less than 55mmHg (7.3kPa), or equal to or less than 59mmHg (7.9kPa) if there is evidence of cor pulmonale or erythrocytosis.[10]

The use of this therapy for patients with other chronic hypoxic lung diseases appears logical, but has yet to be confirmed by controlled trials.[9]

## Assessment of Adequacy of Oxygen Treatment

Although many clinical criteria are listed in textbooks for detecting hypoxaemia and hypercapnia, these are notoriously unreliable even when arterial blood gases are severely abnormal.[11] It is mandatory that an objective measurement of arterial blood gas tensions is made in an appropriate clinical setting. In addition, the interpretation of the arterial $PO_2$ must always be related to the inspired $PO_2$.

Possible methods include the following.

*Arterial*

The best means of assessment of oxygenation is to measure gas tensions in arterial blood. Arterial punctures are relatively atraumatic when 25G needles are used and in general should be performed on radial or brachial arteries where adequate compression is possible to prevent haemorrhage. Modern blood gas analysers require only small volumes of appropriately heparinised blood. However, physicians should be aware of the relatively wide range of reproducibility of some of these measurements.[12]

*Transcutaneous*

Ear oximetry is a non-invasive method for measuring arterial oxygen saturation.[13] It is particularly useful for continuous monitoring, during sleep studies and to assess the effects of therapeutic manoeuvres. Transcutaneous $PCO_2$ and $PO_2$ electrodes are also now available. However, all transcutaneous measurements are subject to doubt in shock states when there is reduced cutaneous blood flow.[13,14]

*Mixed Venous*

Mixed venous $PO_2$ or haemoglobin saturation reflects the balance between oxygen demand and oxygen delivery. Such measurements are used in monitoring patients in the intensive care setting.[15]

The timing and frequency of measurement of blood gas tensions is dependent on the clinical setting. However, in acutely ill patients, arterial $PO_2$ and $PCO_2$ should be measured 15 to 20 minutes after a change in inspired oxygen concentration. The aim of oxygen therapy should be to maintain haemoglobin saturation and thus oxygen delivery at an adequate level while minimising the risk of oxygen toxicity in the lung and other organs.

## Hazards of Oxygen Therapy

### Carbon Dioxide Retention

Some patients with chronic obstructive lung disease have elevated resting arterial $PCO_2$, a compensated respiratory acidosis and arterial hypoxaemia. Much of the ventilatory drive in such patients is derived from hypoxic stimulation of peripheral chemoreceptors. If the arterial $PO_2$ is raised by administration of high oxygen concentrations, the hypoxic ventilatory drive is reduced leading to hypoventilation and further hypercapnia. In addition, any atelectasis (see below) or reversal of compensatory hypoxic vasoconstriction will increase ventilation-perfusion mismatching and hence arterial $PCO_2$. These effects can be minimised by the careful administration of controlled oxygen therapy at inspired concentrations between 24 and 28% and frequent assessment of blood gas tensions.[16]

### Atelectasis

As the inspired oxygen concentration is increased, the likelihood of absorption atelectasis rises. Oxygen displaces the inert gas nitrogen, and when oxygen diffuses from the alveolar airspace into the blood more rapidly than it enters the alveoli by ventilation, the alveoli become smaller and collapse. This impairs gas exchange by increasing shunt. Clearly, this is more likely to occur in lung units with low ventilation-perfusion ratios.[17]

## Oxygen Toxicity

Oxygen is potentially a highly destructive molecule. It has a high affinity for electrons (the third highest after fluorine and chlorine) and liberates energy when it acquires them. If oxidation occurs in a controlled fashion, the energy released can be transformed and used by the cell. However, if oxidation is uncontrolled, with an increased generation of partially reduced oxygen species, called oxygen radicals, then it can lead to cellular and tissue destruction. The free radical theory of oxygen cytotoxicity has been well reviewed.[18-21]

Each atom of the oxygen molecule can potentially accept two electrons, but before this can happen the strong bond between the atoms has to be broken. The addition of the first electron is the essential step of oxygen activation. The activated oxygen molecule is called the superoxide anion. This oxygen species can react with cellular proteins, lipids and nucleotides to disrupt cellular function.[22] It can also accept electrons to form other reactive species, such as the hydroxyl radical, which are even more reactive. Oxygen can be activated by free radicals, ionising radiation and electron-rich metals, notably copper and iron.

### *Defences Against Oxygen*

Under normal conditions almost all of the oxygen consumed by the cell is activated under the control of enzymes involved in oxidative metabolism. The cell has mechanisms to handle activated oxygen in a controlled fashion and enzymes to quench the effects of excess activated oxygen. There are a number of enzymes and enzyme systems that remove activated oxygen species and maintain the homeostatic redox potential. Superoxide dismutases are metalloproteins which accelerate the formation of hydrogen peroxide from superoxide. The hydrogen peroxide itself is disposed of by catalase and glutathione peroxidase. The latter enzyme uses reduced glutathione as a substrate and regenerates it in a reduction reaction requiring glutathione reductase and NADPH. The cell also contains non-protein antioxidants such as vitamin E, ascorbic acid and vitamin A. Thus the cytotoxic effect of oxygen depends on both the dose of oxygen and the levels of antioxidants.

Tolerance to the effects of high concentrations of oxygen can be induced in animals by exposing them to moderate doses of oxidants, such as 85% oxygen or ozone, as well as other chemicals, such as endotoxin. This tolerance appears to be related to an increase in the intracellular enzymes which quench activated oxygen. The relative resistance to high levels of oxygen of some animal species, some strains and younger animals, can be partly explained by high levels of cellular antioxidants.

### *Acute High-dose Oxygen Toxicity*

When supplemental oxygen is administered in disease states, the alveolar cells and the cells lining the respiratory tract are exposed to the highest oxygen concentration. Provided the arterial $PO_2$ is not increased above normal, oxygenation of the other tissues is either normal or remains subnormal. However, during hyperbaric oxygen therapy all tissues may be exposed to high oxygen concentrations.

The earliest effect on the respiratory tract seen after six hours of 90 to 95% oxygen is a decreased clearance of airway mucus and a tracheitis. Twenty-four hours of exposure to this concentration is required before changes in lung function, such as a reduction in vital capacity, are seen. This change may be on the basis of atelectasis. After 24 to 48 hours of 90% or more oxygen the adult respiratory distress syndrome (ARDS) develops.[23,24]

The acute physiological changes include an increase in shunt and dead space, and a decrease in compliance, leading to ventilation-perfusion mismatching and hence hypoxaemia.[25] In animals which survive the acute oxygen toxicity, the lung may return to normal, or it may develop a non-specific fibrotic response. Clinical parallels are seen in neonates exposed to high concentrations of oxygen who subsequently develop bronchopulmonary dysplasia, and in adults who develop pulmonary fibrosis after recovery from ARDS.

These acute and chronic changes can be correlated with distinct cellular changes which have been well described in quantitative morphometric studies in animals.[26] The changes are relatively non-specific to oxygen and are seen in many forms of diffuse lung injury. The histological picture depends upon both the dose of oxygen and the duration of exposure. In patients, the pathology is further complicated by the underlying pulmonary disease and treatment. There are two main processes occurring: (i) the damaging process of oxygen, also called the exudative phase; and (ii) the reparative process by the lung, or proliferative phase.

The earliest damage to the alveoli is seen in the vulnerable endothelial and type 1 epithelial cells.[27] The endothelial cells undergo necrosis, leading to a decrease in overall capillary surface area and lumen, and a leakage of plasma into the interstitial spaces. The necrosis of the attenuated type 1 epithelial cells results in alveolar oedema and leads to alveolar haemorrhage. The filling of alveoli with plasma and blood inactivates pulmonary surfactant leading to alveolar collapse.

The earliest responses to this damage are accumulation of platelets on endothelial cells and infiltration of inflammatory cells in the interstitium. Polymorphonuclear leucocytes are the predominant cell found in the interstitium and alveoli at this time. Lung cells of the endothelium, mesothelium and epithelium can also respond to this injury.[23,24,27] Each cell line has a different tolerance to oxidant damage, with the fibroblasts being the most hardy. The extent and type of response depends upon the degree of damage that these cells have sustained. The stem cell of the epithelium, the type 2 cell, has a characteristic cuboidal appearance with surfactant inclusions and can hypertrophy and proliferate to cover the exposed basement membrane. Subsequently, these cells can differentiate into type 1 cells. However, because the type 2 cell itself can be damaged by oxygen, a florid response is more likely to be seen in animals which have developed tolerance to oxygen, have been exposed to a lower dose of oxygen, or are recovering from high-dose oxygen exposure. If the oxygen dose is too great and the type 2 epithelial cells cannot cover the basement membrane, then fibroblasts hypertrophy and proliferate. This process is not orderly and fibroblasts can proliferate in the vascular space, interstitium and alveoli where they secrete the extracellular matrix, collagen and elastin.

In the terminal bronchioles the non-ciliated secretory (Clara) cells are believed to be the reparative stem cell and proliferate to repair the epithelial damage. Again, if these cells are damaged by the oxidant, the hardier fibroblasts proliferate.

The differences in susceptibility of these cells to oxygen is believed to be due to differences in either the levels or the inducibility of antioxidants.[19,21,22] The importance of the redox state of the cell is further illustrated by the agents or factors which enhance oxygen toxicity. The cytotoxic agents bleomycin, cyclophosphamide and doxorubicin, the pesticide paraquat, the drug nitrofurantoin and ionising radiation are all known to increase the activation of oxygen causing a depletion of the protective enzymes and hence increased oxygen toxicity.

### *Acute Extrapulmonary Effects of High-dose Oxygen*

Premature infants exposed to high concentrations of normobaric oxygen have an enhanced risk of developing retrolental fibroplasia. This is believed to be due to the low levels of the antioxidants such as vitamin E in these tissues.[28]

In hyperbaric oxygen therapy, tissues other than the lung can be exposed to high oxygen tensions and exhibit toxicity. The main toxicity is seen in the central nervous system, when convulsions may occur following exposure to three atmospheres for 35 to 96 minutes.[29]

### *Chronic Low-dose Oxygen Toxicity*

The chronic administration of low concentrations of oxygen (30% or less) to patients is not believed to cause any clinically important pulmonary damage. Postmortem studies on patients receiving continuous ambulatory oxygen at flow rates to maintain the arterial $PO_2$ between 50 and 80mmHg (6.6 and 10.7kPa) for approximately two years[8] have revealed minor proliferative and exudative changes in only some individuals.[30,31]

## References


1. West JB. *Respiratory physiology — the essentials.* 2nd ed. Baltimore: Williams and Wilkins, 1979.
2. Rudolph AM, Nadas AS, Borges WH. Hematologic adjustments to cyanotic congenital heart disease. *Pediatrics* 1953; 11: 454-464.
3. West JB. *Pulmonary pathophysiology — the essentials.* 2nd ed. Baltimore: Williams and Wilkins, 1982.
4. Brown I, McClean P, Boucher R, Zamel N, Hoffstein V. Changes in pharyngeal size with recumbency and the application of continuous positive airway pressure in patients with obstructive sleep apnea (abstract). Proceedings of the Fifteenth World Congress on Diseases of the Chest. Sydney, 1985: 15.
5. Sullivan CE, Issa FG, Berthon-Jones M, Eves L. Reversal of obstructive sleep apnoea by continuous positive airway pressure applied through the nares. *Lancet* 1981; 1: 862-865.
6. West JB. Ventilation-perfusion relationships. *Am Rev Respir Dis* 1977; 116: 919-943.
7. Medical Research Council Working Party. Long-term domiciliary oxygen therapy in chronic hypoxic cor pulmonale complicating chronic bronchitis and emphysema. *Lancet* 1981; 1: 681-686.

8. Nocturnal Oxygen Therapy Trial Group. Continuous or nocturnal oxygen therapy in hypoxemic chronic obstructive lung disease. A clinical trial. *Ann Intern Med* 1980; 93: 391-398.
9. Flenley DC. Long-term home oxygen therapy. *Chest* 1985; 87: 99-103.
10. Timms RM, Kvale PA, Anthonisen NR, Boylen CT, Cugell DW, Petty TL, Williams GW. Selection of patients with chronic obstructive pulmonary disease for long-term oxygen therapy. *JAMA* 1981; 245: 2514-2515.
11. Fraser RG, Pare JAP. Methods in clinical, laboratory and functional investigation. In: *Diagnosis of diseases of the chest.* 2nd ed. Philadelphia: Saunders, 1977: 294.
12. Burki NK. Arterial blood gas measurement. *Chest* 1985; 88: 3-4.
13. Burki NK, Albert RK. Noninvasive monitoring of arterial blood gases. *Chest* 1983; 83: 666-670.
14. Wiedemann HP, Matthay MA, Matthay RA. Cardiovascular-pulmonary monitoring in the intensive care unit (part 2). *Chest* 1984; 85: 656-668.
15. Divertie MB, McMichan JC. Continuous monitoring of mixed venous oxygen saturation. *Chest* 1984; 85: 423-428.
16. Campbell EJM. The management of acute respiratory failure in chronic bronchitis and emphysema. *Am Rev Respir Dis* 1967; 96: 626-639.
17. Dantzker DR, Wagner PD, West JB. Instability of lung units with low $\dot{V}_A\dot{Q}$ ratios during oxygen breathing. *J Appl Physiol* 1975; 38: 886-895.
18. Mustafa MG, Tierney D. Biochemical and metabolic changes in the lung with oxygen, ozone and nitrogen dioxide toxicity. *Am Rev Respir Dis* 1978; 18: 1061-1090.
19. Deneke SM, Fanburg BL. Normobaric oxygen toxicity of the lung. *N Engl J Med* 1980; 303: 76-86.
20. Halliwell B. Oxygen is poisonous: the nature and medical importance of oxygen radicals. *Med Lab Sci* 1984; 41: 157-171.
21. Frank L, Massaro D. Oxygen toxicity. *Am J Med* 1980; 69: 117-126.
22. DiGuiseppi J, Fridovich I. The toxicology of molecular oxygen. *CRC Crit Rev Toxicol* 1984; 12: 315-342.
23. Nash G, Blennerhasset JB, Pontoppidan H. Pulmonary lesion associated with oxygen breathing and artifical ventilation. *N Engl J Med* 1967; 276: 368-374.
24. Gould VE, Tosco R, Wheelis RF, Gould NS, Kapanci Y. Oxygen pneumonitis in man. Ultrastructural observations on the development of alveolar lesions. *Lab Invest* 1972; 26: 499-508.
25. Petty TL. Adult respiratory distress syndrome: definitions and historical perspective. *Clin Chest Med* 1982; 3: 3-7.
26. Crapo JD, Barry BE, Foscue HA, Shelburn J. Structural and biochemical changes in rat lung occurring during exposures to lethal and adaptive doses of oxygen. *Am Rev Respir Dis* 1980; 122: 123-143.
27. Kristler GS, Caldwell PRH, Weibel ER. Development of fine structural damage to alveolar and capillary lining cells in oxygen-poisoned rat lungs. *J Cell Biol* 1967; 33: 605-628.
28. James LS, Lawman JT, eds. History of oxygen therapy and retrolental fibroplasia. *Pediatrics* 1976; 57 (suppl): 591-642.
29. Clark JM, Lambertson CJ. Pulmonary oxygen toxicity: a review. *Pharmacol Rev* 1971; 23: 37-133.
30. Petty TL, Stanford RE, Neff TA. Continuous oxygen therapy in chronic airway obstruction: observations on possible oxygen toxicity and survival. *Ann Intern Med* 1971; 75: 361-367.
31. Jacques J, Cooney TP, Silvers GW, Petty TL, Wright JL, Thurlbeck WM. The lungs and causes of death in the nocturnal oxygen therapy trial. *Chest* 1984; 86: 230-233.

# Chapter 4

# Respiratory Stimulants and Depressants

*S. J. Watt*

## Control of Ventilation

The process of ventilation provides a supply of oxygen to, and removes carbon dioxide from, the alveolar space where gas exchange between air and blood takes place. The level of ventilation (minute volume) must alter to meet the changing requirements of metabolism induced, for example, by exercise. In the normal adult human the minute volume and the rate and pattern of ventilation result from a variety of central nervous influences. The basic rhythmicity of respiration results from spontaneous activity of a number of localised areas in the brainstem and medulla, minute volume is dependent on afferent information from chemoreceptors, whereas the pattern of respiration, the relationship between rate and depth of respiration, and the timing of the components of the respiratory cycle are influenced by afferent information from receptors within the lung.[1] These involuntary controls can readily be over-ridden by cortical influences, for example during speech, coughing or yawning.

The most important control mechanisms responsible for matching the level of ventilation with metabolic requirements are the chemoreceptors. Central chemoreceptors, present within the brainstem, respond to changes in hydrogen ion concentration secondary to changes in carbon dioxide content of arterial blood, whereas peripheral chemoreceptors, present in the carotid bodies and aortic arch, respond to both partial pressure of oxygen and hydrogen ion concentration. Afferent information from the stimulated chemoreceptors results in an increased output from the medullary respiratory centres.[1]

In health and under normal environmental conditions the influence of the arterial partial pressure of oxygen ($PO_2$) is of little importance and the main controlling factor is carbon dioxide ($PCO_2$) acting through the central chemoreceptors. However, in disease or at an altitude where there is a substantial fall in the arterial $PO_2$ the hypoxic drive to respiration becomes of increasing importance. If relative alveolar hypoventilation results in the arterial $PCO_2$ becoming chronically elevated the chemoreceptor response may adopt an elevated set-point with a reduced or absent ventilatory response to a rise in arterial $PCO_2$, and at high levels of arterial $PCO_2$ there may be depression of respiration due to a direct effect of carbon dioxide on the medullary centres.

## Respiratory Stimulants

### Clinical Situations

Clinical indications for therapeutic intervention in the control of respiration are limited. A wide variety of drugs affects the respiratory centres and control mechanisms, and most drugs with a depressant effect on the central nervous system act as respiratory depressants. Likewise, most central nervous stimulants (analeptics) have an action on the respiratory centres, but few drugs have any degree of selectivity and even the most useful agents have a low therapeutic ratio.[2]

Respiratory failure is the most frequent clinical indication for the use of respiratory stimulants, but use of drugs needs to be considered in conjunction with other therapeutic measures such as oxygen therapy and specific treatment of the underlying problem. In practice respiratory stimulants are only of use when the respiratory centres are not already stimulated by the hypoxia or hypercapnia associated with the underlying condition. This limits their possible application to type 2 respiratory failure with hypoxia and hypercapnia due to alveolar hypoventilation, where the increase in arterial $PCO_2$ fails to produce an increase in the drive to respiration. This situation occurs in drug-induced respiratory depression, chronic obstructive airways disease (particularly during exacerbations), and in the primary alveolar hypoventilation and sleep apnoea syndromes.

The management of respiratory depression resulting from drug overdose should not involve the use of respiratory stimulants. Minor degrees of respiratory depression with hypoxia may be corrected with an increase in the inspired partial pressure of oxygen, but if the arterial $PCO_2$ continues to rise, mechanical ventilation is the treatment of choice, allowing the blood gases to be corrected safely. In this situation mechanical ventilation offers a considerably improved prognosis over the use of respiratory stimulants,[2-4] which may be ineffective in subconvulsive doses.

Respiratory failure resulting from an exacerbation of chronic obstructive airways disease is undoubtedly the most frequent indication for the use of respiratory stimulants. The major aim of therapy is correction of hypoxia and the use of raised oxygen concentrations in the inspired gas should be the initial therapy. However, it must be recognised that, in patients with chronically elevated arterial $PCO_2$, even a small increase in inspired oxygen concentration may reduce the hypoxic drive to respiration and result in a reduced minute ventilation and a rising arterial $PCO_2$. Thus careful monitoring of the arterial blood gases is important. When hypoxia cannot be corrected without a reduction in ventilatory drive, respiratory stimulants may be useful by providing an alternative drive.[5] Acute episodes of respiratory failure and cor pulmonale also occur in patients with primary alveolar hypoventilation and require similar management.

In chronic respiratory failure associated with obstructive airways disease,[5] the sleep apnoea syndrome[6] and the alveolar hypoventilation syndrome, where persistent elevation of arterial $PCO_2$ occurs as a result of alveolar hypoventilation, the use of oral respiratory stimulants offers a possible means of controlling some of the complications of chronic hypoxia. A variety of drugs has achieved some popularity. These include carbonic anhydrase inhibitors, progestogens, and the recently introduced peripheral chemoreceptor stimulant, almitrine.

The syndrome of acute mountain sickness occurs on ascent to altitude in normal individuals whose ventilatory response to hypoxia is often less than average. Thus these individuals do not have the same fall in arterial $PCO_2$ at altitude as the unaffected individual. The syndrome is associated with a degree of fluid retention and may be controlled by a diuretic agent, but carbonic anhydrase inhibitors appear particularly useful because they lead to a fall in arterial pH, and a rise in minute ventilation with an associated rise in arterial $PO_2$ in addition to controlling symptoms and fluid retention.[7,8]

Methyl xanthines, in addition to their action as bronchodilators, may also have a respiratory stimulant action. Respiratory muscle fatigue may be important in the pathogenesis of ventilatory failure and it has been suggested that methyl xanthines produce improvement in contractility and fatigue of respiratory muscles,[9] but this is disputed,[10] and the clinical usefulness of the effect is dubious.[11] In type 2 respiratory failure the vasodilator action on the pulmonary vascular bed increases the venous admixture effect and a paradoxical fall in arterial $PO_2$ may result.[12] This is of greater clinical significance than the respiratory stimulant action.

**Central Stimulants**

A variety of non-specific analeptic drugs has been used as respiratory stimulants in the past. These include ethamivan, nikethamide and doxapram. Their mode of action is by direct stimulation of the medullary respiratory centres, though it is possible that they may have some action on the peripheral chemoreceptors in addition.

They must be given by intravenous injection and following a bolus dose the effect on ventilation is transient lasting only a few minutes. The transient nature of the effect is probably related to redistribution of the drug rather than to metabolism, and subsequent doses are likely to produce more widespread stimulation. This limits the usefulness of most of these agents, but doxapram appears to have a wider margin of safety and is undoubtedly the drug of choice in this group.[13,14] Its use is now confined to the management of respiratory failure where the administration of oxygen leads to a rise in arterial $PCO_2$. This situation commonly arises during exacerbations of chronic obstructive airways disease. The use of continuous infusions of doxapram in doses of up to 5mg/min together with oxygen may permit adequate oxygenation to be maintained while the underlying cause (infection, bronchospasm) responds to appropriate therapy.[5] This has allowed many situations to be managed without artificial ventilation and its associated problems in patients with poor respiratory function.

Respiratory stimulants are of no value in the management of respiratory failure resulting from overdosage of sedative agents, or from acute severe asthma, when mechanical ventilation is indicated.

Side effects are predominantly a result of widespread stimulation of the central nervous system and while muscular twitching and more generalised convulsions are the major effects limiting dosage, cardiovascular effects such as hypertension and dysrhythmias and gastrointestinal side effects including vomiting may also cause problems. The use of these drugs results in a rise in oxygen consumption which markedly reduces their value.

Respiratory failure requiring such therapy is clearly a life-threatening situation and contraindications need to be considered in this context. The effect of doxapram is potentiated by monoamine oxidase inhibitor therapy and possibly also by methyl xanthines, which are frequently used in these patients. Pre-existing hypertension and ischaemic heart disease may also deteriorate with doxapram therapy.

## Carbonic Anhydrase Inhibitors

These sulphonamide derivatives which include acetazolamide and dichlorphenamide act by non-competitive inhibition of the enzyme which catalyses the reaction between carbon dioxide and water producing carbonic acid. The enzyme is ubiquitous and requires 99% inhibition to produce a clinical effect. They are mild diuretic agents and cause an alkaline urine with loss of bicarbonate ion in the urine and a metabolic acidosis. This acidosis results in stimulation of chemoreceptors.[15]

They are well absorbed from the gastrointestinal tract and produce a peak plasma level in about two hours. The drugs are heavily bound and hence localised to carbonic anhydrase and are excreted via the kidney. Production of a sustained metabolic acidosis requires frequent doses, such as acetazolamide 250mg three or four times daily in contrast to the usual once-daily diuretic regime.

These drugs have been shown to be of value as respiratory stimulants in several situations. While improvement has been reported in ventilatory failure secondary to obstructive airways disease,[15] this appears of limited value in clinical practice. In primary alveolar hypoventilation some improvement in oxygenation may result in a proportion of patients, but the response is variable.[16] Acetazolamide has been reported as a useful prophylactic agent in the prevention of acute mountain sickness,[7,8] which appears to be associated with a poor ventilatory response to hypoxia. Prophylactic therapy, in addition to prevention of symptoms, has been associated with improved ventilation, lower arterial $PCO_2$ and improved sleep at altitude.

Side effects are uncommon, but in the relatively high doses required some drowsiness and paraesthesiae may occur. Fatigue, irritability and mild gastrointestinal upsets with nausea and vomiting are less common. Hypersensitivity reactions similar to those associated with other sulphonamides including fever, skin reactions and bone marrow depression are rare.

## Almitrine

Although this piperazine derivative is not yet widely available it justifies discussion because of its potential. It acts as a specific stimulator of peripheral chemoreceptors and in both human volunteers and patients with airways obstruction leads to an increase in hypoxic respiratory drive.[17] There is an increase in ventilation, but improvements in arterial $PO_2$ and $PCO_2$ are disproportionate to the change in ventilation. Thus it appears to improve ventilation-perfusion imbalance by an action on the pulmonary circulation though the mechanism is unclear.

The drug is lipid-soluble and may be given by either the intravenous or oral route. It is highly protein-bound and is concentrated in the carotid bodies. Its half-life in plasma is long due to protein binding, but free drug is rapidly metabolised to inactive metabolites which are excreted in the bile.

Almitrine has been used in patients with chronic respiratory failure due to obstructive airways disease,[18,19] as well as primary alveolar hypoventilation and sleep apnoea syndromes.[20] While improvement in blood gases have been maintained for six months there have also been reports of an associated rise in pulmonary arterial pressure,[21] and the precise indications for the use of this drug remain unclear.

Side effects appear to be uncommon, though a number of patients have reported that they find the increase in ventilation distressing, and there have been case reports of a reversible sensory peripheral neuropathy.[22]

### Medroxyprogesterone

Progestogens are responsible for an increase in ventilation during pregnancy and exogenous agents cause a similar rise in ventilation. In normal subjects this results in an increase in minute volume and a fall in arterial $PCO_2$. The mechanism is obscure, but is probably central.[23] The effect on ventilation is of slow onset reaching a maximum after seven days' treatment. The drug may be given either by the sublingual or oral route and is metabolised in the liver.

A number of studies has shown some improvement in oxygenation after treatment with 60 to 120mg of medroxyprogesterone per day in patients with alveolar hypoventilation together with some improvement in other indices including polycythaemia.[24,25] In patients with obstructive sleep apnoea there may be improvement in arterial $PO_2$, but it does not appear to reduce the number of apnoeas.[26] Reports of its use in infants with alveolar hypoventilation have also been encouraging.[27]

Side effects include loss of libido and impotence in male patients and the onset of diabetes mellitus.

### Protriptyline

While not primarily a respiratory stimulant this drug is included, as it appears beneficial in some patients with sleep apnoea. It is a non-sedating tricyclic antidepressant which markedly reduces the amount of REM sleep.

The drug is used in a single oral dose of 20mg at bedtime. It is well absorbed from the gastrointestinal tract and is bound to plasma proteins. It is metabolised to some extent and excreted in the urine.

Protriptyline appears to offer some benefit to patients with obstructive sleep apnoea, with some reduction of total apnoea time and improvement in oxygen saturation. Apnoeas still occur and remain associated with deoxygenation.[28-30] While the drug produces considerable benefit in a few patients, for whom the only alternative may be tracheostomy or mechanical assistance, its effect is variable and unpredictable.

The use of this drug is frequently limited by anticholinergic side effects and these patients appear susceptible. Many patients are older men and urinary retention is a particular problem.

## Respiratory Depressants

A wide variety of drugs has a depressant effect on respiration including opiates, major and minor tranquillisers, hypnotic agents, anaesthetics, psychotropic agents and alcohol. However, the effect on respiration is, under most circumstances, an unwanted side effect and there is virtually no indication for the use of these agents specifically for their depressant action apart from their use in anaesthesia. There are other indications for the use of these agents in the management of patients with respiratory disease when their effect on respiration requires careful consideration.

While detailed pharmacology of all these agents is not justified in this review, some of the indications for the use of these agents will be considered briefly.

**Clinical Situations**

Opiate drugs are widely used for analgesia and also as antitussive agents, especially in the management of malignant disease of the thorax. They may also be used either alone or together with a major tranquilliser for sedative and antitussive action for the procedure of bronchoscopy.[31] In this circumstance the respiratory depression associated with the airway obstruction due to the bronchoscope itself may lead to acute hypoxia despite the administration of oxygen.[32] However, the procedure can be rapidly terminated and the respiratory depression reversed to some extent with naloxone. For this reason some bronchoscopists prefer to use opiates rather than non-reversible alternative tranquillisers.

Minor tranquillisers such as diazepam or midazolam, given intravenously, offer an alternative form of sedation for bronchoscopy; they occasionally lead to severe respiratory depression and rarely transient respiratory arrest, but this can usually be managed with the administration of oxygen alone.

Occasionally patients with chronic respiratory disease may suffer episodes of acute breathlessness due to anxiety often arising from the symptoms of their underlying condition. While sedative agents are normally contraindicated in conditions which may progress to respiratory failure, some of these patients may benefit from minor tranquillisers; if they are prescribed, these drugs should initially be given for a trial period with careful monitoring of the patient.

Apart from the management of concurrent psychiatric disease the indications for the use of a major tranquilliser in the management of a patient with respiratory disease are extremely limited. However, hypoxia may occasionally produce an acute behavioural disorder requiring sedation. In these circumstances intramuscular paraldehyde is possibly the safest agent and may permit correction of hypoxia by effective administration of oxygen.

## References

1. Bradley G. Control of ventilation. In: Scadding JG, Cumming G, eds. *Scientific foundations of respiratory medicine*. London: Heineman, 1981: 162-172.
2. Woolf CR. The use of respiratory stimulant drugs. *Chest* 1970; 58: 49-53.
3. Clemmensen C, Nilsson E. Therapeutic trends in the treatment of barbiturate poisoning — the Scandinavian method. *Clin Pharmacol Ther* 1961; 2: 220-229.
4. Mark LC. Analeptics: changing concepts, declining status. *Am J Med Sci* 1967; 254: 296-302.
5. Rees J. Treatment of pulmonary hypertension in chronic bronchitis and emphysema. *Br Med J* 1984; 289: 1398-1399.
6. Guilleminault C, Tilkian A, Dement WC. The sleep apnoea syndromes. *Ann Rev Med* 1976; 27: 465-484.
7. Gray GW, Bryan AC, Frayser R, et al. Control of acute mountain sickness. *Aerospace Med* 1971; 42: 181-184.

8. Greene MK, Kerr AM, McIntosh IB, Prescott RJ. Acetazolamide in prevention of acute mountain sickness: a double blind controlled cross over study. *Br Med J* 1981; 283: 811-813.
9. Murciano D, Aubier M, Lecocgnic Y, Pariente R. Effects of theophylline on diaphragmatic strength and fatigue in patients with chronic obstructive pulmonary disease. *N Engl J Med* 1984; 311: 349-353.
10. Ethimiou J, Fleming J, Edwards RHT, Spiro SG. Effect of aminophylline on fatigue of the sternomastoid muscle in man. *Thorax* 1986; 41: 122-127.
11. Belman MJ, Sieck GC, Mazar A. Aminophylline and its influence on ventilatory endurance in humans. *Am Rev Respir Dis* 1985; 131: 226-229.
12. Halmagyi DF, Cotes JE. Reduction in systemic blood oxygen as a result of procedures affecting the pulmonary circulation in patients with chronic pulmonary disease. *Clin Sci* 1959; 18: 475-489.
13. Edwards G, Leszczynski SO. A double blind trial of five respiratory stimulants in patients with acute ventilatory failure. *Lancet* 1967; 2: 226-229.
14. Moser KM, Luchsinger PC, Adamson JS, et al. Respiratory stimulation with intravenous doxapram in respiratory failure. *N Engl J Med* 1973; 288: 427-431.
15. Lane DJ, Horwell JB, Stretton TB. The effect of dichlorphenamide on blood and cerebrospinal fluid acid-base state in chronic ventilatory failure. *Clin Sci* 1977; 39: 391-406.
16. White DP, Zwillich CW, Pickett CK, et al. Central sleep apnoea — improvement with acetazolamide therapy. *Arch Intern Med* 1982; 142: 1816-1819.
17. Howard P. Almitrine bismesylate (vectarion). *Bull Eur Physiolpathol Respir* 1984; 20: 99-103.
18. Anonymous. Almitrine in chronic airflow obstruction. *Lancet* 1985; 1: 796-797.
19. Powles ACP, Tuxen DV, Pugsley SO, et al. The effect of almitrine on sleep hypoxaemia in patients with chronic airflow limitation. *Am Rev Respir Dis* 1984; 129: A66.
20. Kreiger J, Mangin P, Kurtz D. Effects of a ventilatory stimulant, almitrine bismesylate in the sleep apnoea syndrome. *Curr Ther Res* 1982; 32: 697-705.
21. Dall WL, Polu JM, Sadoul P. The pulmonary haemodynamic effects of almitrine infusion in man with chronic hypercapnia. *Clin Sci* 1983; 64: 25-31.
22. Chedra R, Nodzenski R, Dunand JF, et al. Peripheral neuropathy during treatment with almitrine. *Br Med J* 1985; 290: 896.
23. Skatrud JB, Dempsey JA, Kaiser DG. Ventilatory response to medroxyprogesterone acetate in normal subjects — time course and mechanism. *J Appl Physiol* 1978; 44: 939-944.
24. Sutton FD, Zwillich CW, Creagh CE, et al. Progesterone for outpatient treatment of pickwickian syndrome. *Ann Intern Med* 1975; 83: 476-479.
25. Strohl KP, Hensley MJ, Saunders NA, et al. Progesterone administration and progressive sleep apnoeas. *JAMA* 1981; 245: 1230-1232.
26. Orr WC, Imes NK, Martin RJ. Progesterone therapy in obese patients with sleep apnoea. *Arch Intern Med* 1979; 139: 109-111.
27. Milerad J, Lagercrantz H, Löfgren O. Alveolar hypoventilation treated with medroxyprogesterone. *Arch Dis Child* 1985; 60: 150-155.
28. Clark RW, Schmidt HS, Schad SF, et al. Sleep apnoea-treatment with protriptyline. *Neurology* 1979; 29: 1287-1292.
29. Brownwell LG, West P, Sweatman P, et al. Protriptyline in obstructive sleep apnoea *N Engl J Med* 1982; 307: 1037-1042.
30. Bradley D, Phillipson EA. The treatment of obstructive sleep apnoea. *Am Rev Respir Dis* 1983; 128: 583-586.
31. Clarke SW, Knight RK. Fibreoptic bronchoscopy Part I. Technique and appraisal. *Practitioner* 1977; 218: 119-122.
32. Credle WF, Smiddy JF, Elliott RC. Complications of fibreoptic bronchoscopy. *Am Rev Respir Dis* 1974; 109: 67-72.

# Chapter 5

# Drugs Which Influence Cough, Mucus and Ciliary Function

*Anthony J. Whelan and Johnathan Rutland*

*In all diseases which affect the lungs . . .*
*. . . sputum should be brought up early.*

*Prognosis,*[1]
Hippocrates.

Cough and sputum production, common symptoms of respiratory disease, often cause patients to seek medical advice for their relief. A variety of proprietary preparations, many containing multiple agents, is available both on prescription and over the counter, intended for symptomatic control of troublesome cough and modification of sputum production. Many of these compounds are traditional remedies of unproven efficacy, but long lineage. However, limitations of methods for assessing these drugs and of published clinical trials performed objectively make evaluation of their clinical impact difficult. Cough does not always require treatment which may, in fact, be counterproductive.

Cough and mucociliary clearance form important parts of the defence mechanisms of the lung, by which unwanted matter is removed from the respiratory tract.[2] The symptoms of cough and expectoration reflect an underlying pathological process and are not disease states in themselves. Treatment should, if possible, be directed towards the underlying disease rather than towards suppression of symptoms alone. In some situations, such as respiratory tract infection after thoracic or abdominal surgery, suppression of cough may be harmful, even though the cough causes the patient pain. However, in other situations, cough or expectoration may be so distressing to the patient that symptomatic measures become important; for example, when definitive treatment is unavailable, as in bronchogenic carcinoma.

## Cough

### Physiology of Cough[3]

Cough consists of three phases. Initially, there is a deep inspiration. This is followed by a compressive phase with active contraction of the expiratory muscles against a closed glottis. During this period, the intrathoracic pressure may exceeed 100mmHg (13.3kPa). The cough is completed by abrupt opening of the glottis with the explosive release of trapped air at speeds approximating the velocity of sound. Vibrations accompanying the expulsion of air loosen secretions adherent to the larynx and major airways. Expulsion of air continues after glottic opening. Airflow is highest and cough-induced clearance most effective where dynamic compression of the airways occurs. As lung volume falls during coughing, the point of such compression moves distally. However, cough is said to be effective only down to approximately the seventh generation of airways.[4] Distal to this, mucociliary clearance (MCC) underlies particle transport.

Receptors which can initiate cough are distributed widely. The cough reflex is mediated by afferent fibres connected to the cough centre and subsequently to efferent pathways. The vagus carries afferent impulses from cough receptors located in the larynx, trachea and bronchi as well as other receptors in the stomach, pleura, and external auditory canal; pharyngeal receptors are connected to the cough centre via the glossopharyngeal nerve; receptors in the nasal cavity and its sinuses are served by the trigeminal nerve and those in the pericardium and diaphragm by the phrenic nerve. The cough centre is located in the dorso-lateral region of the medulla. There are connections with the cerebral cortex (cough is under partial voluntary control), the respiratory centre (which lies adjacent) and to efferents in the phrenic and spinal motor nerves and in the vagus.

## Evaluation of the Patient with Cough

Cough may have many causes and may result from disease occurring wherever the above receptors are located. Some of these causes are listed in Table 5.1. History and physical examination including listening to the character of the cough and observation of sputum usually allow an accurate diagnosis and guide to further investigation and treatment (Table 5.2).

*Table 5.1* Causes of cough

| |
|---|
| *Upper Respiratory Tract* |
| Pharyngitis, laryngitis |
| Postnasal drip: sinusitis |
| Laryngeal tumours |
| *Lower Respiratory Tract* |
| Airways |
| Bronchitis, tracheitis, postviral cough syndrome |
| Bronchiectasis, cystic fibrosis |
| Inhaled foreign body |
| Asthma |
| Bronchogenic carcinoma |
| Aspiration: neurological and oesophageal disease, unconscious states |
| Lung Parenchyma |
| Infections: pneumonia, tuberculosis |
| Malignancy |
| Pulmonary oedema |
| Alveolitis |
| Pleural Space |
| Effusion (large) |
| Bronchopleural fistula |
| Mediastinum |
| Lesions compressing bronchi (enlarged lynph nodes, mediastinal tumours, aneurysms) |
| Pericardial disease |
| Extra-thoracic Disease |
| Ear irritation |
| Subphrenic abscess |
| Psychogenic cough |

*Table 5.2* Diagnosis of cough

| | |
|---|---|
| **Acute Onset Cough** | |
| *Clinical Feature* | *Likely Diagnosis* |
| Pharyngitis, fever, rhinitis, self-limiting course | Viral upper respiratory tract infection |
| Dysphonia | Laryngeal disease |
| 'Bovine' quality | Vocal cord paresis |
| Unproductive, fever, young adult, crepitations | 'Atypical' pneumonia |
| Burning retrosternal pain with cough | Tracheitis |
| Purulent sputum | Acute bronchitis, 'typical' pneumonia |
| **Chronic Cough** | |
| *Clinical Feature* | *Likely Diagnosis* |
| Smoker, mucoid sputum | Chronic bronchitis |
| Haemoptysis | Carcinoma, tuberculosis, bronchiectasis |
| Purulent sputum | Lung abscess, bronchiectasis, complicated chronic bronchitis |
| Weight loss | Carcinoma, tuberculosis |
| Wheeze | Asthma, inhaled foreign body |
| Orthopnoea | Left ventricular failure |
| Dry cough, clubbing, crepitations | Interstitial lung disease |

## Antitussive Agents

### Assessment[5]

Cough suppressants may act centrally or peripherally. These should be used for symptom control only when cough cannot be controlled by treating the underlying disease. In young children antitussives should always be used with caution.

A variety of methods may be used to assess antitussive agents.[5] Despite availability of these methods, comparisons of the effectiveness of antitussive drugs is scanty and little work has been done to assess proprietary preparations containing multiple compounds.

### Antitussives Which Act Centrally

*Narcotics*

Narcotics are the most effective antitussive agents but, because of the development of dependence, should be used only when non-narcotics are ineffective. These drugs have a direct depressant effect on the medullary cough centre as well as on the respiratory centre. Specific antagonists such as naloxone are available. Many of the actions of narcotics are undesirable in the treatment of cough (Table 5.3).

Morphine and other naturally occurring alkaloids, as well as methadone and heroin (both semisynthetic derivatives), are potent antitussives. Because of the potential for addiction and respiratory depression, these agents have limited clinical application. In the patient with advanced malignancy troubled by cough, especially when associated with pain, potent narcotics are indicated. These drugs have been incorporated into many time-honoured mixtures (for example, Brompton Cocktail, Mist. Euphoriens)[6] with good effect in the

Table 5.3 Effects of narcotic drugs

| |
|---|
| *Central Nervous System* |
| Analgesia |
| Sedation |
| Euphoria |
| Addiction |
| *Gastrointestinal* |
| Nausea, vomiting |
| Reduced gastrointestinal motility |
| Smooth muscle spasm |
| *Respiratory* |
| Cough suppression |
| Reduced secretions |
| Respiratory depression |

palliation of advanced malignancy. Short courses may be necessary for cough associated with severe pain in self-limiting conditions such as a fractured rib or pleural pain due to pulmonary infarction or pneumonia. Central respiratory depression may extend to respiratory failure.

Morphine, the parent compound of this group, is absorbed readily by the oral route and via intramuscular or subcutaneous injection. It is distributed widely to the lung, kidney and liver. Excretion and metabolism are by conjugation in the liver to morphine-3-monoglucuronide, and by excretion of this metabolite and a small fraction of unaltered morphine in the urine.[7] As with other drugs in this group, the antitussive dose (2 to 3mg) is less than that required for analgesia.[8]

Codeine (morphine-3-methylether) is a standard antitussive against which others are commonly compared. Codeine has approximately one-quarter of the respiratory depressant effect of morphine,[8] and one-twentieth of the euphoriant effect. Doses ot 10 to 20mg at four to six hourly intervals produce depression of the cough centre equivalent to that of 2 to 3mg of morphine. Codeine is well absorbed orally. The main site of degradation is in the liver — dose adjustment may be necessary in patients with liver disease. Undesirable side effects include sedation, nausea, constipation, and the potential for addiction.

Hydrocodone (dihydrocodeinone), a codeine derivative used widely, has similar antitussive properties to the parent drug. Doses are similar to codeine. This agent is incorporated in many proprietary mixtures.

Normethadone has approximately twice the antitussive effect of codeine, and a longer duration of action (8 to 12 hours) allowing a once or twice daily dosage regimen. Side effects and potential for addiction are similar to codeine.

Pholcodine (morpholinylethylmorphine) is among the most widely used drugs for cough suppression. This agent has little analgesic or euphoriant activity. Pholcodine, in a dose of 15mg, is equivalent to 10mg of codeine. The antitussive effect of pholcodine is potentiated by antihistamines.[9] This agent is suitable for, and widely used in, children. Untoward effects are unusual, although nausea and drowsiness may occur. Because of its efficacy and safety, pholcodine is commonly regarded as the antitussive agent of first choice for benign self-limiting conditions associated with cough where non-narcotic agents are ineffective.

Other narcotic agents, such as pethidine and methadone, are also antitussive, but are rarely used for this purpose alone.

*Non-narcotics*

A diverse group of non-narcotic agents also acts centrally. This group includes dextromethorphan, noscapine and several other agents in use in the USA and Europe. Dextromethorphan (d-3-methoxy-N-methylmorphinan) is used widely (especially in mixtures) and has no analgesic or euphoriant effects. Although an opioid, it has no addictive potential and is considered a non-narcotic antitussive. Efficacy is less than that of codeine. Side effects are unusual. A dose of 15mg every four to six hours is suggested for adults. Metabolic degradation occurs principally in the liver and dose adjustments may be necessary (in common with all opioids) in patients with hepatic insufficiency.

A number of other agents has been used as antitussives in Europe and the USA. Noscapine, a non-narcotic opium alkaloid has antitussive activity equivalent to codeine. Respiratory depression does not occur. Bronchodilation has been reported.[6] Levo-propoxyphene is the levo-isomer of the analgesic dextropropoxyphene. It lacks analgesic effect, but is antitussive in doses of 50 to 100mg every four to six hours. Many other agents such as caramiphen, chlophedianol and carbetapentane are in clinical use in some countries, but clinical efficacy has not been substantiated.[8]

**Antitussives Which Act Peripherally**

Local anaesthetics, bronchodilators and demulcents suppress cough by acting locally on the afferent limb of the cough reflex. (Corticosteroids and cromoglycate, used in patients with airways obstruction, may also act at this level.)

*Local Anaesthetics*

Topical applications of these agents are used to suppress cough prior to bronchoscopy and other instrumentation of the respiratory tract. Prolonged suppression of cough was demonstrated in a small number of patients with intractable symptoms using aerosolised lignocaine 10%.[10] This method has limited application in everyday clinical practice. Other local anaesthetics, notably *p*-aminobenzoate and amethocaine (tetracaine), are incorporated into lozenges used to reduce cough secondary to pharyngeal inflammation such as that due to upper respiratory tract infections.

*Bronchodilators*

These agents may reduce cough secondary to bronchoconstriction. Cough may be the initial or sole manifestation of asthma — here bronchodilators (especially selective beta2-adrenergic agents), not cough suppressants, are indicated. Activation of lung irritant receptors mediates both cough and bronchoconstriction. It has been suggested that bronchoconstriction may be part of the cough reflex.[3,8] Although this is not widely accepted, bronchodilators may assist in cough suppression in some patients without definite asthma. Ipratropium bromide is an anticholinergic bronchodilator which may influence irritant receptor activity and reduce cough independently of its action on bronchomotor tone, but its role in the treatment of cough in non-asthmatic patients has not been established.

*Corticosteroids*

Bronchial hyper-reactivity may result in cough. Systemic or topical (inhaled) corticosteroid agents may suppress such cough. While inhaled corticosteroids are frequently effective in cough which follows viral and other respiratory tract infections, there is little rationale for the use of oral steroids (with their attendant side effects) in this situation. The use of oral steroids in cough due to other causes is rarely justified and usually ineffective.

*Sodium Cromoglycate*

Sodium cromoglycate may also be used in cough secondary to asthma or bronchial hyper-reactivity (see Chapter 7).

*Demulcents*

These are bland substances thought to act by protecting inflamed pharyngeal mucosa. Most are presented as syrups or lozenges; combined preparations containing local anaesthetics, antiseptics and others are in common use, but controlled studies of efficacy are lacking.

### Other Drugs Used As Antitussives

A variety of other drugs such as benzodiazepines and phenothiazines may have antitussive activity. Diazepam and clonazepam suppress cough, but are rarely used for their antitussive effect since sedation limits their usefulness. These agents may be indicated when cough is functional or related to anxiety.

Antihistamines, particularly diphenhydramine, are included in many proprietary cough mixtures. They may potentiate the effects of other cough suppressants, particularly pholcodine[9] and dextromethorphan. Antihistamines may be of use in coughs secondary to nasal allergy with postnasal drip.

'Expectorants' and 'mucolytic' agents have a time-honoured place in many cough mixtures. It seems illogical to stimulate production of secretions in a patient who is being given a cough suppressant and objective evidence of the usefulness of these preparations is lacking.[11]

## Stimulation of Cough

Where cough needs to be stimulated for the removal of retained respiratory secretions (as in bronchiectasis, obtunded and postoperative patients) the use of physical means such as physiotherapy is more appropriate than drug therapy.

# Drugs Acting on Mucociliary Function

## Physiology of Mucociliary Clearance

The respiratory mucosa extends from the proximal trachea to the level of the terminal bronchioles. It consists of pseudostratified columnar epithelial cells which each carry approximately 200 cilia projecting into a layer of secretion lining the airways.[2] Mucus is produced by goblet cells and by mucous glands which lie within the submucosa. These are predominantly under parasympathetic influence. Peripherally, in smaller airways, the numbers of ciliated cells, goblet cells and bronchial glands decline, so that small bronchioles are lined by a relatively uniform layer of low cuboidal non-ciliated cells.

In 1934, Lucas and Douglas[2] proposed that respiratory secretions lining the airways consist of two layers: a fluid layer of low viscosity which surrounds the cilia ('sol' layer or periciliary fluid) and a more viscid 'gel' layer (mucus), 5 to 10μm thick above this (Figure 5.1). The gel layer is composed of secretions arising from goblet cells and mucous glands. There has been considerable controversy as to whether this comprises a continuous layer ('mucous blanket') or 'islands' of gel floating upon and interacting with the cilia in the sol layer.

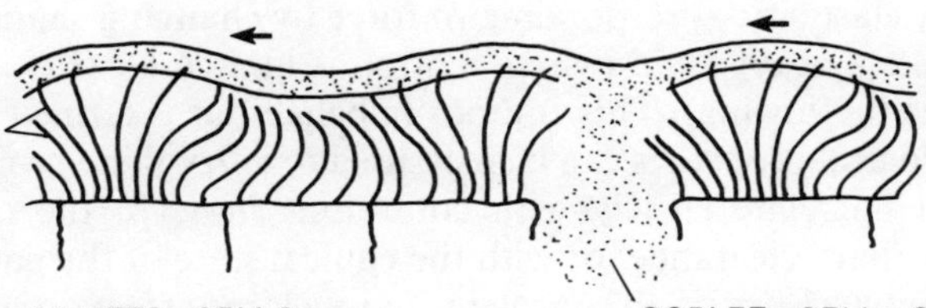


*Figure 5.1* Diagram showing mucus-transporting ciliated epithelium lining the respiratory tract. Cilia penetrate and engage mucus during the effective stroke and retract within the perciliary fluid during the recovery stroke. Arrows indicate the direction of the effective stroke and of mucus movement.

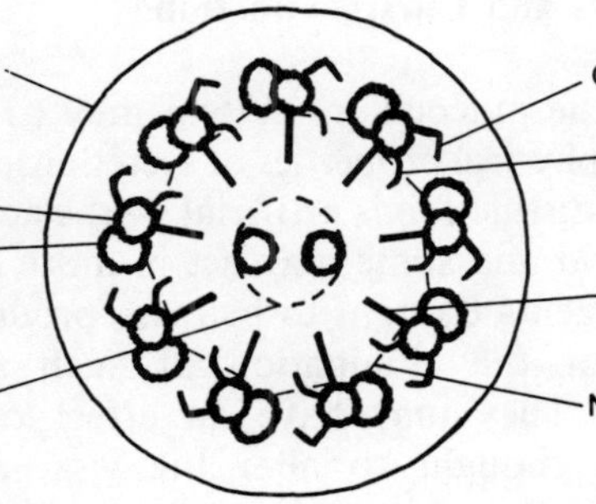


Figure 5.2 Transverse section of a normal cilium. The ciliary membrane surrounds nine peripheral microtubular doublets and two single central microtubules. The central sheath, radial spokes and nexin links form a supporting structure which helps the cilium to regain its shape after each beat.

Cilia beat in a coordinated fasion at a rate of approximately 10 to 15 beats per second.[12] A relatively fast 'effective' stroke during which the cilium engages with and propels overlying mucus forward is followed by a slower 'recovery' stroke when the cilium retracts beneath the layer of mucus. Ciliary ultrastructure is complex[12] and includes a system of longitudinal tubules which provide strength and elasticity (Figure 5.2). There are nine pairs of outer tubules and one central pair. ATPase-containing dynein arms on the A outer tubules attach to adjacent B tubules intermittently after which the arms change shape. This causes some of the tubules to slide relative to others with resultant ciliary bending. Adjacent cilia beat sequentially (probably controlled by hydrostatic forces) so that a wave of ciliary motion proceeds centrally — the metachronal wave (Figure 5.1). The sum of individual ciliary beating (not visible to the naked eye) is central movement of the gel layer producing moving 'rafts' or a 'mucus escalator'.[2] Secretions are carried to the pharynx where they are swallowed or, if excessive, expectorated as sputum.

The greater part of respiratory secretions (over 95%) consists of water. Respiratory mucus contains complex polymers, mucopolysaccharides and proteins. Respiratory secretions are complex mixtures and do not flow in a simple fashion like water. Where secretions exceed the transport capacity of the mucociliary escalator, sputum is produced and expectorated by coughing. Sputum acts in some respects like a semi-solid (motion is determined primarily by elasticity — responding to force by changing shape) and in other respects like a heavy fluid (where motion is limited by viscosity — responding to force by flowing). This composite behaviour is termed visco-elastic. While rheological properties can be measured *in vitro,* these properties of sputum do not correlate closely with conditions *in vivo,* the overall efficiency of mucociliary clearance, or with the clinical state of the patient.[2]

The physical characteristics of glycoproteins have a large effect on sputum viscosity. This is mediated largely by disulphide bonds between adjacent molecules. Splitting disulphide bonds *in vitro* results in decreased sputum viscosity, but the importance of this process *in vivo* is not certain. DNA, derived from leucocytes and bacteria, results in the increased viscosity found in purulent sputum.

## Drug Effects on Mucus and Ciliary Function

Agents which act on the mucociliary system may (i) alter the volume of secretions, (ii) alter the physical properties of secretions, and (iii) affect ciliary function directly. This distinction is artificial — the actions of many agents are not fully understood and some may act in more than one way.

'Expectorants' are agents thought to increase production of respiratory tract secretions and/or the elimination of such secretions from the tracheobronchial tree. They may have an effect on sputum viscosity. 'Mucolytic' drugs are thought to alter the visco-elastic properties of respiratory secretions and, in this respect, may overlap with the effects of expectorants. Other descriptions such as 'mucokinetic' and 'bronchomucotropic' have been used, but so little is known about possible modes of action of some of these agents that such classification is of little help.

## Expectorants: Drugs Thought to Affect Mucus Volume

Hydration plays an important part in mucociliary clearance (MCC). Systemic dehydration, if severe, may impair MCC. Water as steam or mist (from a nebuliser) has been used traditionally to loosen secretions to enhance their removal by expectoration.[13]

Hypotonic and hypertonic solutions have also been used as inhalations.[14] Pavia et al have demonstrated a doubling in the rate of clearance of lung secretions following the nebulisation of hypertonic (7.1%) saline.[13] Hypertonic saline also has a role for inducing the production of sputum for laboratory examination. The administration of these agents is not without risk. Hypotonic or hypertonic inhalations may provoke bronchoconstriction in asthmatic patients.[15]

Several hygroscopic agents have been employed as inhalations because of their ability to absorb water and to resist dehydration of respiratory secretions. Propylene glycol and glycerine have been used alone or as vehicles for nebulised bronchodilator drugs. They are thought to 'stabilise' droplets generated by nebulisation.[14]

Most of the 'expectorants' in proprietary cough medications are thought to act either directly on the bronchial glands, or as gastric irritants which act indirectly by a vagal reflex to alter respiratory secretions. Many of these irritants have an emetic action in higher doses.

Guaiphenesin (glyceryl guaiacolate) is used widely. It may reduce sputum viscosity as well as increasing the volume of respiratory secretions. The doses usually given of 400 to 800mg/day are probably ineffective. Chodosh[16] found the effect of 800mg to be indistinguishable from placebo. Doses of as little as 100 to 200mg are supplied in some proprietary compounds. Although 2400mg/day increases the volume of mucus,[16] the clinical usefulness of guaiphenesin is controversial. Clarke et al.[5,13] found that guaiphenesin improved MCC in patients with chronic bronchitis, but Hirsch[17] found it of little value in the clinical management of this disease.

Organic and inorganic iodides act directly on the bronchial glands. Some preparations are irritant and also act via gastric irritation. The use of iodides results in secretions of reduced viscosity and they may also have a direct action on mucus to split glycoprotein molecules. Iodides have been used for many years for bronchitis and asthma to aid clearance of tenacious secretions, but controlled trials are lacking. Side effects are common and include an unpleasant metallic taste, gastric irritation, increased salivation, acneiform skin eruptions and alterations in thyroid function. The use of iodides cannot be recommended.[18]

A number of vital oils, balsams and vapours play a time-honoured role in the treatment of respiratory disease. When added to hot water a pleasant smelling mist is produced. It is doubtful whether the volatile inhalant confers added benefit over the hydrating effect of water vapour. Boyd[19] found that popular agents such as menthol, compound benzoin tincture (Friar's balsam), camphor and eucalyptus oil had no measurable effect on mucociliary function.

A number of plant extracts, taken orally, have been used as expectorants. These include liquorice, juniper, squill, and garlic — many of which are available from purveyors of alternative medicines. Inorganic ammonium, sodium and potassium salts have been used similarly. Senega and ammonia mixtures have been popular for many years. Proof of efficacy is lacking.

## Mucolytics: Drugs Thought to Alter Sputum Viscosity

Mucolytic drugs act by reducing sputum visco-elasticity. Although this property can be demonstrated *in vitro,* evidence for equivalent activity *in vivo* is lacking for many of these drugs. Acetylcysteine contains a thiol group which breaks the disulphide bridges linking sputum mucoproteins. During this reaction, acetate and cysteine are evolved together with a small amount of hydrogen sulphide resulting in the malodour characteristic of this agent.

Acetylcysteine is given by nebulisation as a 10 to 20% solution; it may also be instilled bronchoscopically or by a tracheostomy as a lavage, particularly in patients with mucous plugging. Effective mucolysis follows direct instillation. When it is given by nebuliser, bronchoconstriction may result and a beta2-agonist bronchodilator agent is commonly added to prevent this. Acetylcysteine is a reducing agent and may cause degradation of rubber or metal parts of respiratory therapy equipment. When given orally, acetylcysteine is well tolerated and well absorbed in daily doses of 200 to 400mg.

Acetylcysteine and its derivatives S-carboxymethylcysteine (S-CMC) and 2-mercaptoethane sodium sulphate produce marked mucolysis *in vitro*. Clinical efficacy is controversial. Multicentre trials from Scandinavia have demonstrated a reduced frequency of acute exacerbations in patients with chronic bronchitis when treated with acetylcysteine for prolonged periods (up to two years).[20] However, the effect of acetylcysteine on lung function was not significant. Even in subjects with viscid sputum, no change was found in lung function after treatment.[21] A series of studies demonstrated subjective and objective thinning of sputum in chronic bronchitis, but no improvement in physical signs, spirometry, or sputum volume.[21] Pulmonary MCC was not improved.[13] The role of acetylcysteine during acute exacerbations of chronic bronchitis remains controversial.

S-CMC is available in the United Kingdom and Japan. Although there has been a suggestion of improvement in lung function,[22] MCC was not affected.[13] Definite clinical usefulness has not been established.

Bromhexine is a mucolytic drug derived from the Indian plant *Adhatoda vasica.* It appears to act directly on the bronchial gland producing depolymerisation of mucopolysaccharides. An action on cholinergic receptors has also been suggested. Bromchitic patients given oral bromhexine produce increased volumes of less viscid sputum. Bromhexine is usually well tolerated in doses of 24 to 48mg/day. Adverse effects include epigastric discomfort, nausea and transient rises in serum transaminase levels without evidence of serious hepatotoxicity. Bromhexine increases the concentration of tetracyclines in respiratory secretions.

Although multiple studies have been conducted into the efficacy of bromhexine, its usefulness is not yet clear. Several studies have suggested subjective improvement in chronic bronchitic patients treated with bromhexine, and it has been shown to produce a small but significant improvement in MCC. The Research Committee of the British Thoracic and Tuberculosis Association found a 'trend' towards improvement in chronic bronchitic patients treated with bromhexine, but was not able to recommend its use routinely in chronic bronchitis.[23] Although some patients may benefit, this group has not been defined.

A number of enzymes has been used by inhalation to enhance liquefaction of sputum. Pancreatic deoxyribonuclease is a beef-derived protease which acts on purulent sputum to break down DNA. This agent has been used in patients with cystic fibrosis, bronchiectasis, lung abscess, and chronic purulent bronchitis who have not responded to optimal antibacterial treatment and physical therapy. Enthusiasm for its use has waned because of doubts about efficacy, high cost and the availability of other mucolytic agents. Trypsin, chymotrypsin, streptokinase and streptodornase have all been used empirically as inhalations to liquefy viscid sputum, but their efficacy is unproven. Trypsin has been used in the treatment of pulmonary alveolar proteinosis via bronchoscopic instillation.

### Drugs Which Act on Cilia

A number of drugs has been shown to affect ciliary function,[24,25] but none is in clinical use solely for this purpose.[2] Drugs which increase ciliary motility are thought to increase MCC, but this will follow only if ciliary beating is coordinated and interacts effectively with overlying mucus. Many drugs which affect ciliary motility also affect mucus visco-elasticity.

Beta-adrenergic agonists are in wide use for the management of airways obstruction. Although bronchodilation overshadows their other respiratory effects, these drugs have been shown to increase ciliary beat frequency and to increase MCC in normal subjects and in patients with chronic bronchitis, asthma and cystic fibrosis.[24] Such actions could be useful by increasing transport of secretions from peripheral to more central airways where cough can be effective. Propranolol (a beta-adrenergic antagonist) impairs ciliary beating *in vitro* and this, in turn, is blocked by fenoterol (a beta-agonist) which itself increases human ciliary beat frequency in the laboratory (Crosby D and Rutland J, unpublished observations).

Other pharmacological agents which may improve human ciliary motility include methyl xanthines and cholinergic agents, but a clinical role has not been demonstrated.

Ciliary beating is decreased by general anaesthetic agents, anticholinergic agents and narcotics. Use of these drugs may contribute to impaired MCC in the postoperative period.

Patients with recurrent respiratory tract disease due to impaired ciliary function have been identified in the last decade.[24] To date, there have been no reports of improved ciliary function following drug therapy.

## Conclusion

Much respiratory disease is self-induced and, in smokers, cessation of smoking is likely to be of more benefit than antitussive and/or mucolytic therapy.

Antitussive agents are in wide clinical use, often as over-the-counter preparations and often in mixtures. Cough is often produced by self-limiting diseases and therapy may be unnecessary. In other situations, such as bronchial suppuration, suppression of cough is inappropriate. Where possible, it is preferable to treat the cause of a cough. Patients should be educated about the possible adverse effects and addictive potential of these drugs, and about the need to seek medical advice to exclude serious disorders rather than embarking on self-prescribed antitussive therapy.

Although used widely, expectorant and mucolytic drugs have a less well defined place in respiratory therapy. Current lack of knowledge about both the effects of many of these agents and their clinical efficacy is reflected in the inverse relationship between the numbers of preparations listed in drug formularies and the space devoted to them in standard textbooks of pharmacology.[6,7] The use of both expectorants and mucolytics remains controversial. The use of other drugs (such as bronchodilators) and physical methods should be explored fully before these agents are used. Routine use of mucolytic drugs such as acetylcysteine, S-CMC and bromhexine cannot be justified, but they may have a role in the prevention of exacerbations in selected patients with chronic bronchitis, in whom a *critical* therapeutic trial may be worthwhile.

Large sums of money are spent each year on antitussive and mucolytic therapy. The clinical role and usefulness of antitussive agents are relatively well understood even though they are overused. However, deficiencies in our knowledge of the mechanisms of action and the clinical efficacy of mucolytics and expectorants preclude firm recommendations about their use and limit their place in respiratory therapy at present.

## References


1. Hippocrates. In: Lloyd GER, ed. *Hippocratic writings.* London: Penguin, 1978: 177.
2. Wanner A. Clinical aspects of mucociliary transport. *Am Rev Respir Dis* 1977; 116: 73-125.
3. Irwin RS, Rosen MJ, Braman SS. Cough. *Arch Intern Med* 1977; 137: 1186-1191.
4. Clarke SW, Thomson ML, Pavia D. Effect of mucolytic and expectorant drugs on tracheobronchial clearance in chronic bronchitis. *Eur J Respir Dis* 1980; 61 (suppl 110): 179-184.
5. Bickerman HA, Rodgers JM. Principles of measurement of cough depressing effect. *Eur J Respir Dis* 1980; 61 (suppl 110): 93-98.
6. Reynolds JEF, ed. *Martindale. The extra pharmacopoeia.* 28th ed. London: The Pharmaceutical Press, 1982.
7. Gilman AG, Goodman LS, Rall TW, Murad F, eds. *The pharmacological basis of therapeutics.* New York: Macmillan, 1985.
8. Bickerman HA. Antitussive drugs. In: Modell W, ed. *Drugs of choice 1982-3.* St Louis: CV Mosby, 1982: 454-470.
9. Edwards GF, Lewis HE, Stafford D. The effect of pholcodine with and without an antihistamine on cough and expectoration. *Br J Dis Chest* 1977; 71: 245-252.
10. Howard P, Cayton RM, Brennan SR, Anderson PB. Lignocaine aerosol and persistent cough. *Br J Dis Chest* 1977; 71: 19-24.
11. Hughes DTD. Cough suppressants, expectorants and mucolytic agents. *Br Med J* 1978; 1: 1202-1203.
12. Sleigh MA. The nature and action of respiratory tract cilia. In: Brain JD, Proctor DF, Reid LM, eds. *Respiratory defense mechanisms.* New York: Marcel Dekker, 1977: 247-288.
13. Pavia D. Effects of pharmacologic agents on the clearance of airway secretions. *Sem Respir Med* 1984; 5: 345-352.
14. Ziment I. *Respiratory pharmacology and therapeutics.* Philadelphia: Saunders, 1978.
15. Schoeffel RE, Anderson SD, Altounyan REC. Bronchial hyperreactivity in response to inhalation of ultrasonically nebulised solutions of distilled water and saline. *Br Med J* 1981; 283: 1285-1287.
16. Chodosh S, Medici TC. Expectorant effect of glyceryl guaiacolate. *Chest* 1973; 64: 543-544.

17. Hirsch SR, Viernes PF, Kory RC. The expectorant effect of glyceryl guaiacolate in patients with chronic bronchitis. *Chest* 1973; 63: 9-14.
18. American Academy of Pediatrics — Committee on Drugs. Adverse reactions to iodide therapy of asthma and other pulmonary diseases. *Pediatrics* 1976; 57: 272-274.
19. Boyd EM. A review of studies on the pharmacology of the expectorants and inhalants. *Int J Clin Pharmacol* 1970; 3: 55-60.
20. Multicenter Study Group. Long term oral acetylcysteine in chronic bronchitis. *Eur J Respir Dis* 1980; 61 (suppl 111): 93-108.
21. Grater WC, Cato A. Double-blind study of acetylcysteine-isoproterenol and saline-isoproterenol in non-hospitalised patients with asthma. *Curr Ther Res* 1973; 15: 660-671.
22. Edwards GF, Steel AE, Scott JK, Jordan JW. S-Carboxymethylcysteine in the fluidification of sputum and treatment of chronic airway obstruction. *Chest* 1976; 70: 506-513.
23. British Thoracic and Tuberculosis Association — Research Committee. A controlled trial of the effects of bromhexine on the symptoms of outpatients with chronic bronchitis. *Br J Dis Chest* 1973; 67: 49-60.
24. Editorial. Pulmonary mucociliary clearance. *Lancet* 1982; 1: 203-204.
25. Sackner MA. Effect of respiratory drugs on mucociliary clearance. *Chest* 1978; 73 (suppl): 958-964.

# Chapter 6

# Bronchodilators

*Claes-Göran Löfdahl and Nils Svedmyr*

## Beta-adrenergic Agonists

Beta-adrenoreceptor stimulants are the most important therapeutic agents in asthmatic disease, and their use has increased over the past decades, as selective beta2-adrenoreceptor stimulants have been developed. Today different effects of alpha and beta1 and beta2-adrenoreceptor stimulants have been verified and several of these effects are important in the treatment of asthma (Table 6.1).[1-3]

### Therapeutic Effects in Asthma Treatment

Of the effects shown for beta2-adrenoreceptor stimulation, the most important in asthma treatment are: (i) bronchial smooth muscle relaxation; (ii) increased mucociliary transport; (iii) inhibition of release of mediators; (iv) suppression of permeability oedema; (v) decreased pulmonary hypertension and increased right ventricular ejection fraction; (vi) improved contractility of fatigued diaphragmatic muscle; and (vii) inhibition of transmission through airway parasympathetic ganglia.

*Table 6.1* Effects of adrenergic receptor stimulation in asthma

| Effect on | Type of receptor stimulated | | |
|---|---|---|---|
| | Alpha | Beta1 | Beta2 |
| Bronchial smooth muscle | Contraction | 0 | Relaxation |
| Bronchial mucosa | Decongestion | 0 | Decongestion |
| Heart rate and tendency to arrhythmias | 0 | Increase | Some increase (mainly reflexogenic) |
| Cardiac output | 0 | Increase | Some increase |
| Resistance of systemic circulation | Increase | 0 | Decrease |
| Urinary bladder muscle | Contraction | 0 | Relaxation |
| Release of endogenous spasmogens | (Increase) | 0 | Decrease |
| Mucociliary transport | ? | ? | Increase |
| Epithelial chloride and water transport | Increase | ? | Increase |
| Mucus secretion | Increase (mainly serous) | Increase (mainly serous) | Increase (mainly serous) |
| Pulmonary artery pressure | ? | 0 | Decrease |
| Diaphragmatic contractility | | | Increase |
| Parasympathetic ganglion transmission | | | Inhibition |

Of these effects the most important seems to be the bronchial smooth muscle relaxation, but the other effects may contribute to the therapeutic effects. Unfortunately, it is difficult to evaluate the clinical significance of these other effects.

### *Bronchial Smooth Muscle Relaxation*

Figure 6.1 gives a schematic representation of intracellular events leading to contraction and relaxation of the smooth muscle. Beta-adrenoreceptor stimulation increases the adenylate cyclase activity and thereby increases the intracellular concentration of cAMP. This relaxes the smooth muscle in several different ways. It activates protein kinases which in turn phosphorylates myosin-light chain kinase, thereby making it less reactive with calcium and calmodulin. Calcium and calmodulin can bind to myosin-light chain kinase and thereby phosphorylate myosin which is a prerequisite for contraction.

Another mechanism for beta2-adrenoreceptor-mediated relaxation is that cAMP increases the internalisation of intracellular calcium into intracellular stores, such as the mitochondria and the sarcoplasmic reticulum. Furthermore, beta-adrenoreceptor stimulation increases the outward flow of calcium from the smooth muscle cell.[4]

As regards *potency,* the maximal bronchorelaxing effect of different beta-adrenoreceptor stimulants and theophylline derivatives is all the same *in vitro* and the relative potency is proportional to the potencies found clinically. Thus, the beta2-agonists are about one thousand times more potent than theophylline.[5] With increased concentrations of contractile agents such as carbachol, it has been shown that the potency difference between isoprenaline and theophylline induced relaxation gradually decreases. O'Donnell and Wanstall[7] have also shown that the relative bronchodilating potency of fenoterol compared to salbutamol is increased in bronchial muscle contracted with high doses of carbachol. The clinical relevance of these experiments is not clear, as clinically beta2-adrenoreceptor stimulants are equally effective. Furthermore, the clinical bronchodilating effect of theophylline is similar to the effect of beta2-adrenoreceptor stimulants.[8]

It has been shown that beta2-adrenoreceptor stimulants relax airway smooth muscle irrespective of what contractile agent (carbachol, histamine, 5-hydroxytryptamine, prostaglandin $F_{2\alpha}$, $LTC_4$, $LTD_4$ or substance P) is used.[9] Thus beta2-adrenoreceptor agonists and also theophylline are effective functional antagonists against the airway constrictor action of a large variety of potential asthma mediators. This functional antagonism at the level of the smooth muscle is probably of importance for the excellent therapeutic effect of beta2-agonists. Their effects are superior to those of anticholinergic agents, which only block acetylcholine and, consequently, only the reflex-mediated bronchoconstriction. The beta2-agonists and xanthines are also more effective than sodium cromoglycate.

As is shown in Table 6.2 adrenaline and ephedrine are potent alpha-adrenoreceptor stimulants, and isoprenaline has beta-adrenoreceptor *selectivity* with equal effect on beta1 and beta2 receptors. Orciprenaline was the first drug with some selectivity for beta2-adrenoreceptor stimulation. The other drugs, fenoterol, rimiterol, salbutamol and terbutaline are equally

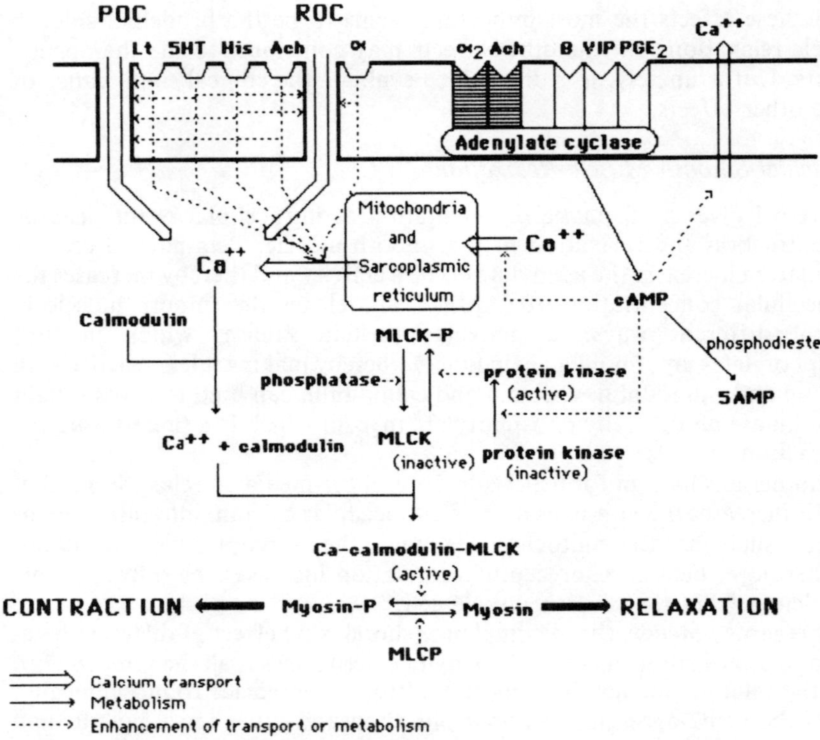


*Figure 6.1* Schematic representation of the biochemistry of the smooth muscle cell and the intracellular events leading to contraction and relaxation. To the left in the figure the factors contributing to contraction are shown and to the right the factors contributing to relaxation. In the upper part of the figure the membrane is shown.

Contraction of the airway smooth muscle occurs when free calcium ($Ca^{++}$) increases due to stimulation by several agonists such as leukotrienes (Lt), 5-hydroxytryptamine (5HT), histamine (His), acetylcholine (Ach) and alpha-adrenoreceptor agonists ($\alpha$). The contraction is dependent upon phosphorylated myosin bound to actin and ATP. The phosphorylation of myosin is catalysed by myosin light chain kinase (MLCK) activated by calcium and calmodulin. Desphosphorylation of myosin-phosphate is catalysed by myosin light chain phosphatase (MLCP) and causes relaxation. One possibility of decreasing the amount of active MLCK is to stimulate protein kinases, which phosphorylate MLCK thereby making it less prone to react with calcium and calmodulin. The protein kinases are dependent on the level of cAMP, which is increased by stimulation of beta-adrenoreceptors on the cellular membrane via activation of adenylate cyclase. An increased level of cAMP also increases the internalisation of calcium into the sarcoplasmic reticulum and the mitochondria. Furthermore, cAMP increases the extrusion of calcium by the calcium extrusion pump and the sodium-calcium exchange. An increased level of cAMP thus decreases the internal level of free calcium and stimulates protein kinases, both of which effects contribute to relaxation. Other agonists besides beta-adrenoreceptor agonists also activate adenylate cyclase — these include VIP and prostaglandin $E_2$ ($PGE_2$). This activation occurs via a stimulating guanine nucleotide-binding protein, whereas inhibition of adenylate cyclase occurs by cholinergic (Ach) and alpha2-receptor ($\alpha$2) stimulation via inhibitory guanine nucleotide binding protein.[87,88]

Another important mechanism regulating intracellular calcium concentration and the contractile status of the bronchial muscle is the phosphatidylinositol (PI) turnover (not shown in the figure). Agonists such as Ach activate PI-breakdown which gives inositoltriphosphate ($PI_3$) which releases calcium from internal stores. Furthermore, diacylglycerol is produced, which activates protein kinase C and is also a precursor of arachidonic acid. Protein kinase increases the sensitivity to calcium ions and thereby activates myosin directly and is especially responsible for sustained contraction of smooth muscle.[4]

*Table 6.2* Relative clinical receptor-stimulating activity of some adrenergic compounds

| Compound | Type of receptor | | |
|---|---|---|---|
| | Alpha | Beta1 | Beta2 |
| Adrenaline (epinephrine) | + + + | + | + + |
| Ephedrine | + + | + | + |
| Isoprenaline (isoproterenol) | (+) | + + + | + + + |
| Orciprenaline (metaproterenol) | 0 | + + | + + + |
| Salbutamol (albuterol) | 0 | + | + + + |
| Terbutaline | 0 | + | + + + |
| Fenoterol | 0 | + | + + + |
| Rimiterol | 0 | + | + + + |

beta2-adrenoreceptor selective. These four drugs are more selective than orciprenaline.[8]

### *Increase in Mucociliary Transport*

Beta2-adrenoreceptor stimulants have been shown to increase mucociliary transport in asthmatic patients, an effect which may contribute to their therapeutic efficacy in asthma.[10] Matthys and co-workers[11] have shown that beta-adrenoreceptor stimulants and theophylline have additive effects on mucociliary transport. A possible explanation for the effect of beta-stimulants on mucociliary clearance could be that beta-stimulants also increase the chloride ion and water secretion into the bronchial lumen.[12,13] One study with inhaled terbutaline did not show any effect on mucociliary transport in mild asthmatics.[14]

### *Inhibition of Anaphylactic Release of Mediators*

Martin and co-workers showed in 1980 that both terbutaline and theophylline given orally to asthmatics protected against antigen-induced bronchoconstriction, and at the same time partly inhibited the release of histamine and neutrophil chemotactic factor. Holgate and Church[16] showed that histamine release from human lung mast cells was more inhibited by beta2-adrenoreceptor agonists than by sodium cromoglycate. Studies with allergic provocation *in vivo* in asthma showed that salbutamol abolished the increase of histamine and neutrophil chemotactic factor at the same time as it inhibited bronchoconstriction. This effect was more pronounced for salbutamol than for sodium cromoglycate or ipratropium bromide.[17] Thus, there are studies indicating that effects on human basophils and mast cells may be of clinical relevance. Other clinical studies throw doubt on the importance of inhibition of mast cell histamine release as a therapeutic effect.[18]

### *Suppression of Permeability Oedema*

The vasconstrictor action of alpha-adrenoreceptor stimulating sympathomimetics is the important mechanism behind their well-known decongestant action. Svensjö et al[19] showed that isoprenaline and terbutaline effectively prevented the mediator-induced extravasation of macromolecules in spite of increased local blood flow.[20] Irrespective of whether the mediator is an amine peptide or a lipid metabolite, beta-adrenoreceptor stimulation is an effective way of preventing the increased vascular permeability. All experiments so far have used high concentrations of beta2-adrenoreceptor agonists to show this effect. After inhaled administration the antipermeability action of these drugs may have increased importance due to higher concentrations in the target tissue. Thus, the effect of inhalation therapy with beta-adrenoreceptor agonists may be due partly to an effect on bronchial venules. However, the clinical relevance of these effects remains to be proven.

*Decrease in Pulmonary Hypertension and Increase in Right Ventricular Ejection Fraction*

Normal doses of beta2-adrenoreceptor stimulants given orally reduce the pulmonary artery pressure and increase the right ventricular ejection fraction in acute tests of patients with hypoxia.[3] These effects can hardly be of any importance in the normal treatment of asthma. However, they may be of importance in patients with chronic obstructive airways disease, in whom pulmonary hypertension and right ventricular failure carry a poor prognosis.[21] These vascular effects cause a further unevenness of ventilation-perfusion ratio resulting in a temporary fall in oxygen tension.

*Improved Contractility of Fatigued Diaphragmatic Muscle*

Beta2-adrenoreceptor stimulants as well as theophylline have in animal studies been shown to augment diaphragmatic muscle activity.[22,23] This effect is additive to the effect by theophylline on this muscle. The effect is probably without clinical relevance in normal asthma treatment. However, it might be of importance when asthmatics are no longer able to breathe and the $PCO_2$ starts to increase; that is, when they need respirator treatment. Recent results in dogs indicate that this effect during hypercapnia only occurs with theophylline.[24] This effect may also be of clinical importance in patients with chronic obstructive airways disease. Clinical evidence for this effect has been described in a patient with systemic lupus erythematosus (SLE), where diaphragm dysfunction restricted ventilatory incapacity. High doses of inhaled salbutamol improved the ventilatory capacity without any effect on bronchial airflow, probably due to an effect on the diaphragmatic muscle.[25]

*Inhibition of Transmission Through Airway Parasympathetic Ganglia*

Beta2-adrenoreceptor agonists block the parasympathetic ganglion transmission in the vagal nerve of ferret trachea.[26] The effect starts with some delay compared with the effect on the bronchial muscle. Whether this effect is of clinical importance is impossible to evaluate at the moment. However, it indicates the possibility that part of the beta-adrenoreceptor agonist effect is mediated via yet another airway target cell apart from the bronchial muscle.

## Side Effects

Skeletal muscle tremor is a dose-limiting factor when beta2-adrenoreceptor agonists are given systemically.[27] Side effects are less pronounced after inhalation of normal doses of all beta2-adrenoreceptor selective agonists.[28,29] Side effects are tachycardia, palpitations, a slight increase of blood glucose and free fatty acid levels, hypokalaemia, and a certain degree of nervousness. These effects are most pronounced when the treatment is started, but the patient develops tolerance towards all these side effects. Inhaled beta2-adrenoreceptor stimulants may cause a temporary fall of $PO_2$ in acute severe asthma. This can be prevented by treatment with oxygen.[1]

### *Skeletal Muscle Tremor*

There is no evidence to date that beta2-adrenoreceptors in skeletal muscle and bronchial muscle are different.[30,31] The effect elicited by beta-adrenoreceptor agonists on skeletal muscle is dependent on the type of fibre involved. In slow-contracting muscle fibres, the tension and degree of fusion in subtetanic contraction are decreased, whereas fast-contracting muscles respond with an increase in these parameters.[32] The depression of slow-contracting muscles is thought to be responsible for the muscle tremor observed. Although there is considerable individual variation in tremor response, the most regular responders may shake so much that fine movements are impossible.[33] Studies by Jenne et al[34] show a close relationship between the initial individual tremor response to beta2-stimulants and the basal tremor. Moreover, the perception of tremor seems to be related to the relative increase over the basal tremor produced by the drug. However, prolonged treatment with beta2-adrenoreceptor agonists makes the skeletal muscle tolerant, whereas the sensitivity of the airway smooth muscle remains essentially unchanged. This has been observed clinically in man[35] and experimentally in the guinea pig.[36] Thus, these drugs should be introduced in a reduced dose until skeletal muscle tolerance develops. Despite this, individuals sometimes cannot tolerate even reduced systemic doses.

### *Cardiovascular Effects*

The cardiac stimulation is mainly reflexogenic through beta2-adrenoreceptor-mediated peripheral vasodilatation.[3] Thus, both tremor and tachycardia are, in principle, beta2-mediated effects and both are dose-dependent

Cardiac side effects when theophyllines are combined with oral beta2-adrenoreceptor stimulants have been discussed recently as an explanation for the increase in sudden death among young asthmatics. An increased rate of arrhythmias was found in patients treated with a combination of theophylline and beta2-adrenoreceptor stimulants given orally in high dosages compared to each drug given alone.[37,38] When the drugs were combined in low dosages, there was no increase in arrhythmias. The combination of oral beta2-adrenoreceptor stimulants and theophylline provides additive anti-asthmatic effects, an additive bronchodilating effect and fewer side effects than with single drugs.[39] However, self-poisoning with high doses of salbutamol (up to 240mg) has caused only moderate symptoms.[40]

## Development of Tolerance

Reports in the late 1960s from Great Britain[41,42] indicated a connection between the sale of beta-adrenoreceptor agonists in spray form (isoprenaline) and an increased mortality from asthma. This soon focused attention on the development of tolerance to these drugs.[43]

The administration of beta2-adrenoreceptor stimulants can cause the development of tolerance in animal studies (*in vitro* and *in vivo*) and in non-bronchial beta2-adrenoreceptor responses in humans (tremor, heart rate, lymphocyte and leucocyte cAMP levels and also down-regulation of the beta-adrenoreceptor number). Development of tachyphylaxis to the bronchodilating effect of beta2-adrenoreceptor agonists in healthy individuals has also been shown, but there was no tachyphylaxis in asthmatic patients under the same test conditions.[44-47] About 40 controlled studies of beta-agonists given both by the oral and the inhaled route in normal doses suggest that asthmatics do not develop tachyphylaxis of clinical importance to conventional doses of beta2-adrenoreceptor agonists.[48-50]

**Pharmacokinetics**

Pharmacokinetic studies of beta-adrenoreceptor agonists have been limited due to the low plasma concentrations achieved by those drugs. Recently, however, new methods especially gas chromatography with mass spectrometry (GCMS) have made it possible to evaluate clinical concentrations of these drugs. Terbutaline has been extensively studied,[51] and studies have also recently been performed with salbutamol.[52] Table 6.3 summarises some of these data.

*Absorption and Bioavailability*

Terbutaline taken orally is absorbed to about 25 to 80%, with a relatively high interindividual variability. Food intake impairs the absorption.[53] For salbutamol data from studies with radiolabelled salbutamol have indicated an absorption of about 100%.[54]

The bioavailability for terbutaline is 10 to 15%; for salbutamol data for absolute bioavailability have not been published.

*Volume of Distribution*

The volume of distribution is about 3L/kg for both terbutaline and salbutamol. Thus, there seems to be an enrichment in tissues which has also been shown in autopsy samples after terbutaline treatment.[55] The protein-binding for both drugs is low in the range of 10%[56] (data on file, Glaxo).

*Metabolism*

For terbutaline the main metabolite in man is the sulphate conjugate; however, about two-thirds is excreted unchanged. The metabolite has no agonistic or antagonistic effects.

For salbutamol the most important metabolite in man is a sulphate conjugate, but 66 to 75% is excreted unchanged. This sulphate metabolite is also without any agonist or antagonist activity.

*Excretion*

The bulk of both drugs is excreted unchanged and the terminal half-life for terbutaline is about 17 hours,[53,57] in spite of earlier reports of about three

*Table 6.3* Some pharmacokinetic parameters for beta2-adrenoreceptor agonists

| Agonist | Absorption (%) | Bioavailability (%) | Clearance (ml/min/kg) | T½ (h) |
|---|---|---|---|---|
| Terbutaline | 25-80 | 10-15 | 3 | 17 |
| Salbutamol | 100 | ? | 3 | ? 5 |

to five hours. This long half-life contributes to almost 40% of the total area under the curve.

For salbutamol the terminal half-life is about five hours in studies with up to 24 hours duration.[52,58]

## Clinical Use of Beta2-adrenoreceptor Stimulants

Patients who have single attacks without any problem between attacks can be given a beta-adrenoreceptor agonist in a metered dose aerosol to be administered when attacks occur. Many asthma patients, however, have a small degree of bronchial obstruction even when they do not experience any problems at all.[59] Therefore, many patients need continuous treatment with a beta2-adrenoreceptor stimulant. Especially if the patients have exercise-related symptoms, or if they are regularly exposed to irritating agents, they may need prophylactic or continuous treatment. The dosage should be individualised. One or two inhalations, in severe cases up to six inhalations, four to six times daily of salbutamol or terbutaline are recommended. For fenoterol half the number of inhalations should be given at every administration. All inhaled beta2-stimulants available today unfortunately have too short a duration to cover the whole night. Patients with pronounced nocturnal asthma may therefore need prolonged treatment with a beta2-adrenoreceptor stimulant by the oral route in a slow-release preparation. Some patients cannot take this treatment because of skeletal muscle tremor, and in those cases theophylline in slow-release form is a better choice.

It is important to instruct the patient that he should contact his doctor or hospital when he experiences acute deterioration. A rule of thumb could be that the patient should contact his doctor if the aerosol dose must be taken with less than three hours' interval. In such cases factors other than muscular spasm, such as mucosal oedema and plugging with mucus, may dominate and therefore other treatment in addition to inhaled beta2-adrenoreceptor agonists may be needed.

The inhalation technique is of utmost importance for the treatment with dose aerosols, and has been fully discussed in Chapter 2.

Several studies have shown that is is very difficult to instruct the patient to follow these recommendations.[60] Therefore, it is very important that the doctor or his personnel carefully instructs the patient how to use a metered dose inhaler (MDI), as this treatment is the cornerstone of asthma treatment today.

During recent years alternative means of inhalation have been developed. Salbutamol as a powder aerosol has in cumulative dose-response studies been shown to be equipotent with the same dose given from an MDI.[61] Another device that decreases the difficulties with inhalation treatment is the extension tube. There are two different kinds of tube, a simple extension tube

(Inhalet) and a pear-shaped extension tube with a valve. Both render cooperation less important, especially the coordination of the firing and the inhalation. Pear-shaped extension tubes give at least the same effect as an ordinary MDI.[62,63] They also decrease deposition of the inhaled drug in the mouth, and thereby decrease the side effects of the inhaled drugs. The pear-shaped tubes are difficult to carry and therefore patients have difficulty using them when they are not at home.

Some patients, such as children and very old people, cannot learn how to use a dose inhaler and a few patients cannot accept this route of administration. They can as an alternative use oral treatment with beta2-adrenoreceptor stimulants at a cost of increasing side effects, the most important of which is skeletal muscle tremor. However, with a gradual increase of the dose, adult patients can stand treatment with salbutamol 4mg tid or terbutaline 5mg tid, or preferably the same doses given twice daily as slow-release formulations.

## Methylxanthines

Methylxanthines have since the middle of the 19th century been used in the management of asthma.[64] The narrow therapeutic range of theophylline and its complicated pharmacokinetics have been a limiting factor in its clincial use. However, during recent years slow-release preparations and reliable theophylline assays have encouraged its use in maintenance treatment.

### Mechanism of Action

For many years phosphodiesterase inhibition was considered to be the mechanism of action for theophylline, as phosphodiesterase inhibition increases intracellular cAMP, and thus relaxes bronchial smooth muscle.[1] However, it has been shown that in therapeutic concentrations theophylline produces only 10 to 20% inhibition of phosphodiesterase activity.[65,66]

Another mechanism which has been thoroughly evaluated is adenosine antagonism.[67] Methylxanthines at low concentrations are inhibitors of extracellular adenosine effects. Adenosine has been shown to cause bronchoconstriction when *inhaled* in asthmatic patients. Theophylline antagonises this effect more effectively than the bronchoconstriction induced by histamine.[68] However, enprofylline, which is devoid of adenosine antagonistic effects and is a weak phosphodiesterase inhibitor is three to four times more potent as a bronchodilator than theophylline.[69] Thus it seems unlikely that adenosine antagonism is the cellular mechanism for methylxanthines' effects on the bronchial smooth muscle.

Other mechanisms involving prostaglandins have been discussed. Methylxanthines have been shown to antagonise the effect of prostaglandins $PGE_2$ and $PGF_2$ on smooth muscle *in vitro*.[70] However, this effect is probably due to the functional antagonistic effect against several bronchocontracting mediators shown recently.[9]

Theophylline also increases endogenous catecholamine release,[71,72] and parts of its effect on the airways are blocked by propranolol.[73] Another proposed mechanism is an effect on intracellular calcium and free calcium ion concentration.[74] Maybe this is the main mechanism for methylxanthines in asthma.

### *Therapeutic Effects*

Theophylline has been shown to have the same effects as beta2-adrenoreceptor stimulation (see above). The only effect which has not been shown for theophyllines is the action on transmission through airway parasympathetic ganglia. Some of the effects are more pronounced for theophylline than for beta2-receptor stimulants. Increased respiratory muscle contractility is better documented for theophylline than for beta2-adrenoreceptor agonists. Theophylline has an effect on respiratory drive, stimulating the respiratory centre, which beta2-stimulants do not have. Studies in normal subjects have shown that this effect is principally due to an increase in hypoxic drive.[75] However, the most important mechanism for the treatment of asthma is the effect on the bronchial muscle.

## Side Effects

The most common side effects or oral treatment are anorexia, nausea, vomiting and mild central nervous system (CNS) stimulation. Nausea is probably both a central effect and a direct toxic effect on the gastric mucosa, as the problem appears to be greater if oral therapy is given. Actual abdominal pain, diarrhoea and rarely also gastric bleeding may occur. In maintenance therapy initial dosage should be low to avoid these gastrointestinal side effects, which seem to occur much more frequently if the initial oral dose is high. A few patients do not, however, tolerate theophylline at all because of this side effect.

There is an increasing number of reports demonstrating that nausea and vomiting might not occur as presenting features of toxicity when theophylline is given by the intravenous route, and that some patients experience more severe complications as a first indication that theophylline in the blood has reached a toxic level.

Mild CNS stimulation is common, especially if the maintenance dose is increased too quickly. The most serious toxic effect is the risk of seizures which have been associated with a mortality rate as high as 50%. Theophylline-induced seizures, however, appear to be rare under a concentration of 220mmol/L (40mg/L).

The cardiovascular side effects are seen mainly with intravenous theophylline. Palpitations, tachycardia and arrhythmias may occur and are relatively common with serum levels in excess of 165mmol/L (30mg/L). Headache, however, is quite common, especially when theophylline therapy is initiated.

Children may have a relatively greater tolerance for theophylline therapy than adults, but reports of sudden death are common in the older paediatric literature. If modern kinetic principles are used, they should not occur.

Acute overdoses of oral theophylline are treated immediately with discontinuation of treatment, followed by use of activated charcoal. Serum concentrations should be measured frequently and intensive care should be considered. Oral treatment with activated charcoal should be repeated, as this decreases the serum concentration also after intravenous theophylline treatment ('gastric dialysis').[76] In severe cases with a risk of seizures, benzodiazepines together with haemoperfusion or haemodialysis should be used.[77] It is important, however, to give high doses, as theophylline antagonises the effect of benzodiazepines on GABA-receptors in the brain (Niemand et al, unpublished). To treat cardiac arrhythmias, lignocaine is the best choice.

Theophylline decreases the plasma potassium concentration which might increase cardiotoxicity. It is therefore important to monitor and supplement potassium during theophylline intoxication.[77]

## Pharmacokinetics

### *Absorption*

Most oral theophyllines used nowadays have 100% bioavailability.[78] Absorption from rectal suppositories is, however, very varying and this route of administration should therefore not be used. Rectal solutions give 100% absorption and the maintenance dose per 24 hours for theophylline is therefore the same for intravenous, oral or rectal treatment. However, it should be pointed out that different salts may give different amounts of theophylline per milligram of the compound, which may be important when calculating the dose.

### *Distribution*

The volume of distribution for theophylline is very constant, around 0.45 within persons and between persons (0.3-0.7L/kg). Therefore, a loading dose of theophylline always gives about the same increase of plasma concentration. (Example: loading dose 6mg/kg increases concentration 6/0.45 = 13mg/L = 74μmol/L.)

### *Metabolism*

Theophylline is metabolised in the liver before being excreted in the urine. Only about 10% is excreted unchanged. The metabolism is mainly dependent on enzymes in the $P_{450}$ cytochrome system. This is the reason why many factors may influence the metabolic clearance of theophylline. Most of the variation is, however, genetically determined, but there are several non-genetic factors influencing theophylline metabolism (Table 6.4).[79]

### *Therapeutic Concentrations*

Theophylline has a very low therapeutic range and a steep dose-response relationship. Mitenko and Ogilvie[80] showed that the effect is very well correlated with the plasma theophylline level. The optimal concentration is 55 to 110μmol/L (10 to 20mg/L). During maintenance treatment of asthma, theophylline is very often combined with a beta2-adrenoreceptor stimulant, and then a concentration of 25 to 50μmol/L (5 to 10mg/L) is enough.[39]

*Table 6.4* Non-genetic factors altering theophylline clearance

| Increased clearance | Decreased clearance |
|---|---|
| Enzyme-inducing drugs | Enzyme-inhibiting drugs |
| ethanol | cimetidine |
| phenobarbitone | ethinyloestradiol |
| rifampicin | propranolol |
| Smoking | erythromycin |
| Marijuana | Methylxanthines (Michelis-Menton kinetics) |
| Barbecued meat | Age |
| Medical coal | Antiviral vaccines |
| High protein, low carbohydrate diet | Viral infections (interferon) |
| Youth | Hepatic cirrhosis |
| Cystic fibrosis | Congestive heart failure |
| | Respiratory insufficiency with cor pulmonale |
| | Fever |

## Clinical Use

The main clinical use of methylxanthines today is as a part of combination treatment with a beta2-adrenoreceptor agonist. It has been shown that it is advantageous to combine inhaled beta2-adrenoreceptor agonists with oral theophylline, as this gives less tremor than combination with an oral beta2-adrenoreceptor stimulant which might give the same bronchodilating effect.[39]

Slow-release preparations of theophylline have a clear advantage in maintenance treatment, as the drug can be given twice daily independently of the individual half-life of the drug. The dosage during oral maintenance treatment is preferably low and could slowly be increased to the following mean doses when combined with a beta2-adrenoreceptor stimulant:

| | |
|---|---|
| Children under 9 years of age | 12mg/kg/24h |
| 9-12 years | 10mg/kg/24h |
| 12-16 years | 9mg/kg/24h |
| Over 16 years | 7mg/kg/24h |

These dosages are related to the ideal body weight, excluding obesity. They usually give a plasma concentration of 30 to 55$\mu$mol/L (5 to 10mg/L). This dosage is to be preferred, if there is no possibility of estimating the plasma concentration. Table 6.5 gives practical recommendations for changes in oral treatment with regard to different plasma concentrations.

It is important that, when oral theophylline is indicated, it should be given as a single drug and the dose should be individualised. Therefore, combination preparations should not be used.

It is also important to teach patients that they should not change the dosage of oral theophyllines even during exacerbations. Patients usually increase their doses of beta2-adrenoreceptor stimulants, but the therapeutic range for theophylline is smaller than for beta2-adrenoreceptor stimulants, and therefore an increased dose of theophylline may cause life-threatening intoxication.

*Table 6.5* Recommended adjustment of dosage during oral maintenance treatment with theophylline combined with a beta2-adrenoreceptor stimulant

| Theophylline (μmol/L) | Concentration (mg/L) | Change of dose |
|---|---|---|
| >190 | >35 | Do not give the next two doses and then decrease the dose 75%. New control is indicated |
| 135-190 | 25-35 | Do not give next dose. Decrease the dose by 66%. |
| 110-135 | 20-25 | Decrease the dose by about 50%. |
| 55-110 | 10-20 | Consider decreasing the dose. The dose could be continued in patients with asthma which is difficult to control, but a prerequisite is plasma concentration measurements. |
| 25-55 | 5-10 | Usually unchanged dose. |
| <25 | <5 | If the disease is under control, the theophylline treatment should be withdrawn. Otherwise the dose should be increased about 100%. |

It is important to check that the patient has taken the drug continuously during the last 48 hours.

### *Intravenous Treatment*

The recommended bolus dose for all, independent of age and other diseases, is 6mg/kg, if the patient has not previously been treated with oral theophylline. This dose usually increases the blood concentration about 66μmol/L (12mg/L). If the patient is on maintenance treatment with oral theophyllines, this bolus dose should be halved (Table 6.6).

Note that intravenous theophylline should always be given via a peripheral vein. Administration via a central venous catheter has probably induced fatal cardiac arrhythmias.

## Anticholinergic Agents

The parasympathetic nervous system via the vagal nerve contributes to the control of the airway calibre, as there is a bronchoconstrictive reflex elicited mainly from irritant receptors in the airways reaching the central nervous system via afferent nerves. In the airways there are paraysmpathetic ganglia modulating the nervous effect. Postganglionic bronchoconstricting effects act via muscarinic receptors on the bronchial smooth muscle as well as by mucus-producing effects on submucosal glands.

Therefore, antimuscarinic substances such as atropine and ipratropium bromide have been shown to have bronchodilating properties.[81,82]

The muscarinic receptors on the bronchial smooth muscle act intracellularly by inhibiting adenylate cyclase, thereby decreasing the intracellular concentration of cAMP. Their stimulation increases the intracellular concentration of calcium ions, by both increased transmembranous calcium flux and release from intracellular calcium stores, and also increases the phosphatidylinositol metabolism which can directly activate myosin.[4]

*Table 6.6* Intravenous maintenance dose of theophylline

| Age of patient | Infusion speed (mg/kg/h) |
|---|---|
| Neonatal period (to treat apnoea) | 0.15 |
| Children 6 months — 9 years | 0.8 |
| Children more than 9 years and adult smokers | 0.65 |
| Adult non-smokers | 0.4 |
| Patients with heart insufficiency or decreased liver function | 0.2 |

As the clearance is very variable it is important to check the plasma concentration within the first 24 hours of theophylline infusion.

## Clinical Use

Ipratropium bromide by the inhaled route has been the most widely used anticholinergic drug. It is a specific muscarinic receptor antagonist. The bronchodilation comes slowly after inhalation of ipratropium bromide and the maximum effect is achieved after about two hours. The duration of the bronchodilating effect is four to six hours (20 to 40μg).

Some studies have used much higher doses, up to 1000μg. It has been shown that 200 to 400μg seems to be an optimal dose, as 750μg gives less bronchodilation than 250μg. Probably this is due to a local irritating effect of the inhaled solution (0.025%).[83,84]

The clinical use of anticholinergic agents has been studied in chronic bronchitis and asthma. It has been shown that some asthmatic patients can have the same bronchodilation with anticholinergic agents as with beta2-adrenoreceptor stimulants. However, many patients with asthma do not have the same response to ipratropium bromide as to beta2-adrenoreceptor stimulants, due to the fact that anticholinergic agents only block acetylcholine-mediated bronchoconstriction, while beta2-agonists and theophyllines are functional antagonists against all asthma mediators.

There are some long-term studies with ipratropium bromide, in which doses of up to 160μg/day have been used for up to six months. A continuous bronchodilating effect without tachyphylaxis has been shown in these studies.[85,86]

The main indication for these drugs is in patients who cannot take inhaled beta2-receptor stimulants because of side effects.

## Side Effects

Ipratropium bromide is poorly absorbed and inhaled treatment is free from systemic side effects. The only practical problem is that patients often do not like the taste of ipratropium; some patients also complain of dryness in the mouth.

As anticholinergic agents have been shown to decrease ciliary movement and to increase the viscosity of sputum, studies have been performed to evaluate these effects. However, doses of up to 200μg of ipratropium bromide have not shown any adverse side effects on mucociliary clearance.[82] However, as these studies have been performed in moderately severe asthmatics with a low parasympathetic tone, the bronchodilating effect of anticholinergic agents is often less effective than that of beta2-adrenoreceptor stimulants.

## References


1. Svedmyr N, Simonsson BG. Drugs in the treatment of asthma. In: Widdicombe J, ed. *Respiratory pharmacology.* Oxford: Pergamon Press, 1981: 657-701.
2. Löfdahl CG. Selectivity of β-adrenoreceptor agonists and antagonists in asthmatics. *Eur J Respir Dis* 1982; 63 (suppl 120): 1-53.
3. Svedmyr N, Löfdahl CG. Physiology and pharmacodynamics of beta-adrenergic agonists. In: Jenne J, ed. *Bronchodilators: theory and practice.* New York: Marcel & Dekker, 1987 (in press).
4. Löfdahl CG, Barnes PJ. Calcium, calcium channel blockade and airways function. *Acta Pharmacol Toxicol* 1986; 58 (suppl 11): 91-111.
5. Svedmyr N. Treatment with β-adrenostimulants. *Scand J Respir Dis* 1977; (suppl 101): 59-70.
6. Karlsson JA, Persson CGA. Influence of tracheal contraction on relaxant effects in vitro of theophylline and isoprenaline. *Br J Pharmacol* 1981; 74: 73-79.
7. O'Donnell SR, Wanstall JC. Evidence that the efficacy (intrinsic activity) of fenoterol is higher than that of salbutamol on β-adrenoreceptors in guinea pig trachea. *Eur J Pharmacol* 1978; 37: 333-340.
8. Svedmyr N. Fenoterol: a $\beta_2$-adrenergic agonist for use in asthma. Pharmacology, pharmacokinetics, clinical efficacy and adverse effects. *Pharmacotherapy* 1985; 5: 109-126.
9. Karlsson JA, Persson CGA. Asthma mediators functional antagonisted by theophylline, enprofylline and terbutaline. Thesis, University of Lund, 1984.
10. Mossberg B, Strandberg K, Philipson K, Camner P. Tracheobronchial clearance in bronchial asthma response to β-adrenoreceptor stimulation. *Scand J Respir Dis* 1976; 57: 119.
11. Matthys H, Köhler D, Daikeler G. Additive actions of bronchodilators on mucous transport. *Respiration* 1984; 46 (suppl 1): 34.
12. AlBazzaz FJ, Cheng E. Effect of catecholamines on ion transport in dog tracheal epithelium. *J Appl Physiol* 1979; 47: 397.
13. Borson DB, Chinn RA, Davies B, Nadel JA. Adrenergic and cholinergic nerves mediate fluid secretion from tracheal glands of ferrets. *J Appl Physiol* 1980; 49: 1027-1031.
14. Bateman JRM, Pavia D, Shenhan NF, Newman SP, Clarke SW. Effects of terbutaline sulphate aerosol on bronchodilator response and lung mucociliary clearance in patients with mild stable asthma. *Br J Clin Pharmacol* 1983; 15: 695-700.
15. Martin GL, Atkins PC, Dynsky EH, Zweiman B. Effects of theophylline, terbutaline and prednisolone on antigen-induced bronchospasm and mediator release. *J Allergy Clin Immunol* 1980; 66: 204.
16. Holgate ST, Church MK. Mediator release from human lung mast cells. *Respiration* 1984; 46 (suppl 1): 22.
17. Howarth PH, Durhem SR, Lee TH, Kay B, Church MK, Holgate ST. Influence of albuterol, cromolyn sodium and ipratropium bromide on the airway and circulating mediator responses to allergen bronchial provocation in asthma. *Am Rev Respir Dis* 1985; 132: 986-992.
18. Hegardt B. Evaluation of the anti-allergic property of the β-adrenoreceptor agonist KWD 2131 in asthmatics. *Eur J Respir Dis* 1981; 62 (suppl 115): 1-154.
19. Svensjö E, Persson CGA, Rutili G. Inhibition of bradykinin-induced macromolecular leakage from postcapillary venules by a $\beta_2$-adrenoreceptor stimulant, terbutaline. *Acta Physiol Scand* 1977; 101: 504.
20. Persson CGA, Svensjö E. Airway hyperreactivity and microvascular permeability to large molecules. *Eur J Respir Dis* 1983; 64 (suppl 131): 183.
21. Wetznblum E, Hirth C, Dulolone A, Mirhom R. Prognostic value of pulmonary artery pressure in chronic obstructive pulmonary disease. *Thorax* 1981; 36: 752.
22. Aubier M, DeTroier A, Sampson M. Aminophylline improves diaphragmatic contractility. *N Engl J Med* 1981; 305: 249.
23. Howell S, Roussos C. Isoproterenol and aminophylline improve contractility of fatigued canine diaphragmae. *Am Rev Respir Dis* 1984; 129: 118.
24. Howell S, Fitzgerald RS, Roussos CH. Effects of aminophylline, isoproterenol and neostigmine on hypercapnic depression of diaphragmatic contractility. *Am Rev Respir Dis* 1985; 132: 241-247.

25. Thompson PJ, Dhillon DP, Ledingham J, Turner-Warwick H. Shrinking lungs, diaphragmatic dysfunction and systemic lupus erythematosus. *Am Rev Respir Dis* 1985; 132: 926-928.
26. Skoogh BE, Svedmyr N. $\beta_2$-Adrenoceptor stimulation inhibits ganglionic transmission in ferret trachea. *Am Rev Respir Dis* 1984; 129 (suppl A232).
27. Formgren H. The therapeutic value of oral long-term treatment with terbutaline (Bricanyl®) in asthma. *Scand J Respir Dis* 1975; 56: 321-328.
28. Thiringer G, Svedmyr N. Comparison of infused and inhaled terbutaline in patients with asthma. *Scand J Respir Dis* 1976; 57: 17-24.
29. Larsson S, Svedmyr N. Bronchodilating effect and side effects of $\beta_2$-adrenoceptor stimulants by different modes of administration (tablets, metered aerosol and combinations thereof). A study with salbutamol and asthmatics. *Am Rev Respir Dis* 1977; 116: 861-869.
30. Löfdahl CG, Bengtsson B, Svedmyr K, Svedmyr N. Two new $\beta_2$-adrenoceptor agonists, D 2343 and QH 25, studied in asthmatic patients. *Allergy* 1982; 37: 351-357.
31. Löfdahl CG, Svedmyr K, Svedmyr N, Andersson P, Bengtsson B, Olsson OAT, Waldeck B. Comparison of $\beta_2$-adrenoceptor stimulation in bronchial and skeletal muscle in experimental and clinical studies. *Eur J Respir Dis* 1984; (suppl 135): 124-127.
32. Bowman WC. Effects of adrenergic activators and inhibitors on the skeletal muscle. In: Szekeres L, ed. *Handbook of experimental pharmacology;* vol 54. Berlin: Springer Verlag, 1981: 47-128.
33. Thiringer G, Svedmyr N. Evaluation of skeletal muscle tremor due to bronchodilator agents. *Scand J Respir Dis* 1975; 56: 93-102.
34. Jenne WK, Ridley DJ, Marcucci RA, Druz WS, Rook JC. Objective and subjective tremor responses to oral $\beta_2$-agents on first exposure. A comparison of metaproterenol and terbutaline. *Am Rev Respir Dis* 1982; 126: 607-610.
35. Larsson S, Svedmyr N, Thiringer G. Lack of bronchial $\beta$-adrenoceptor resistance in asthmatics during long term treatment with terbutaline. *J Allergy Clin Immunol* 1977; 59: 93-100.
36. Holmberg E, Jeppsson AB, Waldeck B. Selective development of tolerance to $\beta$-adrenoceptor agonists in skeletal muscle as compared with airway smooth muscle from the guinea-pig. *Clin Exp Pharmacol Physiol* 1981; 8: 49-56.
37. Laursen LC, Taudorf E, Gnospelius Y, Gymose E, Weeke B. Long-term oral therapy of asthma with terbutaline and theophylline, alone and combined. *Eur J Respir Dis* 1985; 66: 82-90.
38. Conradson TB. An overview of the arrhythmogenic role of theophylline in COPD. In: Isles AF, von Wichert P, eds. *Sustained release theophyllines and nocturnal asthma.* Amsterdam: Excerpta Medica, 1985: 163.
39. Svedmyr K. $\beta_2$-Adrenoceptor stimulants and theophylline in asthma therapy. *Eur J Respir Dis* 1981; 62 (suppl 116): 1-48.
40. Prior JG, Cochrane GM, Raper SM, Ali C, Volans GN. Self-poisoning with oral salbutamol. *Br Med J* 1981; 282: 1932.
41. Speizer FE, Doll R, Heaf P. Observations on recent increase in mortality from asthma. *Br Med J* 1968; 1: 335-339.
42. Speizer FE, Doll R, Heaf P, Strang LB. Investigation in the use of drugs preceding death from asthma. *Br Med J* 1968; 1: 339-343.
43. Conolly ME, Davies DS, Dollery CT, George CF. Resistance to $\beta$-adrenoceptor stimulants (a possible explanation for the rise in asthma deaths). *Br J Pharmacol* 1971; 43: 389-402.
44. Holgate ST, Baldwin CJ, Tattersfield AE. Beta-adrenergic agonist resistance in normal human airways. *Lancet* 1977; 2: 375.
45. Harvey JE, Tattersfield AE. Airway response to salbutamol: effect of regular salbutamol inhalations in normal, atopic, and asthmatic subjects. *Thorax* 1982; 37: 280-287.
46. Van den Berg W, Leferink JG, Fokkens JK, Kreukneit J, Maes RAA, Bruynzeel PLB. Clinical implications of drug-induced desensitization of the beta receptor after continuous oral use of terbutaline. *J Allergy Clin Immunol* 1982; 69: 410-417.
47. Tashkin DP, Conolly ME, Deutsch RI, Kit Hui K, Littner M, Searpace P, Abrass I. Subsensitisation of beta-adrenoceptors in airways and lymphocytes of healthy and asthmatic subjects. *Am Rev Respir Dis* 1982; 125: 185-193.
48. Jenne WK. Reviews. A critic of dosing strategies for $\beta_2$-adrenergic agents and theophylline. *Lung* 1981; 159: 295-314.
49. Tattersfield AE. Bronchodilator drugs. *Pharmacol Ther* 1982; 17: 299-313.

50. Svedmyr N. Is beta-adrenoceptor sensitivity a limiting factor in asthma therapy? In: Morley J, ed. *Perspectives in asthma. II. Beta-adrenoceptors in asthma.* London: Academic Press, 1984: 181-199.
51. Nyberg L, Wood C, eds. Advances in terbutaline pharmacokinetics. *Eur J Respir Dis* 1984; 65 (suppl 134): 1-240.
52. Oxford J. *Applications of gas chromatography and mass spectrometry to drug metabolism.* PhD thesis, Hatfield Polytechnic, Hatfield, Herts, UK, 1979.
53. Nyberg L. Pharmacokinetic parameters of terbutaline in healthy man. An overview. *Eur J Respir Dis* 1984; 65 (suppl 134): 149-160.
54. Evans ME, Walker SR, Brittain RT, Paterson JW. The metabolism of salbutamol in man. *Xenobiotica* 1973; 3: 113-120.
55. Leferink JG, Wagemaker-Engels I, Maes RAA. Determination of terbutaline in postmortem human tissues by gas chromatography -mass spectrometry. *J Anal Toxicol* 1978; 2: 86-88.
56. Ryrfelt A, Ramsay CH. Distribution of terbutaline. *Eur J Respir Dis* 1984; (suppl 134): 63-72.
57. Andersson K-E, Nyberg L. Pharmacokinetics of terbutaline therapy. *Eur J Respir Dis* 1984; 65 (suppl 134): 165-170.
58. Powell ML, Weisberger M, Gural R, Chung M, Patrick J, Radwanski E, Symchowicz SS. Comparative bioavailability and pharmacokinetics of three formulations of albuterol. *J Pharm Sci* 1985; 17: 217-218.
59. Orehek J, Beaupré A, Badier M, Nicoli MM, Delpierre S. Perception of airway tone by asthmatic patients. *Bull Eur Physiopathol Respir* 1982; 18: 601-607.
60. Crompton GK. Problems patients have using pressurized aerosol inhalators. *Eur J Respir Dis* 1982; 63 (suppl 119): 101-104.
61. Svedmyr N, Löfdahl CG, Svedmyr K. The effect of powder aerosol compared to pressurized aerosol. *Eur J Respir Dis* 1982; 63 (suppl 119): 81-88.
62. Cushley MJ, Lewis RA, Tattersfield AE. Comparison of three techniques of inhalation on the airway response to terbutaline. *Thorax* 1983; 38: 909-913.
63. Munch EP, Hidinger KG, Weeke B. Bronchodilation of terbutaline in small doses from a 750 ml spacer. *Allergy* 1983; 38: 487-491.
64. Herrmann G, Agnesworth MB, Martin J. Successful treatment of persistent dyspnoea, "status asthmaticus'. *J Lab Clin Med* 1937; 23: 135-148.
65. Polson JB, Krzanowski JJ, Goldman AL, Szentivanyi A. Inhibition of human pulmonary phosphodiesterase activity by therapeutic levels of theophylline. *Clin Exp Pharmacol Physiol* 1978; 5: 536-539.
66. Bergstrand H. Phosphodiesterase inhibition and theophylline. *Eur J Resp Dis* 1980; 61 (suppl 109): 37-44.
67. Fredholm BB. Theophylline action on adenosine receptors. *Eur J Respir Dis* 1980; 61 (suppl 109): 29-36.
68. Mann JS, Cushley MJ, Holgate ST. Adenosine-induced bronchoconstriction in asthma and its antagonism, by theophylline. In: Herzog H, Perruchoud AP, eds. *Asthma and bronchial hyperreactivity.* Basle: Karger, 1985: 102-105. (Progress in respiration research; vol 19).
69. Lunell E, Svedmyr N, Andersson KE, Persson CGA. A novel bronchodilator xanthine apparently without adenosine receptor antagonism and tremorogenic effect. *Eur J Respir Dis* 1963; 64: 333-339.
70. Horrobin DF, Manku MS, Franks DJ, Hamet P. Methylxanthine phosphodiesterase inhibitors behave as prostaglandin antagonists in a perfused rat mesenteric artery preparation. *Prostaglandins* 1977; 13: 33-40.
71. Poisner AM. Direct stimulant effect of aminophylline on catecholamine release from the adrenal medulla. *Biochem Pharmacol* 1973; 22: 469-476.
72. Snider S, Waldeck B. Increased synthesis of adrenomedullary catecholamines induced by caffeine and theophylline. *Naunyn-Schmiedebergs Arch Pharmacol* 1974; 281: 257-260.
73. Mackay AD, Baldivin CJ, Tattersfield AE. Action of intravenously administered aminophylline on normal airways. *Am Rev Respir Dis* 1983; 127: 609-613.
74. Kolbeck RC, Speir WA, Carrier GO, Bransome ED Jr. Apparent irrelevance of cyclic nucleotides to the relaxation of tracheal smooth muscle induced by theophylline. *Lung* 1979; 156: 173-183.
75. Lakshminarayan S, Sahn SA, Weil JV. Effect of aminophylline on ventilatory responses in normal man. *Am Rev Respir Dis* 1978; 117: 33-38.
76. Mahutte CK, True RJ, Michiels TM, Berman JM, Light RW. Increased serum theophylline clearance with orally administered activated charcoal. *Am Rev Respir Dis* 1983; 128: 820-822.

77. Ahlmén J, Heath A, Herlitz H, Kvist L, Mellstrand T. Treatment of oral theophylline poisoning. *Acta Med Scand* 1984; 216: 423-426.

78. Hendeles L, Iafrate RP, Weinberger M. A clinical and pharmacokinetic basis for the selection and use of slow release theophylline products. *Clin Pharmacokinet* 1984; 9: 95-135.

79. Jonkman JHG, Upton RA. Pharmacokinetic interactions with theophylline. *Clin Pharmacokinet* 1984; 9: 309-334.

80. Mitenko PA, Ogilvie RI. Rational intravenous doses of theophylline. *N Engl J Med* 1973; 289: 600.

81. Massey KL, Gotz VP. Ipratropium bromide, investigational drug, information. *Drug Intell Clin Pharm* 1985; 19: 5-12.

82. Gross NJ, Skorodin MS. Anticholinergic, antimuscarinic bronchodilation. *Am Rev Respir Dis* 1984; 129: 856-870.

83. Dolovich M, Eng P, Jordana G. Atrovert aerosol inhalation in asthmatic adults: a dose-response study. *Allerg Clin Immunol* 1984; 74: 130.

84. Hockley B, Johnson MI. A comparison of three high doses of iptratropium bromide in chronic asthma. *Br J Dis Chest* 1985; 79: 379-384.

85. Laitinen LA, Poppius H, Haahtela T. Comparison of ipratropium bromide and salbutamol in a long term trial in asthmatic and bronchitic patients in a cold climate. *Scand J Respir Dis* 1979; (suppl 103): 163-169.

86. Pierce RJ, Holmes PW, Campbell H. Use of ipratropium bromide in patients with severe airways obstruction. *Aust NZ J Med* 1982; 12: 38.

87. Stiles GL, Caron MG, Lefkowitz RJ. β-Adrenergic receptors: biochemical mechanisms of physiological regulation. *Physiol Rev* 1984; 64: 661-743.

88. Birnbaumer L, Codina J, Mattera R, Rojas RJ, Hildebrandt JD, Rosenthal W, Sunyer T. Structural and regulatory properties of nucleotide binding regulatory N proteins of adenylate cyclase and their effects on hormone receptors. In: Paton W, Mitchell J, Turner P, eds. IUPHAR 9th international congress of pharmacology, London 1984; vol 1. London: MacMillan Press: 279-286.

## Chapter 7

# Drugs Which Affect Chemical Mediators in the Lungs

*J. Paul Seale*

## Chemical Mediators: Release and Effects in the Lungs

For many years it has been known that human lung tissue has the potential to synthesise and release biologically active endogenous substances with potent effects in the lung.[1] Since many of these effects such as bronchoconstriction and exudation resemble various pathophysiological features of asthma, these substances have been considered putative chemical mediators of asthma. However, in addition to demonstrating that lung tissue can synthesise and release a particular mediator, the following criteria should be fulfilled before the mediator can be assigned an important role in pathogenesis.[2]

1. The mediator should be detectable in body fluids during an episode of clinical asthma.
2. Administration of the mediator to man should mimic some or all of the clinical manifestations of asthma.
3. Pharmacological inhibition of its synthesis or antagonism of its actions should abrogate or modify clinical asthma.

At present, none of the potential candidates satisfies all these criteria. Part of the difficulty rests with the fact that many of the mediators are local hormones,[3] being released at, or close to, their sites of action within the lungs. Therefore, determination of concentrations in the peripheral circulation may not reflect substantial changes in concentration at receptor sites within the lung.[2] Furthermore, specific antagonists or inhibitors of the recently discovered mediators (leukotrienes, platelet activating factor, neutrophil chemotactic factor) have not yet been developed. Some of the drugs used in the treatment of asthma simultaneously inhibit the release of a number of mediators or affect their actions, but none is specific for a particular mediator. Thus, these agents may be useful therapeutically, but they do not assist in determining the precise role of an individual mediator in asthma. Current research is directed towards further characterising the action of these putative mediators and their possible interactions and synthesising antagonists and inhibitors so that they may be tested in animal models and undergo clinical evaluation.

### Chemical Mediators

The numerous substances released from lung tissue are divided into preformed mediators and those which are synthesised *de novo* (Table 7.1). The preformed mediators are stored within the cytoplasmic secretory granules of mast cells, packaged in an orderly fashion along the glycosaminoglycan side

*Table 7.1* Chemical mediators released from lung tissue

| Preformed | Newly synthesised |
|---|---|
| Histamine | Arachidonic acid metabolites |
| Chemotactic factors | prostanoids |
| ECF | leukotrienes |
| NCF | hydroxy fatty acids |
| Neutral proteases | |
| Acid hydrolases | Platelet activating factor (PAF) |
| Heparin | |
| Superoxide dismutase | |

ECF = eosinophil chemotactic factor.
NCF = neutrophil chemotactic factor.
PAF = acetyl-glyceryl-ether-phosphoryl-choline (AGEPC).

chains of heparin.[4] When the mast cells are stimulated, the passage of extracellular calcium ions initiates an energy-dependent secretory mechanism in which the perigranular and plasma membranes fuse, facilitating extrusion of the granule contents into the extracellular space.[4]

The newly generated mediators are synthesised at the time of stimulation and released immediately into the extracellular environment. Arachidonic acid, which is released from membrane phospholipids by phospholipase $A_2$ or sequentially by phospholipase C and diglyceride lipase,[5] may be metabolised via the cyclo-oxygenase pathway to thromboxanes ($TxA_2$), prostacyclin ($PGI_2$) and a variety of prostaglandins ($PGD_2$, $PGE_2$, $PGF_2$), or via the 5-lipoxygenase pathway to hydroperoxy and hydroxy derivatives and leukotrienes ($LTB_4$, $LTC_4$, $LTD_4$ and $LTE_4$) (Figure 7.1). Although most cells in the body have the ability to metabolise arachidonic acid via the cyclo-oxygenase pathway, the products vary from one cell type to another. For example, endothelial cells synthesise predominantly $PGI_2$ and platelets synthesise predominantly $TxA_2$.[6]

Human dispersed pulmonary parenchymal mast cells generate mainly $PGD_2$ upon stimulation.[7] Since immunological challenge of human lung fragments results in the release of $PGE_2$, $PGF_{2\alpha}$, 6-keto$PGF_{1\alpha}$ and $TxB_2$,[8] it is inferred that these products are synthesised by cells other than the mast cell.

Research to date has found that a lesser number of cells is capable of metabolising arachidonic acid via the lipoxygenase pathway. $LTB_4$ is synthesised by neutrophils[9] and alveolar macrophages.[10] $LTC_4$, $LTD_4$ and $LTE_4$, which account for the biological actions of slow-reacting substance (SRS-A), are released by pulmonary mast cells.[11] It is possible that additional cell types will be found which are capable of metabolising arachidonic acid to various lipoxygenase products.

Another newly formed mediator is platelet activating factor (PAF) which is also referred to by its chemical name of acetyl-glyceryl-ether-phosphoryl-choline (AGEPC). It is derived from ether-linked phospholipids in cell membranes by a two-stage process. The first is activation of phospholipase $A_2$, which cleaves arachidonic acid from the carbon-2 position of the glycerol backbone yielding an inactive precursor, lyso-PAF. The next stage is catalysed by acetyltransferase, which incorporates an acetyl group in the carbon-2 position, resulting in PAF. A variety of cells, including basophils, neutrophils, eosinophils, macrophages and platelets, generate PAF as a consequence of cellular activation.[12]

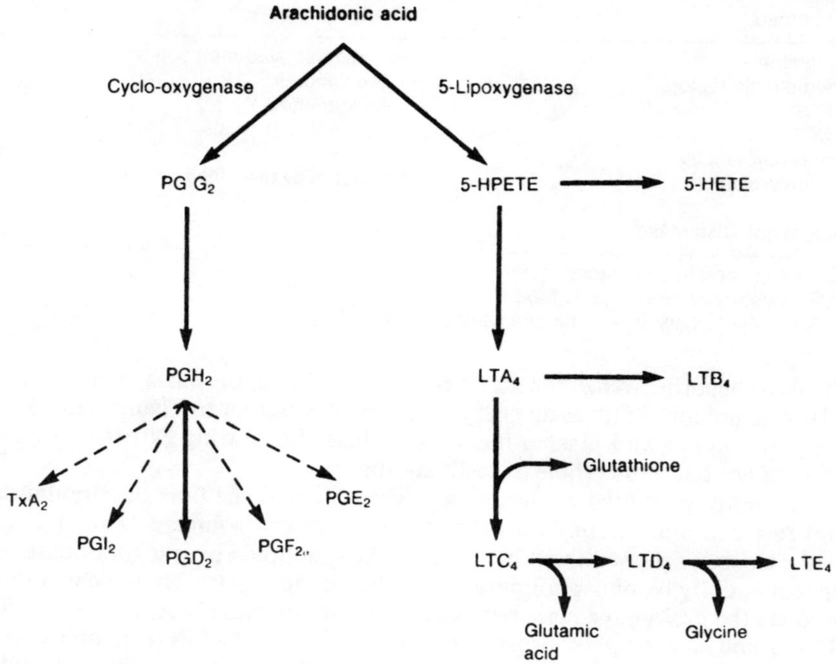


*Figure 7.1* The oxidative metabolism of arachidonic acid within the mast cell by the cyclo-oxygenase and 5-lipoxygenase pathways.

## Mechanisms of Mediator Release

### *Immunological Activation*

Antigen-induced release of mediators from human lung tissue, either passively or actively sensitised, has been the subject of intensive investigation for many years.[5] The process of sensitisation involves the attachment of immunoglobulins to target cells which are thought to be mast cells. Recent techniques for isolation and purification of cells within the lung have facilitated further characterisation of homogeneous cell populations.[13]

Human pulmonary mast cells have surface receptor sites for immunoglobulin E (IgE), which attaches to the mast cell membrane via the Fc fragment (Figure 7.2). Some individuals who respond to foreign substances by synthesising IgE will develop actively sensitised mast cells. In experimental situations, lung tissue may be sensitised passively *in vitro* by incubation in serum with a high IgE titre. The binding of specific antigen to the Fab ends of membrane-bound IgE molecules leads to approximation of Fc receptors (Figure 7.2). This is followed by an influx of calcium ions, which activates the energy-dependent secretory process, involving both preformed and newly generated chemical mediators (Figure 7.2). Although IgE is the usual sensitising antibody, there are some situations in which IgG antibodies have been implicated.[14]

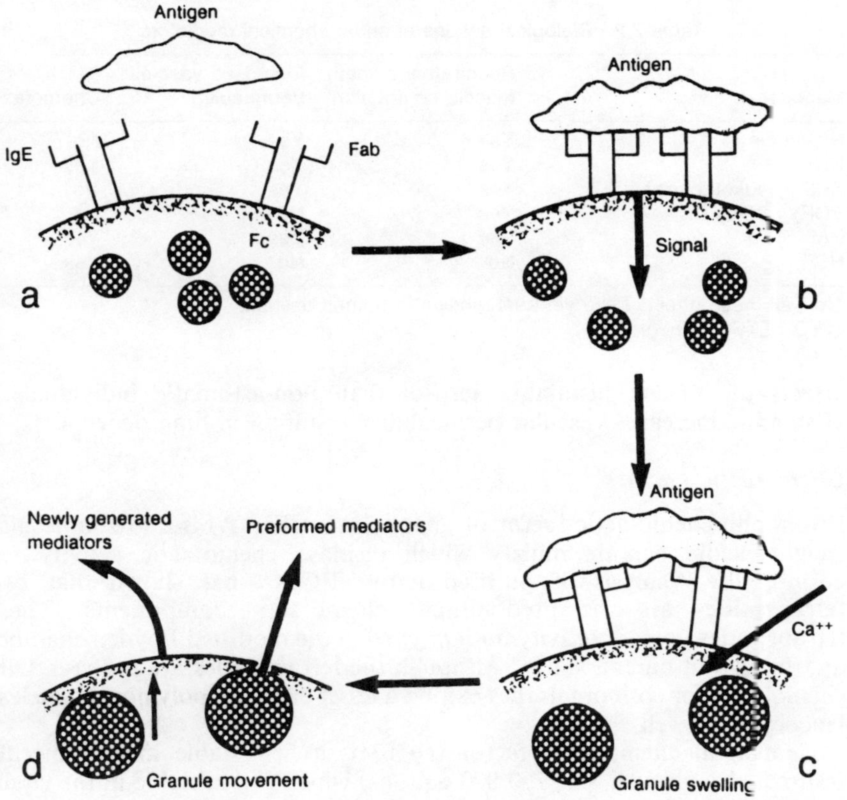


*Figure 7.2* Schematic representation of the cellular events of mast cell degranulation.

### *Non-immunological Activation*

In addition to antigen stimulation, there are other mechanisms of activation, which result in mediator release. The calcium ionophore (A23187) stimulates the release of histamine and leukotrienes from both sensitised and unsensitised human lung tissue.[15] The complement anaphylatoxins (C5a and C5a desarg) release histamine and leukotrienes from guinea-pig lung *in vitro,*[16] and PAF induces leukotriene production in rat isolated perfused lungs.[17]

These findings have indicated that a variety of non-immunological stimuli may initiate the release of chemical mediators, which have previously been considered only in the context of immunological activation. Moreover, it is possible that these mediators may also contribute to the pathogenesis of non-allergic asthma.

## The Mediators and Their Actions

The biological actions of the chemical mediators, which may be relevant to pulmonary pathophysiology, are outlined below (Table 7.2).

### *Histamine*

Histamine contracts respiratory smooth muscle *in vitro* and *in vivo.* Furthermore, asthmatic subjects are more sensitive to the bronchoconstrictor

*Table 7.2* Biological actions of some chemical mediators*

| Mediator | Respiratory smooth muscle contraction | Increased vascular permeability | Chemotaxis |
|---|---|---|---|
| Histamine | Yes | Yes | No |
| $LTB_4$ | Yes | Yes | Yes |
| SRS-A leukotrienes† | Yes | Yes | No |
| $PGF_{2\alpha}$, $PGD_2$ | Yes | No | No |
| PAF | Yes | Yes | Yes |
| NCF | No | No | Yes |

*Not all these effects have yet been shown in human tissues.
†$LTD_4$, $LTC_4$, $LTE_4$.

effects of inhaled histamine aerosol than non-asthmatic individuals.[18] Histamine increases vascular permeability resulting in lung oedema.[19]

### *Chemotactic Factors*

Eosinophil chemotactic factor of anaphylaxis (ECF-A) is a low molecular weight acidic peptide moiety which displays chemotactic activity for eosinophils. Analysis of purified native ECF-A has shown that two tetrapeptides are the predominant chemotactic components. These tetrapeptides possess activity both *in vitro* in the modified Boyden chamber and *in vivo* in human skin.[20] Although the tetrapeptides are preferentially chemotactic for eosinophils they exhibit a lesser effect on polymorphonuclear leucocytes as well.

Neutrophil chemotactic factor (NCF) is a heat-stable macromolecule (estimated molecular size 750 000 daltons) which is detectable in the circulation of asthmatic subjects after inhalation of specific allergen or after exercise-induced asthma.[21] A similar or identical substance is released after immunological challenge of human lung tissue *in vitro*. Further structural characterisation of NCF awaits a chemical method of measurement. NCF induces random, as well as directional, locomotion of neutrophils suggesting a role in the inflammatory response.[21]

### *Heparin Proteoglycan*

Intracellular heparin proteoglycan apparently serves to concentrate other preformed mediators and to determine their orderly arrangement and stability within the mast cell granule.[5] Extracellularly, native heparin proteoglycan inhibits the alternative complement pathway by preventing the formation of amplification convertase.[5] Amongst the various human heparin glycosaminoglycan subunits, only about one-third possess a high affinity for antithrombin III and associated anticoagulant activity.[5]

### *Granule-associated Enzymes*

When human neutral proteases, which are trypsin-like enzymes, are released from the mast cells, as part of an insoluble heparin-protease complex, their possible effects on proteoglycan core peptides, collagen and elastin would be confined to the immediate extracellular milieu. Furthermore, circulating inhibitors such as $\alpha_2$-macroglobulin and $\alpha_1$-antitrypsin would control their activity.[22]

The presence of acid hydrolases (beta-hexosaminidase, beta-glucuronidase and arylsulphatase) in the secretory granules of mast cells indicates that the organelle is a modified primary lysosome where degradation of ingested glycosaminoglycans, glycoproteins and complex glycolipids may occur. Since these enzymes may be released by immunological challenge it is possible that they may augment tissue injury.[5] The superoxide dismutase activity in rat mast cell granules suggests that these cells may be capable of killing ingested micro-organisms.

*Leukotrienes*

$LTB_4$ contracts parenchymal lung strips *in vitro* suggesting that it may contract peripheral airway smooth muscle.[23] Its ability to increase vascular permeability is dependent upon the presence of neutrophils.[24] $LTB_4$ is a potent chemotactic agent for polymorphs.[25] The SRS-A leukotrienes ($LTC_4$, $LTD_4$ and $LTE_4$) contract human airway smooth muscle *in vitro*,[26] induce bronchoconstriction *in vivo*,[27] and increase cutaneous vascular permeability.[28] $LTC_4$ was found to stimulate mucin secretion in anaesthetised cats[29] and $LTC_4$ and $LTD_4$ were reported to increase mucin production from human bronchus *in vitro*.[30]

*Prostaglandins*

Amongst the prostanoids, $PGF_{2\alpha}$ and $PGD_2$ are potent bronchoconstrictors in subjects with asthma.[31] In normal subjects, $PGD_2$ causes small reductions in specific airway conductance, whereas $PGF_{2\alpha}$ has no effect. These findings indicate that $PGD_2$ is more potent than $PGF_{2\alpha}$ in causing changes in airway function. In contrast, $PGE_1$ and $PGE_2$ are bronchodilators.[32] $PGI_2$ is without appreciable affect on airway tone.[33]

*Platelet Activating Factor (PAF)*

The relevant biological actions of PAF have been summarised by Morley et al.[34] PAF induces bronchoconstriction in experimental animals and in man. These acute pulmonary effects of PAF appear to be dependent upon platelet activation because antiplatelet antibodies abolish these changes. Furthermore, PAF contracts in-vitro preparations of respiratory smooth muscle only when platelets are added to the fluid bathing the preparations. PAF increases vascular permeability, but this effect appears to be independent of either platelet or leucocyte activation. PAF stimulates human neutrophils to secrete lysosomal enzymes and PAF is chemotactic for neutrophils.[12]

## Drugs Affecting Chemical Mediators

Pharmacological agents may modify the effects of chemical mediators by inhibiting their synthesis and release or by interfering with their actions on target organs. Some drugs have both these effects (Table 7.3).

*Table 7.3* Action of drugs on the release and effects of chemical mediators in human lung*

| Drug | Mediator Release | Mediator Effects |
|---|---|---|
| Beta-adrenoceptor agonists | Inhibition (H, LT, PG) | Inhibition |
| Theophylline | ± Inhibition (H) | ± Inhibition |
| Calcium antagonists | Inhibition (H, LT) | ± Inhibition |
| Cyclo-oxygenase inhibitors | Inhibition (PG) | Nil |
| Lipoxygenase inhibitors | Inhibition (LT) | Nil |
| Phospholipase $A_2$ inhibitors | Inhibition (LT, PG) | Nil |
| Corticosteroids | ± Inhibition (PG) | ± Inhibition |
| Histamine $H_1$-receptor antagonists | ± Inhibition | ± Inhibition |
| Histamine $H_2$-receptor antagonists | Nil | Nil |
| Disodium cromoglycate (DSCG) | ± Inhibition | ± Inhibition |
| Ketotifen | ± Inhibition | ± Inhibition |

*See text for details. ± = marginal effect. H = histamine, LT = leukotrienes, PG = prostaglandins.

## *Adrenoreceptor Agonists*

Adrenaline, whose anti-anaphylactic effect has been appreciated for many years[35] exerts its pulmonary effects via the stimulation of beta-receptors. Isoprenaline, which is a non-selective beta-adrenoreceptor agonist, relaxes human airway smooth muscle,[36] inhibits the release of histamine and SRS-A from human lung tissue,[1] and reduces histamine-induced increase in vascular permeability.[37] The beta2-selective adrenoreceptor agonists such as fenoterol, salbutamol and terbutaline share the above effects with isoprenaline. Thus, these agents affect mediator release as follows.

### *Inhibition of Mediator Release*

Fenoterol and salbutamol inhibit antigen-induced release of histamine and leukotrienes from human lung tissue *in vitro*.[38,39] This inhibitory effect is exerted via beta2-receptors since the action of fenoterol is reversed by butoxamine, a beta2-receptor antagonist, but not by atenolol, a beta1-receptor antagonist.[38] Although both mediators are inhibited by the beta2-agonists in a dose-related manner, at any given concentration the inhibition of leukotrienes is greater than the inhibition of histamine.[38] The release of prostaglandins from human lung fragments *in vitro* is also suppressed by beta-receptor stimulation,[40] which is thought to inhibit mediator release by increasing intracellular concentrations of cyclic adenosine monophosphate (cAMP).[1] The results of experiments on guinea-pig perfused lungs, showing that activation of phospholipase $A_2$ by certain stimuli may be inhibited by beta-adrenoreceptor agonists[41,42] suggest that phospholipase $A_2$ activity in human lung may also be susceptible to inhibition by beta-adrenoreceptor agonists, resulting in diminished release of both leukotrienes and prostaglandins. Although these inhibitory effects of beta-agonists occur at relatively low concentrations (effective concentration of fenoterol for 50% inhibition of leukotriene release is approximately 6nmol/L) it remains to be shown whether these concentrations are achieved at target cells within the lung in patients using metered dose aerosols of beta-agonists as routine bronchodilator therapy.

Not all stimuli for mediator release are inhibited by beta-receptor activation. Calcium ionophore-induced release of histamine and leukotrienes from human lung tissue was relatively unaffected by fenoterol.[38] It is not yet known whether the release of other mediators (Table 7.1) is inhibited by beta-receptor stimulation.

### *Functional Antagonism*

Beta-adrenoreceptor agonists relax human airway smooth muscle *in vitro*[36] and cause bronchodilation in man. Thus, the contractile effects of histamine and leukotrienes will be reduced by beta-agonists such as salbutamol.[43]

### *Effects on Microvascular Permeability*

When guinea-pigs inhale low concentrations of histamine aerosol for 60 minutes there is an increase in lung weight which is attributed to extravasation of protein and fluid.[19] This effect of histamine is prevented by pretreatment with isoprenaline or terbutaline, suggesting that beta-receptor stimulation counters the action of histamine in the microcirculation of the lung. If this effect of beta-adrenoreceptor agonists also occurs in human lung it may contribute to the 'anti-asthma' activity of these drugs, particularly if it is found that the beta-agonists also inhibit the permeability effects of other mediators such as leukotrienes and PAF.

## Theophylline

Methylxanthines (theophylline, isobutylmethylxanthine) inhibit the release of histamine from human basophils *in vitro*.[44] By inhibiting phosphodiesterase, an enzyme which degrades cAMP, theophylline leads to increased intracellular concentrations of cAMP, which is thought to account for its inhibitory effect on mediator release.[1] However, the concentrations required for this in-vitro effect are approximately 10 times greater than therapeutic plasma concentrations in patients with asthma. Moreover, theophylline does not alter the degree or duration of antigen-induced bronchospasm in asthmatic subjects.[45] Thus, there are no convincing data to suggest that inhibition of mediator release, which is demonstrable with theophylline *in vitro,* operates *in vivo.*

It has been suggested, based on experiments with guinea-pig lung, that theophylline, which is an adenosine receptor antagonist, may suppress adenosine-induced stimulation of histamine release.[46] However, there are major differences in the effects of adenosine between species because adenosine inhibits the antigen-induced release of both histamine and SRS-A in human lung fragments.[47] Theophylline, in concentrations of 50$\mu$mol, which alone had no action on mediator release, reduced the inhibitory effect of adenosine receptor agonists.[47] At higher concentrations theophylline inhibited mediator release in its own right. Thus, if theophylline antagonises adenosine receptors in human lung then it appears that the net effect may be enhanced mediator release.

The anti-permeability effects of theophylline have been investigated in guinea-pigs.[19] Oedema of the lung, produced by inhaling low concentrations of nebulised histamine, was markedly reduced by oral treatment with theophylline (55 to 110mg/kg). It remains to be seen whether this effect of theophylline, which is demonstrable in guinea-pigs, occurs in human lung and whether it contributes to the clinical efficacy of theophylline.

Recently, methylxanthines have been shown to inhibit airway responses which accompany ADP-induced and PAF-induced platelet activation.[34] Since PAF-induced contraction of airway smooth muscle requires the presence of platelets, it is possible that methylxanthines inhibit the release of a factor from platelets which is yet to be identified.[34] Moreover, these results in experimental animals suggest that theophylline may suppress a number of effects of mediators on target organs in the lung.

## Calcium Antagonists

Since the release of histamine and leukotrienes from human lung tissue *in vitro*, stimulated by either antigen or calcium ionophore, is inhibited by depletion of calcium from the incubation medium,[48,49] experiments have been performed to determine the effects of calcium antagonists on mediator release from human lung *in vitro*.[50] Whilst verapamil caused a concentration-dependent inhibition of both histamine and leukotriene release, it had a greater inhibitory action on the release of leukotrienes than on histamine. However, the concentrations of verapamil which produced these inhibitory effects *in vitro* were greater than the plasma concentrations achieved after clinically recommended oral or intravenous doses. Whether other calcium channel blockers affect mediator release from human lung tissue has yet to be determined.

The effects of calcium antagonists on airway responses to some contractile agonists have been determined. Pretreatment of guinea-pig tracheal strips with verapamil or nifedipine resulted in partial protection against $LTD_4$-induced contraction.[51] However, aerosol administration of verapamil to guinea-pigs did not significantly reduce $LTD_4$-induced bronchoconstriction *in vivo*.[51] Clinical trials in subjects with asthma have yielded variable results. Whereas inhalation of verapamil did not alter histamine-induced bronchoconstriction in one study of asthmatic subjects,[52] sublingual nifedipine afforded a small but significant protective effect against histamine challenge in another study.[53] Thus, these studies have shown that calcium antagonists have some effect on the release of leukotrienes and histamine from human lung tissue and they may reduce the responses of airway smooth muscle to histamine and leukotrienes. However, these effects are small, so the currently available calcium channel blockers have not been used in the treatment of asthma.

## Drugs Affecting Arachidonic Acid Metabolism

Although there are many enzymes involved in the metabolism of arachidonic acid, three separate categories of enzyme inhibitors have been investigated extensively.

### *Cyclo-oxygenase Inhibitors*

In view of the potent bronchoconstrictor effects of $PGF2\alpha$ and $PGD_2$[31] it is surprising that inhibitors of the cyclo-oxygenase pathway, such as aspirin or indomethacin, are without appreciable effect in most patients with asthma.

There are rare individuals whose asthma is improved by aspirin and other cyclo-oxygenase inhibitors,[54] suggesting that cyclo-oxygenase metabolites (possibly $PGF_{2\alpha}$ or $PGD_2$) are contributing to bronchoconstriction in these rare individuals. More commonly (in up to 20% of patients with asthma), aspirin and other cyclo-oxygenase inhibitors precipitate attacks of asthma.[55] It is not known whether inhibition of the cyclo-oxygenase pathway reduces the synthesis of a product such as $PGI_2$ which may inhibit mediator release or increases the metabolism of arachidonic acid via the lipoxygenase pathway to bronchoconstricting leukotrienes.[55]

Aspirin and indomethacin have been used successfully to close the patent ductus arteriosus in neonates with cardiac failure, by inhibiting the production of vasodilator prostaglandins ($PGE_2$ and $PGI_2$) within the ductus.[56]

### *Lipoxygenase Inhibitors*

A number of experimental drugs, such as benoxaprofen, BW 755C and U-60257,[57-59] have been found to inhibit the release of sulphidopeptide leukotrienes ($LTD_4$, $LTC_4$, $LTE_4$) from human lung tissue *in vitro*. The efficacy of these agents or similarly acting drugs in clinical asthma and various bronchoprovocation tests is keenly awaited.

### *Phospholipase $A_2$ Inhibitors*

Mepacrine, which inhibited $TxA_2$ release from guinea-pig isolated perfused lungs by a direct effect on phospholipase $A_2$ activity,[60] has been shown to cause a small but statistically significant reduction in leukotriene release from human lung fragments *in vitro*.[61] Inhibitory effects were also noted with chloroquine, which is structurally and pharmacologically similar to mepacrine. The in-vitro concentrations which were required for inhibition (10-100$\mu$mol/L) are greater than the plasma concentrations in patients given these drugs for the treatment of malaria or rheumatoid arthritis. However, since tissue concentrations of these drugs are much higher than plasma concentrations[61] it is possible that the requisite concentrations for inhibition of phospholipase $A_2$ are achieved within the lung. The single case report of a patient who no longer required steroids to control his asthma after commencing treatment with hydroxychloroquine lends credence to the hypothesis that mepacrine and its cogeners may be inhibiting phospholipase $A_2$ *in vivo*.[62]

Anti-inflammatory corticosteroids indirectly inhibit phospholipase $A_2$ in some cell populations by stimulating the synthesis of an effector protein called macrocortin (see below).

### *Prostaglandin and Leukotriene Antagonists*

Whilst it has been established that prostaglandins probably exert their effects through discrete receptors,[31] these has been no major breakthrough of potential therapeutic importance in developing prostaglandin receptor antagonists. Phloretin phosphate compounds such as polyphloretin phosphate (PPP) antagonise the action of prostaglandins on gut and uterine smooth muscle, but these agents have not been applied with any success to pulmonary models of lung disease.

A cromone carboxylic acid, designated FPL 55712, was reported to be a selective target organ antagonist of SRS-A.[63] More recent data have demonstrated that FPL 55712 also inhibits thromboxane synthetase in human platelets.[64] Its short half-life *in vivo* has militated against its useful application in clinical trials. An open study, in which four subjects with asthma were treated with nebulised FPL 55712, failed to draw any definite conclusions on its efficacy.[65]

U-60,257, which is an inhibitor of leukotriene synthesis, also antagonises their contractile effects on the guinea-pig ileum *in vitro*.[59] With further characterisation of receptors for leukotrienes many new compounds will be synthesised for evaluation as receptor antagonists *in vitro* and *in vivo*.

## Corticosteroids

Anti-inflammatory corticosteroids are life-saving drugs in acute asthma and comprise an essential component of drug treatment in many patients with chronic asthma. Despite these unquestionable therapeutic benefits, the underlying mechanisms of their 'anti-asthma' effects remain unclear.

Recent evidence suggests that part of their anti-inflammatory effect is attributable to the synthesis of an effector protein called macrocortin, the synthesis of which involves a number of steps and conforms to the general model of steroid action.[66] According to the model, the steroid molecules enter the cell, bind to cytosolic receptors, and these steroid-receptor complexes interact with nuclear chromatin, resulting in the production of messenger RNA, which then codes for the synthesis of macrocortin by the ribosomes. The model offers an explanation for the latency period for the onset of action which has been observed clinically[67] and experimentally.[68]

### *Effects on Mediator Release*

Inhibition of immunologically-induced histamine release was demonstrated in human basophils incubated with corticosteroids *in vitro* for 12 to 24 hours.[69] However, this effect of corticosteroids was not evident in human lung tissue. Incubation of human lung fragments or human pulmonary mast cells in high concentrations of dexamethasone for 16 to 24 hours failed to significantly reduce immunological histamine release.[68,70]

Experiments with animal models have established that corticosteroids stimulate both the release of preformed macrocortin and the de-novo synthesis of the protein by neutrophils, macrophages and possibly other cell types as well.[66] In guinea-pig isolated perfused lungs, macrocortin inhibited the release of the arachidonic acid metabolite, $TxA_2$, by suppressing the activity of phospholipase $A_2$.[66] By preventing the liberation of arachidonic acid from membrane phospholipids, macrocortin could be expected to inhibit the release of both cyclo-oxygenase products ($TxA_2$ and prostaglandins) and lipoxygenase products (leukotrienes). However, dexamethasone failed to significantly reduce the release of leukotrienes and $PGD_2$ from human lung *in vitro*.[68,70] It was notable that prostaglandins released from non-mast cell sources were inhibited by corticosteroids. Thus, in-vitro experiments have failed to show any inhibitory effect of glucocorticoids on the release of histamine or arachidonic acid products from human pulmonary mast cells.

Whether the suppression of arachidonic acid metabolism in other cell populations within the lung results in anti-inflammatory effects has yet to be determined. The ability of steroids to inhibit serotonin and beta-hexosaminidase release from rat mast cells[71] needs to be investigated in human pulmonary mast cells. Possible inhibitory effects on release of other mediators bears further study. In a preliminary report the production of PAF appeared to be susceptible to inhibition, since alveolar macrophages from steroid-treated patients with asthma were unable to release PAF.[34]

*Functional Antagonism*

Corticosteroids do not relax respiratory smooth muscle so they do not cause acute bronchodilation. Furthermore, there are no available data to suggest that they reduce the bronchoconstrictor effects of histamine or leukotrienes. However, they do suppress leukotriene-stimulated mucus secretion from human airways *in vitro*.[72] In addition, steroids protected mice against the lethal effects of PAF,[73] suggesting that glucocorticoids antagonise some of the actions of PAF.

*Effects on beta-adrenoreceptors*

Corticosteroids increase the density of beta-adrenoreceptors on human lymphocytes and rat lung.[74,75] Furthermore, they attenuate the densensitisation (or tachyphylaxis) associated with chronic beta-receptor stimulation, which is thought to stem from internalisation of receptors and uncoupling from adenylate cyclase.[74] If there is diminished ability of beta-adrenoreceptor agonists to functionally antagonise the actions of chemical mediators during exacerbations of asthma, then it is possible that corticosteroids may help to restore responsiveness to beta-agonists by increasing the density of receptors.

## Antihistamines

Histamine remains a potential candidate as a mediator contributing to the pathogenesis of asthma because inhalation of histamine induces bronchoconstriction in subjects with asthma by stimulating $H_1$-receptors,[76] immunological and non-immunological challenges of human lung fragments *in vitro* release histamine,[1,15] and increased plasma concentrations of histamine are detectable after certain types of provoked asthma, such as exercise-induced asthma.[77] However, histamine $H_1$-receptor antagonists, taken orally, have contributed little to the drug treatment of asthma. The following actions have been ascribed to $H_1$ antagonists.

*Effects on Mediator Release*

A number of $H_1$-receptor antagonists were found to have a biphasic effect on immunologically induced histamine release from human lung *in vitro*.[78] At low concentrations inhibition of histamine release was evident, but higher concentrations directly liberated histamine. Moreover, the potency of these drugs as inhibitors of histamine release was not correlated with their potency as histamine $H_1$-receptor antagonists.[78] It is not known whether this inhibitory effect on histamine release occurs in patients taking oral $H_1$-receptor antihistamines.

*Functional Antagonism*

There has been renewed interest in $H_1$-receptor antagonists based on the fact that when these drugs are taken directly into the lungs by inhalation, they offer some protection against bronchoprovoking stimuli such as inhaled histamine, inhaled allergen and exercise.[79] It would be necessary to know the protective effects of inhaled antihistamines against a number of other stimuli such as methacholine, nebulised water, leukotrienes and sulphur dioxide before making predictions of their potential efficacy in controlling naturally occurring asthma.

Although there is evidence that histamine $H_2$-receptors function as a negative feedback inhibitory mechanism for histamine release from human basophils,[80] no such feedback mechanism is demonstrable in human mast cells, because ranitidine, a histamine $H_2$-receptor antagonist, had no appreciable effect on the antigen-induced release of histamine or leukotrienes from human lung fragments *in vitro*.[81] Furthermore, the histamine $H_2$-receptor antagonist, cimetidine, did not significantly alter the peak flow rates or the degree of exercise-induced asthma in a clinical study involving 10 subjects.[82] From these results it appears that histamine $H_2$-receptor antagonists have no part to play in the drug treatment of asthma.

## Disodium Cromoglycate

The potential therapeutic significance of disodium cromoglycate was apparent after its inhibitory effect on antigen-induced bronchoconstriction in man was noted 20 years ago.[83] Based on experiments in rats, in which disodium cromoglycate was found to inhibit passive cutaneous anaphylactic reactions and to suppress histamine release from peritoneal mast cells, its protective action against allergic bronchoconstriction in man was ascribed to a similar mechanism. The subsequent course of experimental and clinical research has revealed that this assumption was incorrect.[84]

*Effects of Mediator Release*

The demonstrable inhibitory effect of disodium cromoglycate on passive cutaneous anaphylactic reactions in the rat was attributed to 'mast cell stabilisation', because disodium cromoglycate was found to inhibit antigen-induced degranulation and the associated histamine release from rat peritoneal mast cells. Initial experiments suggested that a similar inhibitory action of disodium cromoglycate could be demonstrated in human lung tissue.[84] However, more detailed studies with human lung have revealed some inconsistencies. In some specimens of human lung disodium cromoglycate failed to inhibit histamine release and in other specimens its activity was variable.[85] In general it was a weak inhibitor of both histamine and SRS-A release from human lung.[86]

Structural analogues, which are more potent than disodium cromoglycate in suppressing histamine and SRS-A release, have been synthesised,[85,87] but these analogues have been disappointing in clinical trials, casting grave doubt upon the notion that the clinical efficacy of disodium cromoglycate is due to inhibition of mediator release from the lung.[84]

### *Functional Antagonism*

Although there have been rare exceptions,[88] most studies have failed to show any bronchodilator effect of disodium cromoglycate.

There are conflicting data on the ability of disodium cromoglycate to reduce airway responses to inhaled methacholine and histamine.[89] Some studies have reported no changes in response to histamine after pretreatment with disodium cromoglycate,[79] but other studies have noted that it afforded complete protection against histamine-induced bronchoconstriction.[90] Some insight into these apparent discrepancies was provided by Woenne et al,[89] who found marked variation between subjects, so that disodium cromoglycate afforded substantial protection for some subjects and was ineffective in others. Thus, there are some subjects whose airway responses to inhaled chemical mediators are attenuated by disodium cromoglycate.

No mechanism which satisfactorily accounts for this effect has been advanced. Current research endeavours are focused on neural pathways which may be susceptible to inhibition by disodium cromoglycate. Support for these lines of investigation has come from the observation that airway responses to sulphur dioxide, which are reflexly mediated, are inhibited by disodium cromoglycate.[91] Furthermore, studies in dogs have revealed the existence of disodium cromoglycate-sensitive left ventricular afferent receptors within the endocardium, which mediate reflex bronchoconstriction to histamine.[92]

It is evident that further investigations are necessary to unravel the mechanism of action of this drug, which is of proven efficacy in the treatment of asthma.

### Ketotifen

Ketotifen was developed in the search for an orally effective disodium cromoglycate-like anti-allergic drug. Although it has antihistamine activity, its ability to inhibit passive cutaneous anaphylactic reactions in the rat suggests that it may possess additional properties because clemastine, a histamine $H_1$-receptor antagonist, is without effect on rat passive cutaneous anaphylactic reactions. In common with other $H_1$-receptor antagonists, ketotifen inhibits histamine release from human lung tissue *in vitro* at low concentrations and stimulates histamine release at higher concentrations.[78]

Clinical studies have shown that ketotifen reduces histamine-induced bronchoconstriction to the same extent as clemastine.[79] Its effects on allergen challenge in subjects with asthma are variable.[79] However, in those individuals for whom ketotifen does provide some protection against antigen-induced bronchoconstriction, it is not known whether the drug is inhibiting mediator release or antagonising the effects of the mediators on target organs.

## Conclusions

Amongst the numerous drugs which affect the release or actions of chemical mediators in the lungs, many have been valuable in the treatment of clinical asthma. The discovery and chemical characterisation of the leukotrienes and PAF have introduced a new era in research on asthma and its underlying mechanisms. The development of specific inhibitors and specific antagonists of these recently described chemical mediators should lead to a better understanding of the pathogenesis of asthma and more effective drug treatment.

## References


1. Orange RP, Austen WG, Austen KF. Immunological release of histamine and slow-reacting substance of anaphylaxis from human lung. I. Modulation by agents influencing cellular levels of cyclic 3 ', 5 '-adenosine monophosphate. *J Exp Med* 1971; (suppl 134): 136-138.
2. Anonymous. Inflammatory mediators of asthma. *Lancet* 1983; 2: 829.
3. Bakhle YS, Vane JR. Pharmacokinetic function of the pulmonary circulation. *Physiol Rev* 1974; 54: 1007-1045.
4. Holgate ST, Church MK. Control of mediator release from mast cells. *Clin Allergy* 1982; 12: 5.
5. Lewis RA, Austen KF. Mediation of local homeostasis and inflammation by leukotrienes and other mast cell-dependent compounds. *Nature* 1981; 293: 103-108.
6. Moncada S, Vane JR. Unstable metabolites of arachidonic acid and their role in haemostasis and thrombosis. *Br Med Bull* 1978; 34: 129-135.
7. Lewis RA, Soter NA, Diamond PT, Austen KF, Oates JA, Roberts JL. Prostaglandin $D_2$ generation after activation of rat and human mast cells with anti IgE. *J Immunol* 1982; 129: 1627.
8. Schulman ES, Newball HH, Demers LM, Fitzpatrick FA, Adkinson NF. Anaphylactic release of thromboxane $A_2$, prostaglandin $D_2$ and prostacyclin from human lung parenchyma. *Am Rev Respir Dis* 1981; 124: 402-406.
9. Borgeat P, Samuelsson B. Arachidonic acid metabolism in polymorphonuclear leukocytes: unstable intermediate in the formation of dihydroxy acids. *Proc Natl Acad Sci USA* 1979; 76: 3213-17.
10. Fels AO, Pawlowski NA, Cramer EB, King TKC, Cohn ZA, Scott WA. Human alveolar macrophages produce leukotriene $B_4$. *Proc Natl Acad Sci USA* 1982; 79: 7866-7870.
11. MacGlashan DW, Schleimer RP, Peters SP, Schulman ES, Adams GK, Newball HH, Lichtenstein LM. Generation of leukotrienes by purified human lung mast cells. *J Clin Invest* 1982; 70: 747-751.
12. Pinckard RN, McManus LM, Halonen M, Hanahan DJ. Immunopharmacology of acetyl-glyceryl-ether-phosphoryl-choline (AGEPC). In: Newball HH, ed. *Immunopharmacology of the lung*. New York: Marcel Dekker, 1983: 73-107.
13. Caulfield JP, Lewis RA, Hein A, Austen KF. Secretion in dissociated pulmonary mast cells. Evidence for solubilization of granule contents before discharge. *J Cell Biol* 1980; 85: 299.
14. Bryant DH. The role of IgG in human asthma. In: Lichenstein LM, Austen KF, eds. *Asthma: physiology, immunopharmacology and treatment*. New York: Academic Press, 1977: 315-327.
15. Seale JP, Piper PJ. Chemical mediators and non-allergic asthma. *Lancet* 1978; 2: 1265.
16. Stimler NP, Bach MK, Bloor CM, Hugli TE. Release of leukotrienes by C5a desArg anaphylatoxin. *J Immunol* 1982; 128: 2247-2252.
17. Voelkel NF, Worthen S, Reeves JT, Henson PM, Murphy RC. Nonimmunological production of leukotrienes induced by platelet-activating factor. *Science* 1982; 318: 286-288.
18. Boushey HA, Holtzman MJ, Sheller JR, Nadel JA. Bronchial hyperreactivity. *Am Rev Respir Dis* 1980; 121: 389-413.
19. Persson CGA, Ekman M, Erjefalt I. Vascular anti-permeability effects of $\beta$-receptor agonists and theophylline in the lung. *Acta Pharmacol Toxicol* 1979; 44: 216-220.
20. Lewis RA, Austen KF. Nonrespiratory functions of pulmonary cells: the mast cell. *Fed Proc* 1977; 36: 2676-2683.
21. Kay AB, Lee TH. Neutrophil chemotactic factor of anaphylaxis. *J Allergy Clin Immunol* 1982; 70: 317-320.
22. Lagunoff D. Neutral proteases of the mast cell. In: Becker EL, Simon AS, Austen KF, eds. *Biochemistry of the acute allergic reactions*. New York: Liss Press 1981: 89-101.

23. Sirols P, Borgeat P, Jeanson A. Comparative effects of leukotriene $B_4$, prostaglandins $I_2$ and $E_2$, 6-keto-$PGF_1$, thromboxane $B_2$ and histamine on selected smooth muscle preparations. *J Pharm Pharmacol* 1981; 33: 466-468.
24. Wedmore CV, Williams TJ. Control of vascular permeability by polymorphonuclear leukocytes in inflammation. *Nature* 1981; 289: 646-650.
25. Ford-Hutchinson AW, Bray MA, Doig MV, Shipley ME, Smith MJH. Leukotriene B, a potent chemokinetic and aggregating substance released from polymorphonuclear leukocytes. *Nature* 1980; 286: 264-265.
26. Hanna CJ, Bach MK, Pare PD, Schellenberg RR. Slow-reacting substances (leukotrienes) contract human airway and pulmonary vascular smooth muscle *in vitro*. *Nature* 1981; 290: 343-344.
27. Barnes NC, Piper PJ, Costello JF. Comparative effects of inhaled leukotriene $C_4$ and leukotriene $D_4$ and histamine in normal subjects. *Thorax* 1984; 39: 500-504.
28. Peck MJ, Piper PJ, Williams TJ. Effect of leukotrienes $C_4$ and $D_4$ on the microvasculature of guinea-pig skin. *Prostaglandins* 1981; 21: 315-321.
29. Peatfield AC, Piper PJ, Richardson PS. The effect of leukotriene $C_4$ on mucin release into the cat trachea *in vivo* and *in vitro*. *Br J Pharmacol* 1982; 77: 391-393.
30. Shelhamer JH, Marom Z, Sun F, Bach M, Kaliner M. The effects of arachinoids and leukotrienes on the release of mucus from human airways. *Chest* 1982; 81: 365-375.
31. Hardy CC, Robinson C, Tatterfield AE, Holgate ST. The bronchoconstrictor effect of inhaled prostaglandin $D_2$ in normal and asthmatic men. *N Engl J Med* 1984; 311: 209-213.
32. Smith AP, Cuthbert MF, Dunlop LS. Effect of inhaled prostaglandins $E_1$, $E_2$ and $F_{2\alpha}$ on the airway resistance of healthy and asthmatic man. *Clin Sci Mol Med* 1975; 48: 421-430.
33. Szczeklik A, Gryglewski RJ, Nizankowska E, Nizankowski R, Musial J. Pulmonary and anti-platelet effects of intravenous and inhaled prostacyclin in man. *Prostaglandins* 1978; 16: 651-660.
34. Morley J, Sanjar S, Page CP. The platelet in asthma. *Lancet* 1984; 2: 1142-1144.
35. Schild HO. Histamine release and anaphylactic shock in isolated lungs of guinea pigs. *Quart J Exp Physiol* 1936; 26: 165-179.
36. Goldie RG, Paterson JW, Wale JL. Pharmacological responses of human and porcine lung parenchyma, bronchus and pulmonary artery. *Br J Pharmacol* 1982; 76: 515-522.
37. Green VL. The antiinflammatory effect of catecholamines in the peritoneal cavity and hind paw of the mouse. *Br J Pharmacol* 1972; 45: 322-332.
38. Hughes JM, Seale JP, Temple DM. Effect of fenoterol on immunological release of leukotrienes and histamine from human lung *in vitro:* selective antagonism by β-adrenoceptor antagonists. *Eur J Pharmacol* 1983; 95: 239-245.
39. Butchers PR, Fullarton JR, Skidmore IF, Vardey CJ, Wheeldon A. Characterisation of the receptor mediating the anti-anaphylactic effects of adrenoceptor agonists in human lung *in vitro*. *Br J Pharmacol* 1980; 71: 663.
40. Strandberg K, Mathé AA, Ten S-S. Release of histamine and formation of prostaglandins in human lung tissue and rat mast cells. *Int Arch Allergy Appl Immunol* 1977; 53: 520-529.
41. Seale JP, Ozols S. Activation of arachidonic acid metabolism in guinea-pig lungs by leukotriene $E_4$ and its inhibition by beta adrenoceptor agonists. In: Piper PJ, ed. *Leukotrienes and other lipoxygenase products*. Chichester: John Wiley & Sons, 1983; 188-197.
42. Compton MR, Seale JP, Shaw J. A possible mechanism in the anti-anaphylactic effect of beta adrenoceptor agonists in guinea-pig lungs. *Arch Int Pharmacodyn Ther* 1985; 276; 112-119.
43. Armour CL, Nicholls IJ, Schellenberg RR. The effects of salbutamol, theophylline and FPL 55712 on leukotriene contraction of guinea-pig trachea. *Eur J Pharmacol* 1982; 82: 229-232.
44. Lichtenstein LM, Margolis S. Histamine release in vitro: inhibition by catecholamines and methylxanthines. *Science* 1968; 161: 902-903.
45. Bleeker EF, Mason PL, Nissim JE, Norman PS. The effect of chronic aminophylline therapy on methacholine and antigen airways reactivity in asthma. *Am Rev Respir Dis* 1981; 123: 53.
46. Fredholm BB. Theophylline actions on adenosine receptors. *Eur J Respir Dis* 1980; 61 (suppl 109): 29-36.
47. Hillyard PA, Nials AT, Skidmore IF, Vardey CJ. Characterisation of the adenosine receptor responsible for the inhibition of histamine and SRS-A release from human lung fragments. *Br J Pharmacol* 1984; 83: 337-345.

48. Hutchcroft BJ, Orange RP. The role of calcium in the generation of intracellular SRS-A in passively sensitised human lung challenged with antigen. *Clin Allergy* 1980; 10: 565-573.
49. Lee VY. *Effects of drugs on mediator release from the lung: potential relevance to asthma.* BSc(Med) Thesis, University of Sydney, 1981.
50. Lee VY, Hughes JM, Seale JP, Temple DM. Verapamil inhibits mediator release from human lung *in vitro*. *Thorax* 1983: 386-387.
51. Weichman BM, Tucker SS, Muccitelli RM. Effect of calcium antagonists on the pulmonary actions of the peptidoleukotrienes. *Prostaglandins* 1984; 28: 611-613.
52. Patel KR. The effect of verapamil on histamine and methacholine-induced bronchoconstriction. *Clin Allergy* 1981; 11: 441-447.
53. Barnes PJ, Wilson NM, Brown MJ. A calcium antagonist, nifedipine, modifies exercise-induced asthma. *Thorax* 1981; 36: 726-730.
54. Szczeklik A, Nizankowska E. Asthma improved by aspirin-like drugs. *Br J Dis Chest* 1983; 77: 153-158.
55. Szczeklik A. Analgesics, allergy and asthma. *Br J Clin Pharmacol* 1980; 10: 401S-405S.
56. Coceani F, Olley PM, Lock JE. Prostaglandins, ductus arteriosus, pulmonary circulation: current concepts and clinical potential. *Eur J Clin Pharmacol* 1980; 18: 75-81.
57. Lee VY, Hughes JM, Seale JP, Temple DM. Effect of benoxaprofen on release of slow-reacting substances from human lung tissue *in vitro*. *Clin Sci* 1982; 63: 219-221.
58. Armour CL, Hughes JM, Seale JP, Temple DM. Effect of lipoxygenase inhibitors on release of slow-reacting substances from human lung. *Eur J Pharmacol* 1981; 72: 93-96.
59. Bach MK, Brashler JR, Smith HW, Fitzpatrick FA, Sun FF, McGuire JC. 6,9-deepoxy-6,9 (phenylimino)-6,8-prostaglandin I, (U-60,257), a new inhibitor of leukotriene C and D synthesis: in vitro studies. *Prostaglandins* 1982; 23: 759-771.
60. Blackwell GJ, Flower RJ, Nijkamp FP, Vane JR. Phospholipase $A_2$ activity of guinea-pig isolated perfused lungs: stimulation and inhibition by anti-inflammatory steroids. *Br J Pharmacol* 1978; 62: 79-89.
61. Kench JG, Seale JP, Temple DM, Tennant C. The effects of phospholipase $A_2$ on leukotriene and histamine release from human and guinea-pig lung. *Prostaglandins* 1985; 30: 199-208.
62. Goldstein JA. Hydroxychloroquine for asthma. *Am Rev Respir Dis* 1983; 128: 1100-1101.
63. Chand N. FPL55712 — an antagonist of slow reacting substance of anaphylaxis (SRS-A): a review. *Agents and Actions* 1979; 9: 133-140.
64. Welton AF, Hope WC, Tobias LD, Hamilton JG. Inhibition of antigen-induced histamine release and thromboxane synthetase by FPL 55712, a specific SRS-A antagonist. *Biochem Pharmacol* 1981; 30: 1378-1382.
65. Lee TH, Walport MJ, Wilkinson AH, Turner-Warwick M, Kay, AB. Slow-reacting substance of anaphylaxis antagonist FPL55712 in chronic asthma. *Lancet* 1981; 2: 304.
66. Blackwell GJ, Carnuccio R, Di Rosa M, Flower RJ, Parente L, Persico P. Macrocortin: a polypeptide causing the anti-phospholipase effect of glucocorticoids. *Nature* 1980; 287: 147-149.
67. Rebuck AS, Read J. Assessment and management of severe asthma. *Am J Med* 1971; 1: 788-798.
68. Schleimer RP, Schulman ES, Maglashan DW, et al. Effects of dexamethasone on mediator release from human lung fragments and purified human lung mast cells. *J Clin Invest* 1983; 71: 1830-1835.
69. Schleimer RP, Lichtenstein LM, Gillespie E. Inhibition of basophil histamine release by antiinflammatory steroids. *Nature* 1981; 292: 454-455.
70. Seale JP. Effects of corticosteroids in asthma is not due to suppression of leukotriene release. *N Engl J Med* 1983; 308: 846.
71. Marquardt DL, Wasserman SI. Modulation of rat serosal mast cell biochemistry by in vivo dexamethasone administration. *J Immunol* 1983; 131: 934.
72. Marom Z, Shelhamer JH, Sun F, Kaliner M. The effects of corticosteroids on mucous glycoprotein secretion from human airways *in vitro*. *Am Rev Respir Dis* 1984; 129: 62.
73. Myers A, Ramey E, Ramwell P. Glucocorticoid protection against PAF-acether toxicity in mice. *Br J Pharmacol* 1983; 79: 595.
74. Lefkowitz RJ. Mechanisms for regulation of $\beta$-adrenergic receptor function in desensitisation. In: Turner P, ed. *World congress on clinical pharmacology and therapeutics.* London: Macmillan, 1980: 145-153.

75. Mano K, Akbarzadeh A, Townley RG. Effect of hydrocortisone on beta-adrenergic receptors of lung membranes. *Life Sci* 1979; 25: 1925.
76. Eiser NM, Mills J, Snashall PD, Guz A. The role of histamine receptors in asthma. *Clin Sci* 1981; 60: 363-370.
77. Anderson SD, Bye PTP, Schoeffel RE, Seale JP, Taylor KM, Ferris L. Arterial plasma histamine levels at rest, and during and after exercise in patients with asthma: effects of terbutaline aerosol. *Thorax* 1981; 36: 259.
78. Church MK, Gradidge CF. Inhibition of histamine release from human lung *in vitro* by antihistamines and related drugs. *Br J Pharmacol* 1980; 69: 663-667.
79. Phillips MJ, Ollier S, Gould CAL, Davies RJ. Effect of antihistamines and antiallergic drugs on responses to allergen and histamine provocation tests in asthma. *Thorax* 1984; 39: 345-351.
80. Lichtenstein LM, Gillespie E. The effects of the $H_1$ and $H_2$ antihistamines on 'allergic' histamine release and its inhibition by histamine. *J Pharmacol Exp Ther* 1975; 192: 441-450.
81. Hughes JM, Seale JP, Temple DM. Ranitidine does not potentiate mediator release from human lung *in vitro*. *Br J Clin Pharmacol* 1985; 19: 711-712.
82. Leopold JD, Hartley JPR, Smith AP. Effects of oral $H_1$ and $H_2$ receptor antagonists in asthma. *BrJ Clin Pharmacol* 1979; 8: 249-251.
83. Altounyan REC. Inhibition of experimental asthma by a new compound, disodium cromoglycate, 'Intal'. *Acta Allergologica* 1967; 22: 487.
84. Stokes TC, Morley J. Prospects for an oral Intal. *Br J Dis Chest* 1981; 75: 1-13.
85. Church MK, Gradidge CF. The activity of sodium cromoglycate analogues in human lung *in vitro:* a comparison with rat passive cutaneous anaphylaxis and clinical efficacy. *Br J Pharmacol* 1980; 70: 307-311.
86. Butchers PR, Fullarton JR, Skidmore IF, Thompson LE, Vardey CJ, Wheeldon A. A comparison of the anti-anaphylactic activities of salbutamol and disodium cromoglycate in the rat, the rat mast cell and in human lung tissue. *Br J Pharmacol* 1979; 67: 23-32.
87. Armour CL, Hughes JM, Seale JP, Temple DM. Effects of sodium cromoglycate analogues on the immunological release of slow reacting substance of anaphylaxis and histamine from human and guinea-pig lung *in vitro*. *J Pharm Pharmacol* 1982; 34: 401-402.
88. Chung JTN, Jones RS. Bronchodilator effect of sodium cromoglycate and its clinical implications. *Br Med J* 1979; 2: 1033-1034.
89. Woenne R, Kattan M, Levison H. Sodium cromoglycate-induced changes in the dose-response curve of inhaled methacholine and histamine in asthmatic children. *Am Rev Respir Dis* 1979; 119: 927-932.
90. Kerr JW, Govindaraj M, Patel KR. Effect of alpha-receptor blocking drugs and disodium cromoglycate on histamine hypersensitivity in bronchial asthma. *Br Med J* 1970; 2: 139.
91. Harries MG, Parkes PEG, Lessof MH, Orr TSC. Role of bronchial irritant receptors in asthma. *Lancet* 1981; 1: 5-7.
92. Dixon M, Jackson DM, Richards IM. The action of sodium cromoglycate on 'C' fibre endings in the dog lung. *Br J Pharmacol* 1980; 70: 11-13.

# Chapter 8

# Corticosteroid Therapy

*G.M. Cochrane*

Following the first report in 1949 of the beneficial effects of cortisone in the treatment of rheumatoid arthritis, corticosteroids were used for the treatment of asthma. The value of corticosteroids in asthma was recognised more rapidly than the alarming and extensive array of side effects which develop after prolonged administration. These side effects led to a reduced usage of corticosteroids in the 1960s especially for asthma and sarcoidosis. The more recently developed topical steroids have led to a resurgence in the use of corticosteroids in asthma, but topical steroids are unsuitable for sarcoidosis and fibrosing alveolitis. Even 37 years later there remains considerable controversy and uncertainty as to the correct role of corticosteroids in the management of respiratory diseases.

## History and Development

Initial interest in corticosteroids occurred in the early 1930s after it had been noticed that women with rheumatoid arthritis had a remission during pregnancy. It was believed that this was due to the increase in naturally occurring adrenocortical secretions. Despite considerable research efforts on the isolation and characterisation, the synthesis of corticosteroids took nearly 20 years. In 1948 sufficient quantities of Kendall's compound 'E' (cortisone) was produced and used in a clinical trial. A single patient with rheumatoid arthritis was given a series of injections with dramatic improvement after two days of treatment with 100mg. Hench et al[1] extended this study and also used adrenocorticotrophic hormone (ACTH). As a result of this success, ACTH was tried on five patients with asthma and a dramatic improvement was noticed, within 4 to 48 hours. Over the next few years corticosteroids were used in a variety of diseases including tuberculosis and sarcoidosis. The trials were poorly controlled and patients, once on the drug, did not wish to stop even high doses of cortisone or the repeated injections of ACTH. However, by 1953 the serious side effects of long-term use were becoming apparent and the panacea drug rapidly became considered an evil drug which should not be used.

New analogues were synthesised in an attempt to separate the beneficial from the unwanted side effects. In 1954 prednisone and prednisolone were developed and found to have more potent anti-inflammatory properties. Unfortunately, neither of these drugs separated beneficial effects from side effects so other corticosteroids were looked for with the development of methylprednisolone and triamcinolone acetate in 1957 and dexamethasone and betamethasone in 1959. During these years various trials had been conducted using inhaled versions of these drugs for the management of asthma; although they were effective they had little benefit over systemic therapy as they did not appear to reduce side effects. The potency of these various new compounds was correlated with their ability to produce local vasoconstriction in human skin, and this gave a useful indication of potential topical activity. In the early 1960s betamethasone valerate and beclomethasone dipropionate were produced, and because of a high level of topical activity were particularly useful in the treatment of skin diseases. Because of this topical activity beclomethasone dipropionate was further developed for inhaled use, but unfortunately the initial study showed little effect on airways obstruction, which was perhaps not surprising as most of the patients had irreversible airflow obstruction. However, it was noted that there was little evidence of adrenal suppression. Inhaled corticosteroids with their high topical activity with minimal systemic effects in standard therapeutic doses are now accepted therapies for asthma, but many respiratory diseases still require systemic therapy (Table 8.1). The aims of this chapter are to show that due consideration of the pharmacokinetics and drug interactions may allow safer use of systemic steroids, and to demonstrate why topical inhaled steroids are associated with fewer systemic side effects.

*Table 8.1* Examples of the use and routes of administration of corticosteroids in some respiratory diseases

| Oral | Parenteral | Topical |
|---|---|---|
| Sarcoidosis | Acute asthma | Asthma |
| Cryptogenic fibrosing alveolitis | Adult respiratory distress syndrome | Trial of reversibility of airflow obstruction |
| Extrinsic allergic alveolitis | Bronchospasm induced by inhalational pneumonia | Allergic rhinitis |
| Severe intractable asthma | | |
| Trial of reversibility of airflow obstruction | Severe hayfever | |

## Basic Structure and Chemistry of Corticosteroids

Corticosteroids utilised in the treatment of respiratory disease should ideally have a high degree of anti-inflammatory activity and a low degree of mineralocorticoid activity. The majority of corticosteroids now used are synthetic analogues of the naturally occurring adrenal corticoid hormone, cortisol, but developed to increase acute inflammatory activity and to reduce mineralocorticoid action. The various alterations in the molecular structure of hydrocortisone developed have, however, affected the relative potencies of the steroids with some alteration in both their pharmacological and pharmacokinetic properties. However, despite these molecular changes all corticosteroids are capable of binding to glucocorticoid receptors and thus of mimicking the effects of hydrocortisone. Thus the synthetic analogue corticoids can have profound effects on carbohydrate and protein metabolism, and on cellular kinetics with alterations in cellular function and immune reactions and inflammatory response, as well as on the hypothalamic-pituitary-adrenal (HPA) axis.

Chemically, corticosteroids consist of a basic cyclopentenophenanthrane ring with varying side groups which form a 21-carbon molecule. Naturally occurring corticosteroids or glucocorticoids have a double bond between C-4 and C-5, ketone groups at C-3 and C-20, and hydroxyl groups at C-11 and C-21 (Figure 8.1). Structural changes in corticosteroid analogues can alter absorption, distribution, metabolism and receptor affinity of the compounds. Highly topically active drugs have also been developed for skin diseases. The important variations in basic structure are highlighted in Table 8.2. Although the improved anti-inflammatory properties have been useful, the increase in duration of biological activity has not always been appreciated.

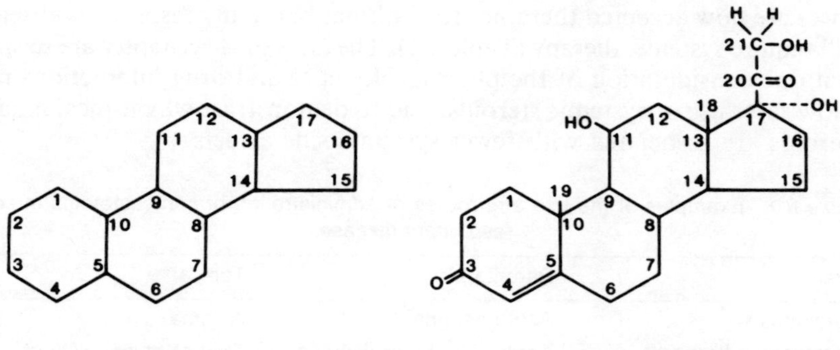


*Figure 8.1* Steroid nucleus showing positions of the carbon atoms and the configuration of hydrocarbons.

*Table 8.2* Effect of varying the chemical structure of corticosteroid analogues

| Corticosteroid | Structural variation | Therapeutic significance |
|---|---|---|
| Cortisone<br>Prednisone | Ketone group C-11 | Biologically inactive until ketone group hydroxylated (by the liver) |
| Prednisone<br>Prednisolone | Double bond between C-1 and C-2 | Increases anti-inflammatory properties with some reduction in sodium retention |
| Dexamethasone<br>Betamethasone | Both drugs contain fluoride atom at C-9; additional methyl group at C-16 | Increases anti-inflammatory properties; eliminates virtually all salt-retaining properties. |
| Beclomethasone dipropionate | Esterification with two propionate groups at C-17 and C-21 | Enhances topical action |
| Triamcinolone acetonide | Acetonation | Prolongs duration of action and increases anti-inflammatory properties |

## Anti-inflammatory and Anti-allergic Effects of Corticosteroids

The mechanism of action of corticosteroids in respiratory diseases is believed to be their ability to suppress inflammatory processes. They suppress virtually every step of the inflammatory reaction by numerous biochemical and cellular effects. Almost all cell types in the body respond in one way or another to corticosteroids.

### Biochemical Effects

Corticosteroids enter the cell by passive diffusion and combine with class-specific soluble cytoplasmic protein receptors to form a receptor-steroid complex.[2] This complex migrates to the cell nucleus and binds to nuclear chromatin. This derepresses a section of the genome producing messenger RNA with consequent protein synthesis; it is these proteins which are responsible for the expression of glucocorticoid activity. One of the new proteins synthesised is lipomodulin, a protein with a molecular weight of 40 000. A smaller protein macrocortin (molecular weight 15 000) has also been characterised, but this is thought to be a phosphorylated part of lipomodulin. Lipomodulin is a selective inhibitor of phospholipase A2, the rate-limiting enzyme, and therefore important in the production of mediators from membrane-derived arachidonic acid.[3] Corticosteroids also stimulate the extracellular release of preformed lipomodulin and induce resynthesis of the protein within the cells. Lipomodulin is also found in a prestored form in neutrophils and macrophages. (Figure 8.2).

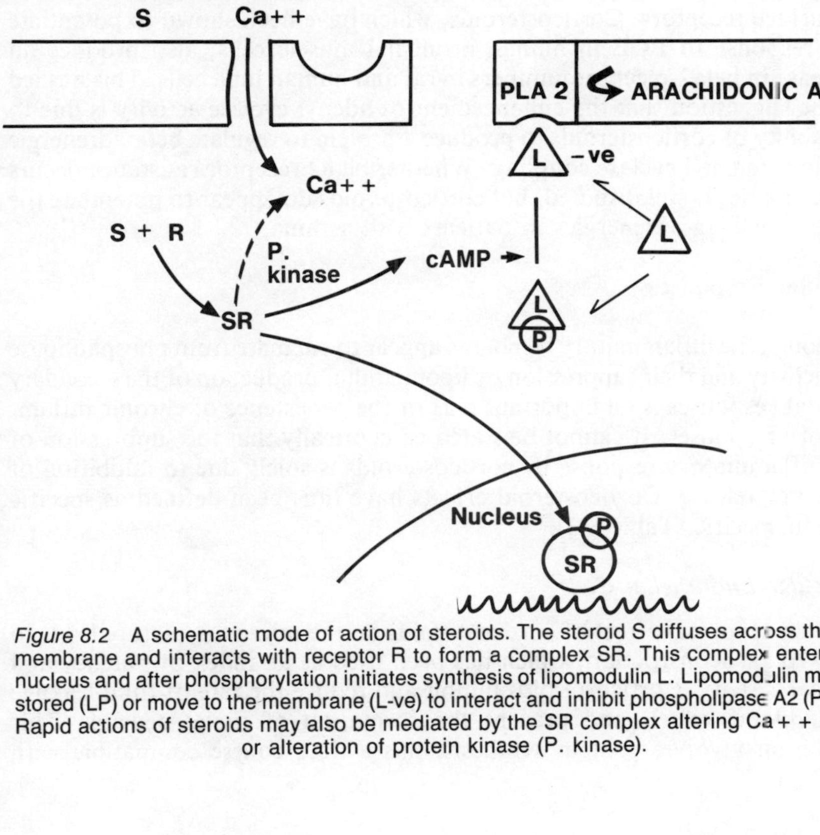


*Figure 8.2* A schematic mode of action of steroids. The steroid S diffuses across the cell membrane and interacts with receptor R to form a complex SR. This complex enters the nucleus and after phosphorylation initiates synthesis of lipomodulin L. Lipomodulin may be stored (LP) or move to the membrane (L-ve) to interact and inhibit phospholipase A2 (PLA2). Rapid actions of steroids may also be mediated by the SR complex altering Ca++ influx or alteration of protein kinase (P. kinase).

Inhibition of phospholipase A2 activity inhibits both the membrane-delivered and granule-associated mediator secretion from inflammatory cells, and corticosteroids are the only anti-inflammatory drugs which inhibit both sources of mediators derived from arachidonic acid (see Chapter 7). With reduction in phospholipase activity cell activation signals, such as neutrophil chemotactic factor, are reduced. Lysolecithin production will be reduced and thus its potent fusagen activity will be curtailed with a reduction in the release of lysosomal and stored mediators from inflammatory cells. Reduced phospholipase A2 activity by lipomodulin appears to be the general mechanism of action of corticosteroids in suppressing inflammatory responses in lung disease. This action, although complicated on an intracellular basis, appears also to be the extracellular action. An endogenous protein inhibitor, with similar actions to lipomodulin, has been observed in human serum by Saed et al,[4] and this protein exhibits increased activity in samples taken after administration of corticosteroids.

Interestingly, suppression of naturally occurring lipomodulin activity could perhaps be a factor in disease itself. This concept has been supported by the finding of an antoantibody to lipomodulin in patients with rheumatic diseases such as systemic lupus erythematosus.[5]

## Effect of Corticosteroids on the Adenyl Cyclase System

Prostaglandin $E_1$ and (more importantly in the context of asthma) beta-adrenergic drugs, act by increasing the membrane-bound adenyl cyclase linked to surface receptors. Corticosteroids, which have been shown to potentiate this response to PGE in human bronchial muscle cells, also produce an increase in beta2-receptor numbers in rat and human lung cells. This has led to the suggestion that the enhancement of adenyl cyclase activity is due to the ability of corticosteroids to produce a protein to regulate beta-adrenergic receptor/adenyl cyclase coupling. Whether beta2 receptor resistance occurs in asthmatics is still disputed, but corticosteroids do appear to potentiate the actions of beta-adrenergics in patients with asthma.

## Cellular Responses

Although the inflammatory responses appear to emanate from phospholipase A2 activity and their suppression by lipomodulin, production of the secondary cellular responses is an important part of the persistence of chronic inflammatory responses. It cannot be stated categorically that the suppression of the inflammatory response by corticosteroids is solely due to inhibition of mediator release. Corticosteroid effects have thus been defined as specific or non-specific (Table 8.3).

### *Vascular Endothelial Cells*

The direct topical effect of corticosteroids on the microvasculature leads to marked vasoconstriction, which has been used as an index of potency and topical activity. Corticosteroids inhibit and reduce the rate of fluid leakage from blood vessels and prevent the formation of tissue oedema. This inhibition involves protein synthesis, has a time course compatible with specific receptor-mediated corticosteroid action, and appears to be separate from inhibitory effects of steroids on cell function. The exact mechanism for the vascular changes, however, remains unclear.

*Table 8.3* Characterisation of specific and non-specific corticosteroid effects

| Specific | Non-specific |
|---|---|
| Occur at low concentrations | Occur at high concentrations |
| Related to potency of drug | No rank order of potency |
| Dose-response effects | No dose-response relationships |
| Inhibited by:<br>RNA synthesis inhibitors<br>Protein synthesis inhibitors | Not inhibited by:<br>RNA synthesis inhibitors<br>Protein synthesis inhibitors |
| Onset delay and action prolonged after drug stopped | Respond only to presence of steroid |
| Living cell required | Membranes only required |

### *Neutrophils*

Corticosteroid administration in man leads to a circulating neutrophilia but paradoxically it inhibits the migration of neutrophils into an inflamed site. It is suggested that steroids inhibit the adherence of neutrophils to the vascular endothelial surfaces with additional accelerated release from the bone marrow and a reduction in neutrophil tissue stores. However, whether corticosteroids reduce inflammatory activity of neutrophils still attached to tissues is unknown, but there is certainly a reduction in local neutrophil numbers at sites of inflammation.

### *Lymphocytes*

Lymphocytopenia mainly due to redistribution of T cells and modulation of lymphoid tissue follows corticosteroid administration. However, suppression of antibody synthesis in man only occurs following high doses of corticosteroids and then only in specific diseases where in-vitro studies have shown an increase in antibody production. The precise effect of corticosteroids on lymphocyte function is further confused by differing responses between antigen and mitogen stimulation and species variation especially between rodents (frequently used in experimental situations) and man.

### *Macrophages, Mast Cells and Eosinophils*

Reduced migration to inflammatory sites and a profound monocytopenia occur following corticosteroid administration. Corticosteroid receptors have been found in subcultured murine cells and the inhibition of secretion of elastase, collagenase and plasminogen activator appears to be a specific glucocorticoid effect. Rodent macrophage prostaglandin production can also be reduced by relatively low concentrations of corticosteroids. The macrophage appears to be an important cell in the chronic inflammatory reaction, and corticosteroids inhibit migration, activity and mediator production of the macrophage.

Eosinopenia is a marked feature of corticosteroid administration and is due to cellular redistribution rather than cytolysis, although inhibition of chemotactic responses only occurs at high doses. Corticosteroids have no apparent specific effect on mast cells in pharmacological concentrations, although inhibition of histamine release and stabilisation of mast cell membranes occur as non-specific effects.

## Pharmacology of Corticosteroids

The pharmacology of corticosteroids is complex, not just because of the large numbers of synthetic analogues with different anti-inflammatory potencies, but because of the variations in pharmacokinetics between each drug and the route of administration. The route will determine different absorption characteristics between drugs, although once absorbed, the distribution within the tissues is similar, but can be qualitatively different between the naturally occurring corticosteroids and the synthetic analogues. Many factors will affect elimination and alter both the plasma and the biological half-life. Variation in the biological half-life between preparations has only just been recognised as a possible cause for increased incidence of side effects with administration of betamethasone and dexamethasone.

### Absorption (Other Than Topical Steroids)

Corticosteroids may be given orally, intravenously or intramuscularly in order to achieve a systemic effect. Topical administration, often as a skin cream or as an inhaled aerosol, is usually a route chosen to deliberately reduce systemic absorption and its associated side effects. Topical inhaled steroids will be covered later.

In order to improve water solubility most corticosteroid preparations are conjugated to various esters, with some also having a phosphate group as this will further improve absorption from any site. Therefore, with the exception of deoxycortisone, almost all corticosteroid analogues are rapidly absorbed from the gastrointestinal tract or muscle. In fact, although peak plasma levels are slightly slower with oral administration of corticosteroids,[6] because of the delay in producing specific biological corticosteroid actions the difference in time of clinical response between oral and intramuscular administration is barely detectable. Intravenous administration, however, will produce slightly earlier clinical responses than oral or intramuscular administration, although the intravenous route is usually used in acute severe asthma to be sure that the steroid is absorbed, as there is theoretically reduced gastrointestinal absorption in the presence of hypoxia, and reduced intramuscular absorption in severely ill asthmatics. Cortisone acetate and prednisone, although well absorbed, are inactive until converted by hepatic hydroxylation.

Gastrointestinal absorption of corticosteroids (in particular the most frequently studied prednisolone) appears not to be affected by antacids or H2-blockers. However, enteric-coated preparations will have delayed peak plasma levels compared to plain tablets, although the total amount of drug available is not reduced. Erratic absorption of enteric-coated preparations has not been reported as a consistent finding in patients with respiratory disease, although this has been noted in patients with ileostomies.[7] Intramuscular injections tend to have erratic absorption and therefore have not been regularly used, although recently triamcinolone acetonide has been suggested in the treatment of chronic severe asthma. The pharmacology of this intramuscular preparation is poorly determined and, although its absorption characteristics, peak plasma levels and duration of biological action are unclear, they are prolonged.[8]

## Distribution of Systemically Absorbed Corticosteroids

Following absorption, lipid solubility, tissue binding and plasma protein binding will determine the distribution and availability of free corticosteroids and thereby influence the amount of hormone which is free to enter the cell. Naturally occurring circulating cortisol is approximately 75% bound to a cortisol-binding globulin (transcortin, an alpha2 globulin) while a further 15% is bound to albumin. The bound steroid is relatively resistant to degradation and excretion. Transcortin has a high affinity but a low binding capacity, while albumin has a high binding capacity but a low affinity. Patients with a low serum albumin or liver disease will therefore have higher levels of free steroid. The protein-bound hormone is inactive and serves as a store in equilibrium with the free hormone. Approximately 5 to 10% of the circulating cortisol is therefore in a free metabolically active form. There is a diurnal variation in transcortin-binding capacity with least binding during the morning resulting in higher daytime free cortisol. With increasing corticosteroid concentrations therapeutically effective steroid plasma protein binding may be exceeded. A small increase in steroid administration can lead to a much greater increase in metabolically active steroid. This may explain why comparatively small doses of corticosteroids, especially if they have a lower transcortin-binding affinity and a comparatively high potency, may lead to such devastating side effects. Prednisolone has a relatively high affinity for transcortin, but dexamethasone has a very low affinity for transcortin with less than 1% bound to transcortin, allowing a much greater quantity of metabolically active drug to be circulating.

## Elimination and Degradation of Systemic Steroids

Naturally occurring steroids are rapidly inactivated in the liver by hydroxylation and conjugation to a glucuronide which is then mainly excreted in the urine. The synthetic analogues have structural changes which interfere with hydroxylation and glucuronide conjugation and therefore degradation is by alternative pathways, with both metabolically active and inactive metabolites circulating in the blood and free unchanged steroids excreted in the urine. Less than 3% of a dose of hydrocortisone is excreted unchanged in the urine, but as much as 20 to 40% of a dose of prednisolone is excreted as a free steroid in the urine. Systemic corticosteroids, unlike topical steroids, have a low biliary excretion (less than 10%).

Clearance of corticosteroids is affected by a number of factors. Thyrotoxicosis increases hepatic clearance whereas myxoedema reduces clearance as does severe liver disease. Chronic renal disease may reduce clearance of synthetic analogues. Drugs causing hepatic enzyme induction such as phenobarbitone, phenytoin, ephedrine and rifampicin will lead to considerable reductions in the pharmacological (plasma) half-life of administered corticosteroids.[9] It has been estimated that in patients receiving rifampicin a doubling of the dose of prednisolone is required to obtain the same glucocorticoid action.[10] Antibiotics such as erythromycin cause an increase in circulating methylprednisolone levels. The subtle structural changes in the chemistry of the steroid analogues significantly alter not only the affinity for the intracellular receptors, but also the metabolism and clearance of the drug, and thus, other drug interactions may occur (Table 8.4).

*Table 8.4* Factors affecting corticosteroid metabolism either by increasing metabolism or changing rate of excretion

| Reduced corticosteroid levels | Increased corticosteroid levels |
|---|---|
| Thyrotoxicosis | Myxoedema |
| Ephedrine | Cirrhosis |
| Phenytoin | Renal failure |
| Phenobarbitone | Erythromycin (methylprednisolone) |
| Oestrogens | |

## Plasma Half-lives, Biological Half-lives and Relative Potencies

The plasma half-life of the naturally occurring hydrocortisone is short, as is its biological half-life when assessed in terms of hypothalamic-pituitary-adrenal axis suppression. However, many of the synthetic corticosteroid analogues have a comparatively short plasma half-life but, as mentioned previously, their degree of protein binding may significantly increase their biological effects (Table 8.5). The discrepancy is most strikingly shown by the recommended six to eight hourly administration of dexamethasone, a drug with an intermediate plasma half-life but a biological half-life measured in terms of two to three days. Any comparison between corticosteroid

*Table 8.5* Comparison of commonly used corticosteroids

| Compound | Relative anti-inflammatory effect | Equi-effective doses (mg) | Relative sodium-retaining properties | Plasma half-life (h) | Biological half-life (h) |
|---|---|---|---|---|---|
| Hydrocortisone | 1 | 20 | 1 | 1.5-2 | 8-12 |
| Prednisolone | 4 | 5 | 0.25 | 3 | 18-36 |
| Methyl-prednisolone | 5 | 4 | 0.1 | 4 | 18-36 |
| Triamcinolone | 5 | 4 | ± | 1-2 | 18-36 |
| Triamcinolone acetonide | 50-75 | 0.3 | ± | Unknown | Unknown but up to 28 days after single injection |
| Betamethasone | 25-30 | 0.6 | 0 | 6 | 36-54 |
| Dexamethasone | 25 | 0.8 | 0 | 2-5 | 36-54 |

analogues must also take into account their glucocorticoid potency usually assessed in terms of anti-inflammatory response. In the UK triamcinolone acetonide injection has been recommended for persistent severe asthma.[11] Here the 10 to 15 times increase in anti-inflammatory property of the acetonide preparation compared to triamcinolone base was ignored. The protracted drug level was considered an advantage with no account taken of the useful diurnal variation of transcortin binding, which can be protective if a single morning dose of an intermediate biological half-life corticosteroid such as prednisolone is used. Previous workers who suggested the use of triamcinolone acetonide for asthma[12] have since noted considerably greater side effects,[13] and have concluded that the drug is unsuitable for long-term use because of its pharmacodynamics.

## Inhaled Topically Active Corticosteroids

The logical route in the treatment of airways disease meant that inhaled corticosteroids were tried in the early 1950s. However, initially only systemically active drugs were tried and they had little beneficial effect. Topical corticosteroids with high topical activity relative to systemic effect or absorption were developed for the treatment of skin diseases. It was only when such drugs as beclomethasone dipropionate and betamethasone valerate were developed for inhalation that the advantages of the inhaled over the systemic route were realised. Since then other similarly topically active drugs have been developed, in particular budesonide. The topical potency of these drugs is demonstrated by their ability to cause vasoconstriction on human skin; the topically active drugs being 500 to 1000 times more potent than even potent systemic corticosteroids such as dexamethasone[14,15] (Figure 8.3).

### Do Topically Active Corticosteroids Have a Similar Mechanism of Action to 'Systemic' Steroids?

The clinically beneficial effects of topical steroids have a similar time course of action to systemic steroids and behave in asthma similarly, being unable to prevent immediate bronchoconstrictor responses to acute challenge, but preventing the late responses.[16] Corticosteroid receptor sites are present in human fibroblasts and epidermal cells, and have a high affinity for topical steroids. Whether their high topical solubility or large ester groupings alter intracellular transport or binding is unknown, but no obvious differences in dose requirements or responses have been documented when corticosteroid potency has been taken into account. It would appear that, in patients with asthma, topical corticosteroids work in a similar fashion at the cellular level to systemic steroids, although they appear to have fewer non-specific corticosteroid effects such as neutrophilia and eosinopenia.[17] The pharmacokinetics at lung level are poorly understood although rapid absorption from the lung has been documented for both beclomethasone dipropionate and budesonide.[18,19] Lung metabolism is different for these two compounds, beclomethasone being de-esterified locally with a potential decrease in systemic effects, while budesonide is not hydrolysed within lung tissue, but 100% metabolism by the liver prevents systemic effects. However,

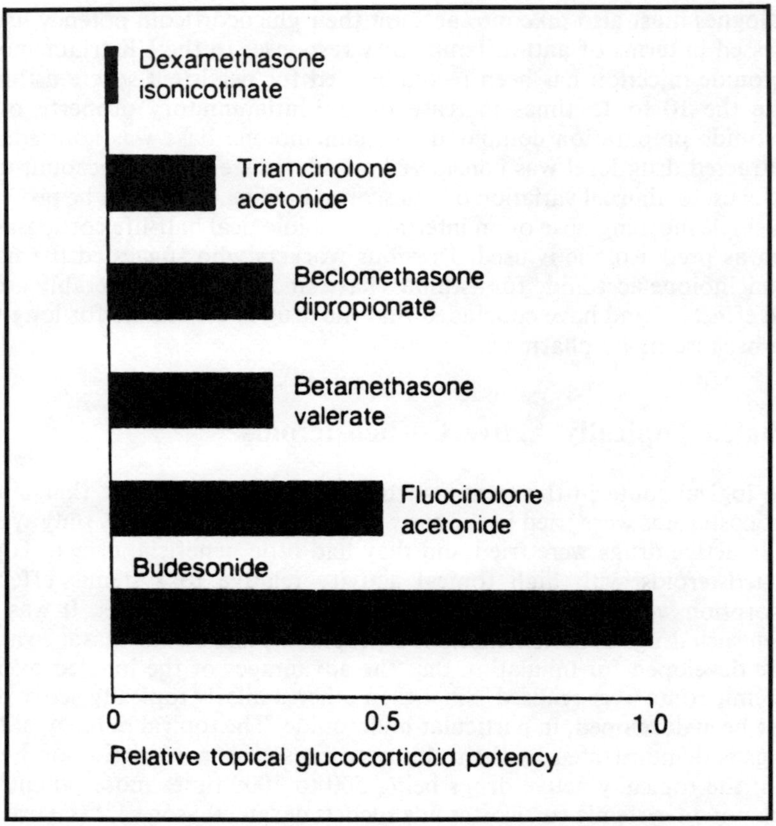


*Figure 8.3* Relative topical glucocorticoid potency as assessed by human skin vasoconstriction effect.[30]

there appears to be no significant difference in local kinetic behaviour in the lung between 'topical' steroids and 'systemic' steroids to account for the marked reduction in unwanted side effects (especially on the pituitary adrenal axis in man) between topical and systemic steroid therapy in the treatment of asthma.

## Mechanisms to Account for the Limited Side Effects of Topical Steroids

The majority of any inhaled drug, whether delivered by metered dose aerosol, dry powder delivery or as a nebulised spray, is swallowed and at best approximately 10% of the dose will reach the lung. The other 90% of the dose of inhaled aerosol will be absorbed via the gastrointestinal tract in a similar fashion to an orally administered steroid. The difference in side effects of systemic corticosteroids and inhaled topical steroids is due to different handling after gastrointestinal absorption of the oral systemic steroid compared with the swallowed portion of the topical steroid. Absorption of systemic steroids is almost complete as (contrary to common belief) is absorption of the topical steroids. All drugs, once absorbed, are transported to the liver and undergo metabolism. Bioavailability can be determined by comparing oral and intravenous dosing with the corticosteroid; prednisolone and dexamethasone have an 80% bioavailability of the oral preparation, but the topical preparations show less than 20% such bioavailability. Oral topical steroids have a very high order of first-pass time metabolism and interestingly enough have high levels of biliary excretion.[20]

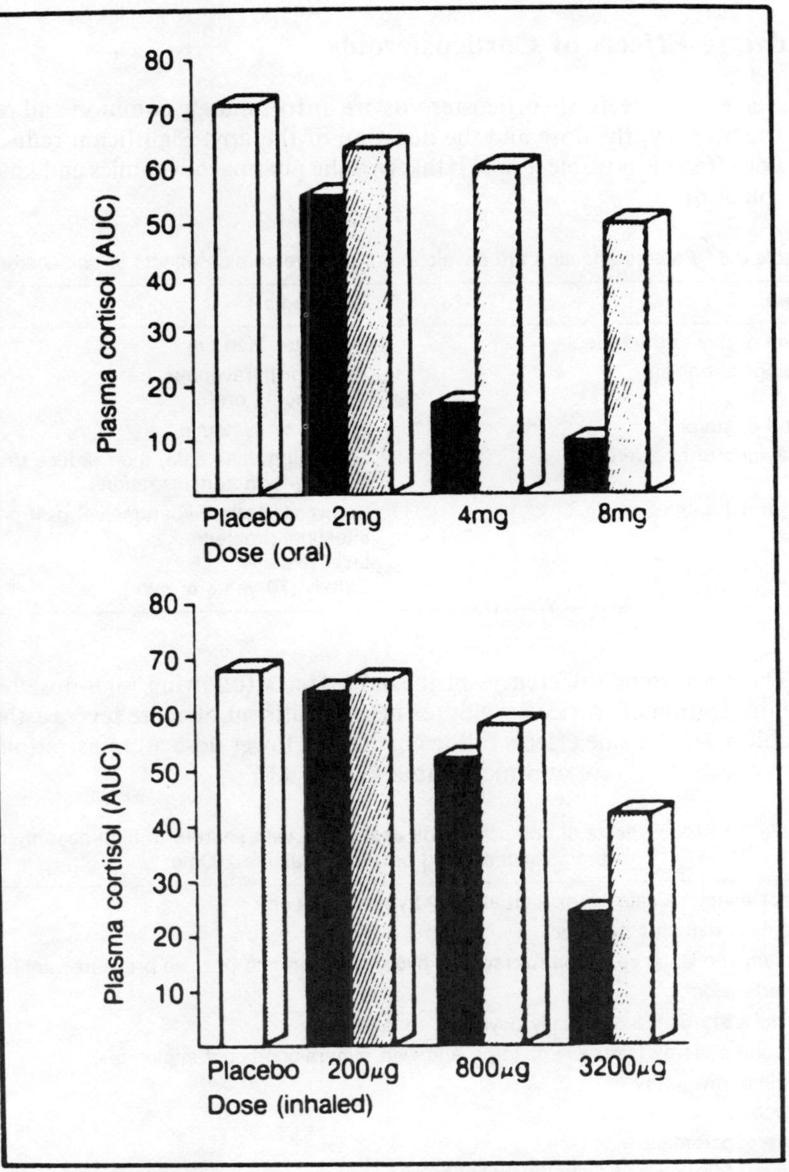


*Figure 8.4* An index of plasma cortisol suppression after oral administration and inhalation of budesonide (hatched columns) and beclomethasone dipropionate (closed columns).[30]

Figure 8.4 shows the doses of beclomethasone dipropionate and budesonide which cause significant adrenal suppression from the effects of lung absorption, or the small percentage of drug avoiding first-pass metabolism when given orally. The usually recommended inhaled maximal doses, however, are less than 2mg/day, a level where adrenal suppression is chemically detectable, but may not appear to be of clinical significance.

## Adverse Effects of Corticosteroids

Adverse side effects of corticosteroids are unfortunately common and relate to the potency, the dose and the duration of therapy. Significant reduction in side effects is possible if note is taken of the pharmacodynamics and kinetics (Table 8.6)

*Table 8.6* Factors affecting the development of adverse side effects to corticosteroids

| Dose | Comments |
|---|---|
| Time of day and frequency | am better than pm |
| Biological half-life | Short for intravenous<br>18-36 hours oral |
| Type of steroid | Topical or systemic |
| How long drug given | Short high dose safe, then reduce drug for long-term administration |
| Other risk factors | Known diabetic, hypertensive, gastro-intestinal problems<br>Liver disease<br>Elderly (70 years or over) |

There are some differences in the side effects following high-dose acute administration of corticosteroids (as in the treatment of acute severe asthma) (Table 8.7), and side effects following chronic lower dose administration for sarcoidosis or severe chronic asthma (Table 8.8).

*Table 8.7* Side effects of corticosteroids associated with short-term high-dose therapy (prednisolone 40mg or hydrocortisone 200mg)

| |
|---|
| Hypokalaemic alkalosis (exacerbated by hyperventilation) |
| Chemical diabetes mellitus |
| Sodium and water retention (worse with hydrocortisone and positive pressure ventilation) |
| Hypertension |
| Mental disturbance especially psychotic reactions |
| Cerebral oedema (worse in children and with mineralocorticoid analogues) |
| Proximal myopathy |
| Glaucoma |
| Acute pancreatitis |
| Peptic ulceration and gastrointestinal haemorrhage |
| Catabolic state |

*Table 8.8* Side effects of corticosteroids more likely to be associated with long-term administration (10-20mg prednisolone or equivalent)

| |
|---|
| Suppression of hypothalamic-pituitary-adrenal axis |
| Growth failure in children and adolescents |
| Osteoporosis with vertebral compression and multiple bone fractures |
| Aseptic necrosis of bone |
| Cerebral atrophy |
| Latent epilepsy activated |
| Variations in mood: depression, anxiety and increased lability of mood |
| Posterior subcapsular cataracts |
| Hyperlipidaemia with increased incidence of gallstones |
| Obesity: centripetal (lemon-on-a-toothpick appearance) |
| Secondary amenorrhoea |
| Reduced immune response with increased vulnerability to bacterial and opportunistic organisms |
| Impaired wound healing with subcutaneous tissue atrophy |

*Acute side effects may also occur (see Table 8.4).

## Side Effects Associated with Acute High-dose Corticosteroids

Side effects to acute administration of corticosteroids are usually uncommon and reversible. The acute fall in serum potassium level is associated with metabolic alkalosis; it is induced by mineralocorticoid activity of the corticosteroid and is frequently exacerbated in acute respiratory illness by the associated alveolar hyperventilation and respiratory alkalosis. Diabetes mellitus is due to enhanced gluconeogenesis and simultaneous antagonism of the action of insulin. Sodium and water retention with associated hypertension are dependent on the precise molecular structure of the corticosteroid used, hydrocortisone being much more likely to cause fluid retention than dexamethasone. However, the greater mineralocorticoid activity tends to inhibit the fluid shift from extracellular to intracellular compartments. Vasopressin production is decreased with enhanced destruction and a reduction in its action on the kidney.

Cerebral oedema in children and sudden mental disturbances, usually an acute psychosis in adults, are uncommon side effects. The mechanism is poorly understood, but increased neuronal excitability with a reduction in the reuptake of cerebral catecholamines has been implicated. Proximal myopathy is associated with acute high-dose and long-term low-dose corticosteroid therapy and appears to be far more common with fluorinated steroids such as triamcinolone acetonide.[21] This may be due to the greater potency, longer tissue half-lives and glycolytic and oxidative changes in metabolism, which produce an overall catabolic effect causing muscle wasting and atrophy.[22] Glaucoma and pancreatitis are accepted complications of acute therapy, but the mechanisms are obscure. Dyspepsia, peptic ulceration and gastrointestinal haemorrhage are associated with any episode of severe stress and are even more frequent during acute respiratory illnesses. Corticosteroids are associated with increased production of gastric acid by increasing gastric secretion, but there is still debate as to the clinical significance of steroid-induced gastrointestinal problems. The clinical signs of gastrointestinal problems will be masked by steroids and prophylactic use of the H2-blocker, cimetidine, although effective, may prolong the half-life of other drugs such as theophylline which are frequently used in respiratory diseases. Ranitidine, a newer H2-blocker does not have this problem.[23] Ways that side effects may be reduced in the acute situation have been suggested in a review by Cochrane.[24]

## Side Effects Associated with Chronic Low-dose Corticosteroids

The most significant side effect of chronic endogenous corticosteroid administration is the suppression of the hypothalamic-pituitary-adrenal axis. Endogenous synthesis of cortisol is by the adrenal cortex which is stimulated by ACTH. Pituitary corticotrophin is stimulated by corticotrophin releasing factor (CRF), a peptide produced by the hypothalamus which travels via the portal circulation from the hypothalamus to the anterior pituitary. There is a feed-back control system where cortisol levels will reduce CRF and ACTH secretion and vice versa. The circadian variations in cortisol are hypothalamic-related. Exogenous corticosteroids, by increasing plasma corticosteroid levels, suppress CRF release by the hypothalamus, which in turn depresses ACTH secretion. Because of reduced levels of ACTH over long periods, atrophy of the adrenal cortex occurs as well as some atrophy of the hypothalamic-pituitary axis. Usually the adrenal cortex is slowest to recover, but occasionally permanent hypothalamic-pituitary atrophy does occur. Short courses of prednisolone (40mg/day for three weeks) are associated with only a few days' suppression,[25] but lower doses (15mg/day) for three months may lead to suppression for up to nine months or more.[26]

Chronic steroid administration is also associated with retarded growth in children. Although adrenal suppression is important if the corticosteroids are to be stopped, in some respiratory diseases chronic administration for life is necessary. In such patients the direct side effects may be severe and demand a balance between the disease process and the possible side effects.

Decreased production of cartilage and bone with severe osteoporosis associated with anti-vitamin D activity leads to renal loss of calcium and increased renal stone formation. Osteoporosis in the elderly can be devastating with vertebral compression or multiple fractures especially of the ribs on coughing. In younger people aseptic necrosis of bone occurs, although the damaging effects of altered fat distribution with reduced protein synthesis leading to centripetal obesity, skin striae and limb muscle wasting are frequently more troublesome to the patient. Vulnerability to opportunistic infection or recurrence of pulmonary tuberculosis is rarely a problem with patients with asthma, but may occur in other conditions where the immune system is already altered, as in rheumatoid arthritis. Poor wound healing, increased incidence of gallstones due to changes in fat metabolism, and chronic dyspepsia are all associated with exogenous systemic steroid administration.

## Adverse Effects of Topical Corticosteroids

Side effects associated with the topical corticosteroid used in the treatment of respiratory diseases are limited, especially in the doses usually prescribed.

Higher inhaled doses are associated with systemic effects (especially on the adrenal cortex, Figure 8.4) from the systemically absorbed drug from the lung and the small proportion not removed by the liver with first pass metabolism.

Oral candidiasis is uncommon with very low doses of inhaled topical steroids and leads to clinical problems in only about 5% of patients[27] and responds readily to local treatment. Hoarse voice has been noted and is considered to be due largely to muscle myopathy,[28] and although usually trivial may be helped by a reduction in dose. Systemic side effects from inhaled corticosteroids may be expected if a dose of over 2mg/day of beclomethasone dipropionate is used, and possibly even higher doses of budesonide are needed before clinically significant systemic side effects will occur.

## Corticosteroid Therapy, Which, What Dose and When?

There now appears no place for the use of ACTH or synthetic analogues which will suppress pituitary function, have increased actions on the adrenal cortex and have been associated with anaphylactic reactions.

### Acute Treatment

Hydrocortisone, with its shorter half-life, rapid onset of action and ease with which a dose equivalent to maximal adrenal stimulation can be achieved and maintained, appears most suitable for the emergency treatment of respiratory disease especially asthma. The lack of evidence to support the use of very high dose therapeutic regimes even in the adult respiratory distress syndrome[29] means that the more potent but slower in onset prednisolone is not required. Either continuous infusion or six hourly administration is usually recommended.

### Chronic Systemic Treatment

Prednisolone (not prednisone) should be used for chronic systemic therapy with corticosteroids and should be given in the early morning as a single dose. Short courses (less than two weeks) may be stopped abruptly (as regards the HPA axis), but longer courses must be reduced more slowly. Enteric coating will delay the peak absorption and may lead to an increase in systemic side effects. Highly potent corticosteroids with long biological half-lives should not be used. Triamcinolone acetonide should not be used for chronic administration although as a single injection each year it may possibly have a place in the treatment of seasonal allergic rhinitis.

### Chronic Topical Treatment

The introduction of beclomethasone dipropionate and the more recent addition of budesonide have led to a profound change in the morbidity of patients with asthma not always from the disease, but frequently from the side effects of systemic corticosteroid treatment. The substitution of topical steroids should be considered with chronic systemic steroids in all patients with asthma.

## References


1. Hench PS, Kendall EC, Slocumb CH, Polley HF. The effect of a hormone of the adrenal cortex (17-hydroxy-11-dehydrocortico-sterone, compound E) and of pituitary adrenocorticotropic hormone on rheumatoid arthritis. *Mayo Clin Proc* 1949; 24: 181.
2. Baxter JD, Rousseau GG, eds. *Glucocorticoid hormone action*. Berlin, Heidelberg, New York: Springer-Verlag, 1979 (Monographs in endocrinology).
3. Blackwell GJ, Carnuccio R, Rossa MD, Flower RJ, Parente L, Persico P. Macrocortin: a polypeptide causing the antiphospholipase effect of glucocorticosteroids. *Nature* 1980; 287: 147.
4. Saed SA, McDonald, Gibson WJ, et al. Endogenous inhibitor of prostaglandin synthesis. *Nature*1977; 270: 32.
5. Hirata F, Carmine RD, Nelson CA, Axelrod J. Presence of autoantibody for phospholipase inhibitory protein lipomodulin in patients with rheumatic disease. *Proc Natl Acad Sci USA* 1981; 78: 3.
6. Gambertoglio JG, Amend WJC, Benet LZ. Pharmacokinetics and bioavailability of prednisolone and prednisone in health volunteers and patients. A review. *J Pharmacokinet Biopharmacol* 1980; 3: 1-52.
7. Al-Habet SM, Kinsella HC, Rogers HJ, Trounce JR. Malabsorption of prednisolone from enteric coated tablets after ileostomy. *Br Med J* 1980; 281: 843.
8. Kusama M, Sakanchi W, Kamaska SR. Studies of plasma levels and urinary excretion after intramuscular injection of triamcinolone acetonide. *Metabolism* 1971; 20: 590-596.
9. Liddle GW. The adrenals. In: Williams RH, ed. *Textbook of endocrinology*. 6th ed. Philadelphia: WB Saunders, 1981.
10. McAllister WAC, Thompson PJ, Al-Habet SM, Roger HJ. Rifampicin reduces effectiveness and bioavailability of prednisolone. *Br Med J* 1983; 286: 923.
11. McLeod DT, Capewell SJ, Law J, Maclaren W, Seaton A. Intramuscular triamcinolone acetonide in chronic severe asthma. *Thorax* 1985; 40: 340.
12. Willey RF, Ferguson RJ, Godden DJ, Crompton GK, Grant IWB. Comparison of oral prednisolone and intramuscular depot triamcinolone in patients with severe chronic asthma. *Thorax* 1984; 39: 390.
13. Willey RF, Fergusson RJ, Godden DJ, Crompton GK, Grant IWB. Comparison of oral prednisolone and intramuscular depot triamcinolone in patients with chronic severe asthma. *Thorax* 1985; 40: 208.
14. Harris DM. Some properties of beclomethasone dipropionate and related steroids in man. *Postgrad Med J* 1975; 51 (suppl 4): 20.
15. Clissold SP, Heel RC. Budesonide. A preliminary review of its pharmacodynamic properties and therapeutic efficacy in asthma and rhinitis. *Drugs* 1984; 28: 485.
16. Pepys J, Davies RJ, Breslin AB, Hendrick DJ, Hutchcroft BJ. The effect of inhaled beclomethasone dipropionate (Becotide) and sodium cromoglycate on asthmatic reaction to provocation tests. *Clin Allergy* 1974; 4: 13.
17. Willey RF, Godden DJ, Carmichael J, Preslin P, Frame M, Crompton GK. Comparison of twice daily administration of new corticosteroid budesonide with beclomethasone dipropionate four times daily, in the treatment of chronic asthma. *Br J Dis Chest* 1982; 76: 61.
18. Martin LE, Tanner RJN, Clark TJH, Cochrane GM. Absorption and metabolism of orally administered beclomethasone dipropionate. *Clin Pharmacol Ther* 1982; 15: 267.
19. Brattsand R, Kallstrom L, Nilsson E, Ryrfeldt A, Tonnesson M. The lung disposition of budesonide in guinea pig and rats. *Eur J Respir Dis* 1982; 63 (suppl 122): 263.
20. Martin LE, Harrison C, Tanner RJN. Metabolism of beclomethasone dipropionate by animals and man. *Postgrad Med J* 1975; 51 (suppl 4): 11.
21. Peake MD, Cayton RM, Howard P. Triamcinolone in corticosteroid resistant asthma. *Br J Dis Chest* 1979; 73: 39.
22. Mandel S. Steroid myopathy. Insidious cause of muscle weakness. *Postgrad Med* 1982; 72: 207.
23. Breen KJ, Bury R, Desmond PV, Mashford ML, Morphett B, Westwood B, Shaw RG. Effects of cimetidine and ranitidine on hepatic drug metabolism. *Clin Pharmacol Ther* 1982; 31: 297.

24. Cochrane GM. Systemic steroids in asthma. In: Clark TJH, ed. *Steroids in asthma.* Auckland; ADIS Press, 1983; 103-120.
25. Webb J, Clark TJH. Recovery of plasma corticotrophin and cortisol levels after a three week course of prednisolone. *Thorax* 1981; 36: 22.
26. Rogers HJ, Sepctor RG, Trounce JR, eds. *A textbook of clinical pharmacology.* London: Hodder and Stoughton, 1981.
27. Milne LJR, Crompton GK. Beclomethasone dipropionate and oralpharyngeal candidiasis. *Br Med J* 1974; 3: 797.
28. Williams AJ, Baghat MS, Stableforth DE, Cayton RM, Schennoi PM, Skinner C. Dysphonia caused by inhaled steroids; recognition of a characteristic laryngeal abnormality. *Thorax* 1983; 38: 11, 818.
29. Flick MR, Murray JF. High dose corticosteroid therapy in the adult respiratory distress syndrome. *JAMA* 1984; 252: 1054.
30. Johansson SA, Anderson KE, Brattsand R, Gruvstad E, Hedner P. Topical and systemic glucocorticoid potencies of budesonide and beclomethasone dipropionate in man. *Eur J Clin Pharmacol* 1982; 22: 523.

# Chapter 9

# Pneumonia

*Allan R. Glanville and Graham E. Marlin*

The clinical manifestations of pneumonia are as diverse as its aetiological agents are numerous (Table 9.1). However, it is still possible to broadly divide most pneumonias into a 'typical'[1] or 'atypical'[2] syndrome. Typical pneumonias present with a productive cough, fever, rigors, dyspnoea and frequently haemoptysis and pleurisy. The most common agent implicated is the bacterium *Streptococcus pneumoniae.* Atypical pneumonias often have an insidious onset with a non-productive cough and prominent systemic symptoms such as malaise, confusion, prostration, myalgia, arthralgia and diarrhoea. *Mycoplasma pneumoniae* and *Legionella pneumophila* are the commonest causes of this syndrome except during times of influenza virus epidemics.

Several factors influence the aetiological agent and hence the ultimate choice of antimicrobial therapy. Firstly, whether the pneumonia is community-acquired or nosocomial. An infection should be considered nosocomial if the patient acquires the pneumonia within hospital or has attended hospital within the previous month. Secondly, whether the patient was previously healthy or had impaired local or systemic host defence mechanisms, that is, was 'at risk'. Unusual and opportunistic infections occur more frequently in the at-risk group depending upon the nature of the underlying host defence abnormality (Table 9.2). Infections in this group are commonly polymicrobial and often refractory to standard therapy. Certain occupations are associated with unusual and exotic infections (Table 9.3). Apart from these groups, community-acquired pneumonia in the healthy host is most commonly due to *S pneumoniae, M Pneumoniae* and influenza virus infection, less frequently to *Staphylococcus aureus* and *Mycobacterium tuberculosis.* There are many conditions which closely mimic pneumonia or may coexist with pneumonia (Table 9.4). Although certain radiological appearances are suggestive of a particular cause, none is diagnostic.

## Diagnostic Features

These are shown in Table 9.5.

Antimicrobial prescription in pneumonia depends on accurate aetiological diagnosis. Unfortunately the history, physical signs and radiological appearance give the clinician no more than a general guide to aetiology, and specific diagnostic tests should be undertaken (Figure 9.1).

The role of sputum analysis in the diagnosis of pneumonia remains a controversial area. Factors which may influence the growth of organisms in sputum samples include the presence of chronic bronchial infection, recent

*Table 9.1* Aetiological agents of pneumonia

| Common | Less common | Rare |
|---|---|---|
| **Typical Pneumonia** | | |
| *Streptococcus pneumoniae* | *Mycobacterium tuberculosis* | *Acinetobacter calcoaceticus* |
| *Staphylococcus aureus* | *Klebsiella pneumoniae* | *Actinomyces israelii* |
| *Haemophilus influenzae* | *Klebsiella* spp. | *Nocardia asteroides* |
| | *Proteus mirabilis* | α-haemolytic streptococci |
| | *Serratia marcescens* | *Corynebacteria* spp. |
| | *Escherichia coli* | *Branhamella catarrhalis* |
| | *Enterobacter* spp. | *Yersinia pestis* |
| | | *Streptococcus pyogenes* |
| | | *Pseudomonas pseudomallei* |
| | Anaerobes | |
| | *Bacteroides fragilis* | *Neisseria meningitidis* |
| | *Bacteroides melaninogenicus* | *Pasteurella multocida* |
| | *Bacteroides oralis* | *Salmonella typhi* |
| | *Bacteroides ruminicola* | *Salmonella paratyphi* |
| | *Bacteroides ureolyticus* | *Mycobacterium avium-intracellulare* |
| | *Fusobacterium nucleatum* | |
| | *Fusobacterium necrophorum* | *Listeria monocytogenes* |
| | *Peptostreptococcus* spp. | *Citrobacter* spp. |
| | *Peptococcus* spp. | *Proteus* spp. |
| | Microaerophilic vibrios | *Staphylococcus epidermidis* |
| | *Veillonella* spp. | *Brucella abortus* |
| | | *Brucella melitensis* |
| **Atypical Pneumonia** | | |
| *Mycoplasma pneumoniae* | *Chlamydia psittaci* | *Bacillus anthracis* |
| *Legionella pneumophila* | *Chlamydia trachomatis* | *Francisella tularensis* |
| Influenza A virus | *Coxiella burnettii* | *Legionella bozemanii* |
| Influenza B virus | *Legionella micdadei* | *Legionella dumoffii* |
| | Cytomegalovirus | *Legionella longbeachae* |
| | Adenovirus | *Legionella wadsworthii* |
| | Respiratory syncytial virus | *Legionella oakridgensis* |
| | Parainfluenza virus | *Legionella jordanis* |
| | *Aspergillus fumigatus* | Herpes simplex virus |
| | *Candida albicans* | Varicella/zoster virus |
| | *Cryptococcus neoformans* | *Blastomyces dermatitidis* |
| | *Pneumocystis carinii* | *Coccidioides immitis* |
| | *Toxoplasma gondii* | *Torulopsis glabrata* |
| | *Histoplasma capsulatum* | *Paracoccidioides brasiliensis* |
| | | *Sporothrix schenckii* |
| | | *Entamoeba histolytica* |
| | | Measles virus |

antibiotic therapy, altered oropharyngeal flora due to severe illness or alcoholism, and the method of collection and processing. The sample should be collected by deep coughing in the presence of a medical attendant and examined promptly to confirm the abundance of polymorphonuclear leucocytes and the absence of buccal mucosal cells (which imply gross oropharyngeal contamination — some contamination is inevitable). The sample is then submitted for Gram stain and culture plus special stains and cultures for *M tuberculosis,* fungi and *Pneumocystis carinii* where appropriate. Even using these methods, sputum culture does not reliably reflect the flora of the lower respiratory tract. Barrett-Connor[3] found concordant sputum cultures in only 50 of 100 patients with bacteraemic

*Table 9.2* Pneumonia in the at-risk patient

| Host defence | Likely infection |
|---|---|
| **Local and Mechanical** | |
| Impaired nasopharyngeal filtration (tumour, polyps, tracheostomy or endotracheal intubation) and/or altered level of consciousness (epilepsy, alcoholism, stroke, narcotic usage) | Aspiration pneumonia<br>mixed anaerobes<br>enterobactericeae |
| Altered oropharyngeal microbial flora (antibiotics, severe illness, hospitalisation, viral infection, diabetes mellitus, oral sepsis) | Gram-negative bacilli<br>*Staphylococcus aureus* |
| Ciliary dyskinesia | Gram-negative bacilli |
| Breach of intravascular compartment (haemodialysis, Hickman's line, intravenous narcotic abuse) | *Staphylococcus aureus* |
| **Immunodeficiency States** | |
| Granulocytopenia | Gram-negative bacilli<br>Fungi |
| Hypogammaglobulinaemia | *Streptococcus pneumoniae*<br>*Haemophilus influenzae* |
| Asplenia and hypocomplementaemia | *Streptococcus pneumoniae*<br>*Haemophilus influenzae*<br>*Neisseria meningitidis* |
| Reduced cell-mediated immunity (combined immunodeficiency, Wiskott-Aldrich syndrome, Di George syndrome, ataxia telangiectasia, chronic mucocutaneous candidiasis, acquired immune deficiency syndrome (AIDS),* lymphoma, cytotoxic chemotherapy, organ transplantation) | *Mycobacterium* (typical and atypical)<br>*Nocardia asteroides*<br>*Legionella pneumophila*<br>*Pneumocystis carinii*<br>Fungi and viruses, (especially cytomegalovirus, herpes simplex virus) |
| Pulmonary alveolar macrophage dysfunction (pulmonary alveolar proteinosis, cyclophosphamide, glucocorticoids and chronic granulomatous disease of childhood) | As above |

*AIDS may be defined by the reliable diagnosis of a disease at least moderately predictive of a defect in cell-mediated immunity in the absence of an immunosuppressive disease or treatment.

pneumococcal pneumonia. Other organisms were grown in 25 patients and the remainder had no sputum or no growth, confirming the observation that many ill or debilitated patients with bacterial pneumonia are not able to produce sputum. A positive sputum culture, however, does reliably localise the source of a bacteraemia in the pneumonic patient and strongly implies pathogenicity when an unusual organism is isolated, such as *M tuberculosis, Cryptococcus neoformans, Nocardia asteroides* and *Pseudomonas pseudomallei.*

Blood cultures should be performed on all patients with pneumonia regardless of their temperature or recent antimicrobial usage. Pneumococcal pneumonia is associated with bacteraemia in 25 to 40% of cases and this

*Table 9.3* Pneumonia: occupational and occasional risks

| Occupation or occasion | Organism (disease) |
|---|---|
| Meat worker, slaughterman | *Coxiella burnettii* (Q fever) |
| Bird fancier, petshop owner, poultry farmer | *Chlamydia psittaci* (psittacosis)<br>*Cryptococcus neoformans* |
| Residence or travel in the tropics | *Pseudomonas pseudomallei* (melioidosis)<br>*Mycobacterium tuberculosis* |
| Flea or animal bite | *Yersinia pestis* (plague)<br>*Pasteurella multocida*<br>*Francisella tularensis* |
| Air conditioning, cooling towers | *Legionella pneumophilia* (Legionnaire's disease) |
| Institutions, colleges, military barracks | *Mycoplasma pneumoniae*<br>*Legionella pneumophila*<br>Adenovirus |
| Post-influenza | *Staphylococcus aureus*<br>*Haemophilus influenzae*<br>*Streptococcus pneumoniae*<br>*Streptococcus pyogenes* |
| Homosexuals, bisexuals or partners, haemophiliacs, Haitians and illicit IV drug users | *Pneumocystis carinii*<br>Atypical mycobacteria |
| Farmworker, handlers of animal hair, hides or carcasses | *Bacillus anthracis* (anthrax) |
| Infants (1-6 months) | *Chlamydia trachomatis*<br>Respiratory syncytial virus |

IV = intravenous.

*Table 9.4* Pneumonia: differential diagnosis

| Diagnosis | Features |
|---|---|
| Pneumonitis | Cryptogenic organising pneumonitis<br>Irradiation<br>Drug toxicity (for example, bleomycin)<br>Aspiration of blood/gastric contents |
| Fibrosing alveolitis | Cryptogenic<br>Associated connective tissue disease |
| Pulmonary infarction | |
| Cardiogenic pulmonary oedema | |
| Adult respiratory distress syndrome | |
| Malignancy | Bronchogenic carcinoma<br>Alveolar cell carcinoma<br>Lymphangitis carcinomatosis<br>Lymphoma |
| Pulmonary haemorrhage | Pulmonary haemosiderosis<br>Goodpasture's syndrome<br>Systemic lupus erythematosus<br>Rapidly progressive glomerulonephritis |
| Non-infectious granulomata | Sarcoidosis<br>Extrinsic allergic alveolitis<br>Allergic bronchopulmonary aspergillosis<br>Wegener's granulomatosis<br>Lymphomatoid granulomatosis<br>Churg-Strauss disease |

*Table 9.5* Pneumonia: diagnostic criteria

| Type of pneumonia | Absolute | Presumptive |
|---|---|---|
| Bacterial | Isolation of organism from<br>• blood and sputum<br>• fine needle aspirate<br>• sterile catheter (>$10^3$ colony-forming units/ml) | Isolation from<br>• blood alone<br>• transtracheal aspirate<br>• sputum (unusual organisms, see text) |
| Viral | Fourfold rise in complement fixation antibody titres.<br>Presence of viral inclusion bodies plus cytopathogenic effect in pulmonary tissue or exfoliated cells | Widespread viral inclusion bodies in pulmonary tissue or exfoliated cells |
| Legionnaire's disease | Demonstration within pulmonary tissue or secretions via Dieterle silver stain or fluorescent antibody testing plus a fourfold rise in complement fixation titres | Fourfold rise in complement fixation titres alone, or single titre ≥1/128 |
| Mycoplasma | Fourfold rise in complement fixation titres | Single titre ≥1/256 |
| Fungal | Demonstration of invasion of pulmonary tissue | Culture from pulmonary secretions in absence of other organisms and response to antifungal therapy |
| *Pneumocystis carinii* (PCP) | Demonstration within pulmonary tissue or secretion | Fourfold rise in titres |

carries an increased mortality rate. Bacteraemia is less common in staphylococcal pneumonia (10 to 15%) where it often implies that the primary locus of infection is extrathoracic, for example, an infected arteriovenous fistula used for haemodialysis, a furuncle or deep-seated abscess, osteomyelitis and occasionally endocarditis). Gram-negative bacillary bacteraemia is often associated with circulatory collapse.

In clinical practice, there is often a pressing need to commence antimicrobial therapy before the results of blood and sputum cultures are available. Although sputum Gram stains may be useful, the principal decision is whether to commence empirical therapy based on the likely agents, as outlined above, or to proceed to further diagnostic manoeuvres. We favour procedures in the following groups:[4] (i) patients at risk; (ii) nosocomial infection; (iii) fulminant pneumonia; (iv) history of aspiration; and (v) treatment failure.

The consideration in an individual patient must always be whether the known risk of further investigation outweighs the potential gain from the diagnostic procedure. On balance, it is usually worth proceeding given the high morbidity and mortality rate of pneumonia in these groups, the diversity of possible infecting agents and the toxicity of complicated empirical antimicrobial regimes.

In general, we prefer a step-wise method of investigation, performing fibreoptic bronchoscopy prior to consideration of open lung biopsy wherever

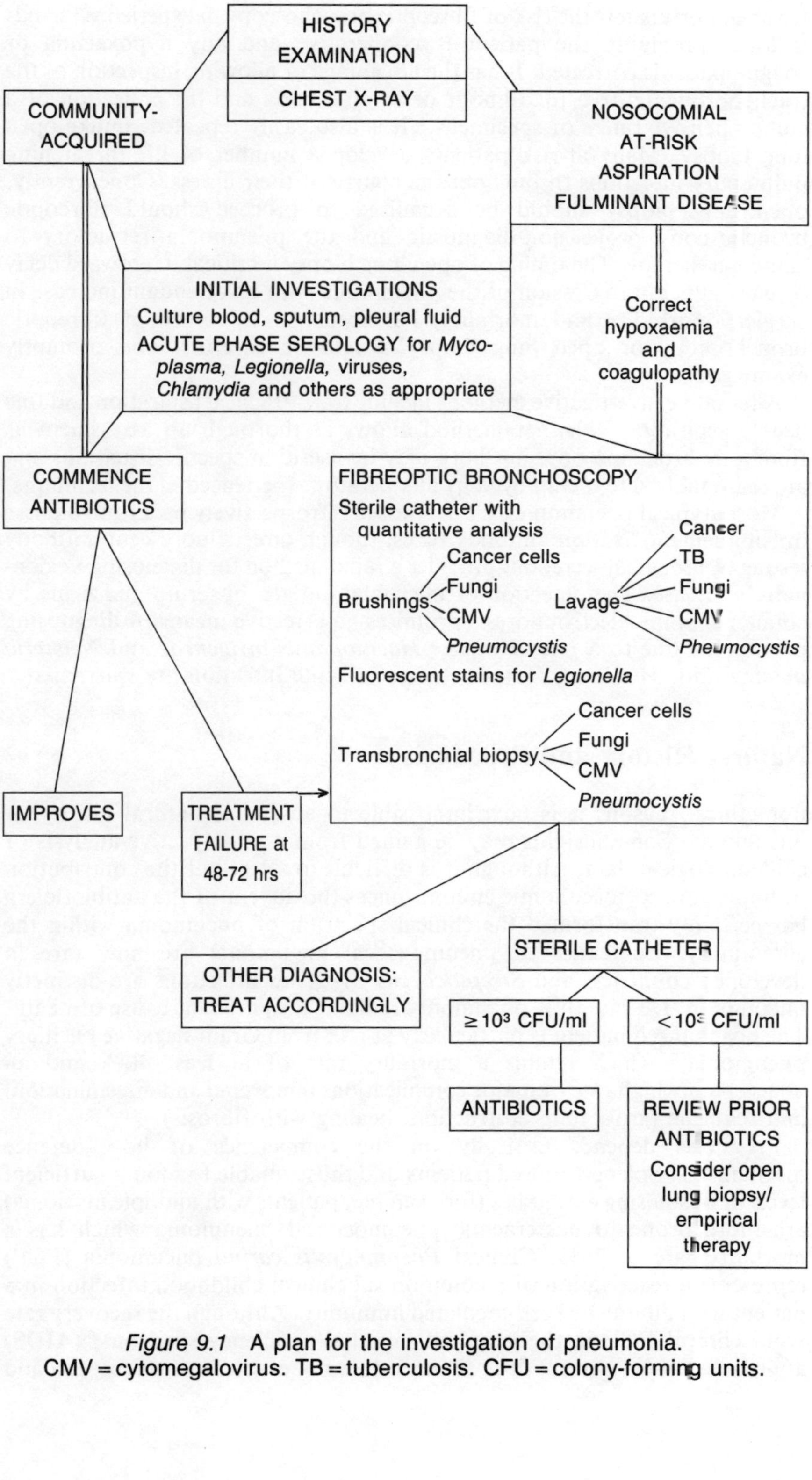


*Figure 9.1* A plan for the investigation of pneumonia.
CMV = cytomegalovirus. TB = tuberculosis. CFU = colony-forming units.

feasible. Fortunately the risk of fibreoptic bronchoscopy in experienced hands is low,[5] providing the patient is cooperative and any hypoxaemia or coagulopathy is corrected. It has the advantage of allowing inspection of the tracheobronchial tree for tumour or foreign body and the collection of a comprehensive range of specimens.[6] It is also easily repeated, unlike open lung biopsy. Many at-risk patients develop a number of life-threatening pulmonary infections throughout the course of their illness. Concurrently, open lung biopsy should be organised to proceed should fibreoptic bronchoscopy prove non-diagnostic and the pneumonia refractory to empirical therapy. The timing of open lung biopsy is critical. Untoward delay often results in progression of the pneumonia with an attendant increase in surgical morbidity and mortality. All specimens obtained at fibreoptic bronchoscopy or open lung biopsy should be carefully and promptly examined.

Alternative investigative methods include trans-tracheal aspiration and fine needle aspiration.[7] Neither method allows as thorough an assessment as fibreoptic bronchoscopy, but both may be useful in specific situations and are reasonably safe if employed by an operator experienced in the technique.

Most atypical pneumonias are diagnosed retrospectively by a fourfold rise in complement fixation antibody titres, though direct fluorescent antibody testing of bronchial secretions provides a rapid method for diagnosing Legionnaire's disease. The detection of microbial antigen in serum and urine by counter-immunoelectrophoresis promises an effective means of diagnosing pneumonia due to *S pneumoniae,*[8] *Haemophilus influenzae* and *Neisseria meningitidis*. However, further studies in acute infection are warranted.

## Natural History and Prognosis

For ethical reasons it is now impossible to study the natural history of pneumonia. Some insights may be gained from a retrospective analysis of epidemiological data. Although it is difficult to select out the contribution of improving socioeconomic circumstances the advent of the antibiotic era has certainly transformed the clinical spectrum of pneumonia within the community. Epidemics of pneumococcal pneumonia are now rare in developed countries, and *Streptococcus pyogenes* infections are distinctly uncommon. Despite this, pneumonia remains a significant cause of death. The hospitalised patient is particularly at risk from Gram-negative bacillary pneumonia,[9] which retains a mortality rate of at least 40% and an unacceptably high rate of major complications (empyema and dissemination) and sequelae (gross lung destruction, healing with fibrosis).

Prognosis depends critically on the competence of host defence mechanisms. Splenectomised patients and those unable to mount sufficient levels of opsonising antibodies (for example, patients with multiple myeloma) are more prone to bacteraemic pneumococcal pneumonia which has a mortality rate of 25%. Clinical *Pneumocystis carinii* pneumonia (PCP) represents a reactivation of a common subclinical childhood infection in a patient with diminished cell-mediated immunity. Although the recovery rate from clinical PCP in the acquired immune deficiency syndrome (AIDS) approaches 60%, current drug therapy does not eradicate the protozoa and some 40% of survivors will die from recrudescent PCP. Fortunately, the outlook in community-acquired *Mycoplasma pneumoniae* infection is generally benign. Tetracyclines have been shown in a double-blind study in military recruits to hasten the resolution of fever, cough, the clearing of 'crackles', systemic symptoms and radiological abnormalities.[10] The macrolide antibiotics, erythromycin and josamycin, have been shown to be equally effective.[11,12] In general, pneumonia carries a poor prognosis in the at-risk group, in nosocomial infection, in fulminant disease with bacteraemia, or where diagnosis and appropriate therapy are delayed.

## Goals of Treatment

The aim of therapy of pneumonia is to preserve life and maintain lung function. Acute-phase therapy should be designed to treat bacteraemic shock, respiratory failure and abscess and empyema formation, with an awareness of potential toxicity of drug and oxygen therapy. Effective bronchopulmonary toilet with early diagnosis and appropriate antimicrobial therapy may avoid the long-term complications of bronchiectasis and fibrosis. Attention to predisposing conditions is vital to prevent recurrence, as is the recognition of sentinel cases within a community or hospital population which may herald a serious outbreak, such as nosocomial Legionnaire's disease.[13]

## Treatment

Even apparently simple community-acquired pneumonia may rapidly deteriorate with profound hypoxaemic respiratory failure. For this reason it is preferable to manage all patients with pneumonia in hospital, at least until a favourable therapeutic response is obtained. The initial resuscitation and correction of hypoxaemia, use of bronchodilator therapy where appropriate, and mobilisation of secretions via effective chest physiotherapy all play an important role in the management of pneumonia; however, we will concentrate here on antimicrobial therapy.

In general, the preferred route of administration of antimicrobial agents is intravenous, as this provides the most reliable means of obtaining adequate serum and tissue concentrations. With intermittent intravenous therapy, higher peak serum concentrations will result in higher tissue concentrations and at steady-state conditions, equilibrium will develop between blood and tissues. In view of the nature of lung parenchyma where there is enormous surface area contact between alveolar walls and capillaries, serum antibiotic concentrations are likely to approximate closely to those in lung parenchyma. On the other hand, the bronchial mucosa is the site of infection in acute exacerbations of chronic bronchitis and eradication of infection will depend upon the antibiotic concentration achieved at this site as well as natural defence mechanisms.[14-18] The significance of penetration of antimicrobial agents into pulmonary secretions is uncertain, but poor penetrance into thick purulent secretions may in part explain the difficulty in eradicating certain organisms such as *Pseudomonas aeruginosa* from the tracheobronchial tree.[18,19] The duration of effect of the antimicrobial agent will depend upon the exposure time and the concentration of the drug achieved in serum and tissue, which should at least be greater than the minimal inhibitory concentration against the range of organisms concerned. The dosing interval will depend upon the half-life of the drug. Careful and regular inspection of venous sites used for administration is mandatory to avoid thrombophlebitis. The use of in-line filtration has been shown to reduce the incidence of thrombophlebitis occurring with some antimicrobial agents, such as erythromycin,[20] cephalothin,[21] and amphotericin B.[22] It is also known that commercial intravenous preparations contain particulate matter which may mechanically or chemically injure the venous epithelium.[23] Intravenous therapy avoids the erratic absorption of enteral or intramuscular therapy in the ill patient. The latter route is painful and potentially hazardous in the wasted patient.

When antibiotics are administered orally after the initial intravenous therapy, instructions regarding timing of dose with meals must be carefully followed. In some instances bioavailability of certain antibiotic formulations, such as erythromycin,[24] may be markedly impaired by food. Absorption may also be affected by drug chelation in the gut; for example, tetracyclines with magnesium or aluminium salts contained in antacid preparations. Oral doses of antimicrobial agents may often be limited by adverse gastrointestinal symptoms. However, larger doses are not necessarily more effective as more antibiotic will be inactivated or excreted. All too frequently excessive doses of antibiotics are used and this may lead to unnecessary drug toxicity and costs.

The duration of therapy should be tailored to suit the individual infection. The end point of therapy is usually determined by the resolution of symptoms, radiological improvement and the inability to culture viable organisms from pulmonary secretions. There are notable exceptions to these basic guidelines, however. A lung abscess usually requires at least six weeks' therapy as does Gram-negative bacillary pneumonia. Pulmonary tuberculosis requires protracted therapy (see Chapter 12) and nocardiosis may require more than one year's treatment. *Pseudomonas pseudomallei* often recurs with resistant strains if initial therapy is given for less than 30 days.[25] Serious fungal infections may take several months to clear. Radiological resolution occurs at variable rates. Pneumococcal pneumonia should show marked clearing within 7 to 10 days. Lack of clearing or progression of the radiological lesion after two weeks' therapy is an indication for fibreoptic bronchoscopy to exclude the possibility of endobronchial obstruction due to a neoplasm or foreign body.

Antibiotic therapy may be divided into two broad groups: firstly, where the aetiological agent is known or strongly suspected (Table 9.6); and secondly, where empirical therapy is employed (Table 9.7)

## Empirical Therapy

The intention of empirical therapy[26,27] is to cover the most likely infecting organisms based on an understanding of any underlying host defence abnormality and the community or hospital origin of the infection. In the previously healthy host with a typical community-acquired pneumonia, *S pneumoniae* should be covered, for example with penicillin. In an atypical syndrome,

*Table 9.6* Antimicrobial therapy of pneumonia

| Aetiological agent | Drug of first choice<br>(daily dose, frequency, route) | Alternatives<br>(daily dose, frequency, route) |
|---|---|---|
| **Gram-positive Cocci** | | |
| *Staphylococcus aureus*<br>• methicillin sensitive | Cloxacillin 4-12g q4-6h IV<br>or oxacillin 4-12g q4-6h IV<br>or methicillin 4-12g q4-6h IV<br>or nafcillin 4-12g q4-6h IV | Cefamandole 2-12g q4-6h IV<br>Cefotaxime 2-12g q4-6h IV<br>of cefuroxime 2.25g q8h IV<br>or flucloxacillin 4-8g q6h po/IV |
| • methicillin resistant | Vancomycin 2g q6h IV | Rifampicin 600mg d po<br>or chloramphenicol 50mg/kg q6h po/IV |
| *Staphylococcus epidermidis* | (as above) | (as above) |
| *Streptococcus pneumoniae* | Penicillin G 2-20 megaU q4-6h IV | Erythromycin 1-2g q6h po/IV<br>or cefamandole 2-12g q4-6h IV<br>or cefuroxime 2.25g q8h IV |
| α-Haemolytic streptococci | Penicillin G 2-20 megaU q4-6h IV | Erythromycin 1-2g q6h po/IV |
| *Streptococcus pyogenes* | Penicillin G-2-20 megaU q4-6h IV | Erythromycin 1-2g q6h po/IV |
| **Gram-negative Cocci** | | |
| *Neisseria meningitidis* | Penicillin G 2-20 megaU q4-6h IV | Erythromycin 1-2g q6h po/IV |
| *Branhamella catarrhalis* | Cefamandole 2-12g q4-6h IV<br>or cefoxitin 2-12g q4-6h IV<br>or cefotaxime 2-12g q4-6h IV<br>or cefuroxime 2.25g q8h IV | Amoxycillin 1500mg q8h po<br>+<br>Clavulanic acid 750mg q8h po |
| **Gram-positive Bacilli** | | |
| *Bacillus anthracis* | Penicillin G 20 megaU q6h IV | Erythromycin 2-4g q6h IV<br>Tetracycline 2g q6h IV |
| *Corynebacterium* spp. | Erythromycin 2g q6h IV/po | Penicillin G 2-20 megaU q4-6h IV |
| *Corynebacterium JK* | Vancomycin 2g q6h IVI | Teichomycin 2g q6h IV |

*Table 9.6* Continued

| Aetiological agent | Drug of first choice (daily dose, frequency, route) | Alternatives (daily dose, frequency, route) |
|---|---|---|
| **Enteric Gram-negative Bacilli** | | |
| *Enterobacter* spp.<br>*Escherichia coli*<br>*Klebsiella pneumoniae*<br>*Proteus* spp.<br>*Serratia* spp.<br>*Citrobacter* spp.<br>*Listeria monocytogenes* | Gentamicin 2-5mg/kg q8h IV<br>or tobramycin 2-5mg/kg q8h IV<br>or amikacin 15mg/kg q8-12h IV | Ceftizoxime 2-8g q4-6h IV<br>Ceftazidime 1-6g q6-8h IV<br>Cefotaxime 2-12g q4-6h IV<br>or latamoxef 2-12 g q4-6h IV |
| *Salmonella* spp. | Chloramphenicol 50mg/kg q6h po | Trimethoprim 960mg q12h IV<br>Sulphamethoxazole 4800mg q12h IV |
| *Yersinia pestis* | Streptomycin 30mg/kg q12h IM<br>+<br>Tetracycline 2g q6h IV | Chloramphenicol 50mg/kg q6h po/IV<br>or doxycycline 200mg stat po<br>100mg d po |
| **Other Gram-negative Bacilli** | | |
| *Acinetobacter calcoacetius* | Gentamicin 2-5mg/kg q8h IV<br>or tobramycin 2-5mg/kg q8h IV | Latamoxef 2-12g q4-6h IV<br>or cefotaxime 2-12g q4-6h IV |
| *Brucella abortus*<br>*Brucella melitensis* | Tetracycline 2g q6h IV/po<br>±<br>Streptomycin 15mg/kg d IM | Chloramphenicol 50mg/kg q6h po/IV<br>±<br>Streptomycin 15mg/kg d IM |
| *Francisella tularensis* | Streptomycin 15mg/kg d IM | Tetracycline 2g q6h IV |
| *Haemophilus influenzae* | Ampicillin 4-6g q4-6h IV | Amoxycillin 1500mg q8h po<br>Cefuroxime 2.25g q8h IV<br>Cefotaxime 2-12g q4-6h IV<br>Latamoxef 2-12 q4-6h IV |

*Table 9.6* Continued

| Aetiological agent | Drug of first choice (daily dose, frequency, route) | Alternatives (daily dose, frequency, route) |
|---|---|---|
| *Legionella pneumophila*<br>*Legionella* spp. | Erythromycin 2-4g q4h IV<br>±<br>Rifampicin 600mg d po | Doxycycline 200mg stat po<br>100 mg q12h po<br>100mg d po<br>±<br>Rifampicin 600mg po |
| *Pseudomonas aeruginosa* | Tobramycin 2-5mg/kg q8h IV<br>or gentamicin 2-5mg/kg q8h IV<br>or amikacin 15mg/kg q8-12h IV<br>+<br>Azlocillin 18g q4h IV<br>or ticarcillin 18g 4qh IV<br>or piperacillin 18g q4h IV<br>or mezlocillin 18g q4h IV | Ceftazidime 1-6g q8-12h IV<br>Ciprofloxacin 1g q12h po |
| *Pseudomonas pseudomallei* | Trimethoprim 960mg q12h po/IV<br>Sulphamethoxazole 4800mg q12h po/IV | Doxycycline 200mg stat po<br>100mg d po<br>± Rifampicin 600mg d po<br>± Chloramphenicol 50mg/kg q6h po/IV |
| **Anaerobic Bacteria** | | |
| *Bacteroides* spp. (except *B fragilis*) | Penicillin G 6-20megaU q6h IV<br>or clindamycin 0.9-2.5g q6-8h IV | Metronidazole 15-30mg/kg q6h IV/po |
| *B fragilis* | Metronidazole 15-30mg/kg q6h IV/po | Clindamycin 0.9g q8h po<br>Cefoxitin 2-12g q6h IV<br>Latamoxef 2-12g q6h IV |
| **Actinomycetes** | | |
| *Actinomyces israelii* | Penicillin G 20megaU q6h IV | Doxycycline 200mg stat po<br>100mg d po |

*Table 9.6* Continued

| Aetiological agent | Drug of first choice (daily dose, frequency, route) | Alternatives (daily dose, frequency, route) |
|---|---|---|
| *Nocardia asteroides* | Trimethoprim 960mg q12h IV<br>Sulphamethoxazole 4800mg q12h IV | Sulfisoxazole 6-12g q6h IV/po<br>or sulfadiazine 6-12g q6h IV/po |
| **Chlamydia** | | |
| *Chlamydia psittaci* | Doxycycline 200mg stat po<br>100mg d po | Chloramphenicol 50mg/kg q6h po/IV<br>Erythromycin 1-2g q6h IV |
| *Chlamydia trachomatis* | Erythromycin 2-4g q6h po/IV | Sulfisoxazole 6-12g q6h IV<br>or sulfadiazine 6-12g q6h IV |
| **Mycoplasma** | | |
| *Mycoplasma pneumoniae* | Erythromycin 1-2g q6h IV | Doxycycline 200mg stat po<br>100mg d po |
| **Fungi** | | |
| *Aspergillus* spp. | Amphotericin B (as below) d IV | |
| *Blastomyces dermatitidis* | " | Miconazole 1800-2400mg q8-12h IV |
| *Candida* spp. | " | ± Flucytosine 50-150mg/kg q6h po |
| *Cryptococcus neoformans* | " (1mg test dose, | ± Flucytosine 50-150mg/kg q6h po |
| *Coccidioides immitis* | " increase by | ± Flucytosine 50-150mg/kg q6h po |
| *Histoplasma capsulatum* | " 5-10mg/d to | Miconazole 1800-2400mg q8-12h IV |
| *Paracoccidioides brasiliensis* | " 0.3-0.8mg/kg/d) | |
| *Sporothrix schenckii* | " | |
| *Torulopsis glabrata* | " | (Ketoconazole 200-800mg d po as 2nd line for *Blastomyces/Candida/Cryptococcus/Coccidioides* and *Histoplasma)* |
| **Protozoa** | | |
| *Pneumocystis carinii* | Trimethoprim 20mg/kg q6h IV<br>Sulphamethoxazole 100mg/kg q6h IV | Pentamidine 4mg/kg d IM/IV |

*Table 9.6* Continued

| Aetiological agent | Drug of first choice (daily dose, frequency, route) | Alternatives (daily dose, frequency, route) |
|---|---|---|
| *Toxoplasma gondii* | Pyrimethamine 50mg d po for 3 days<br>25mg d po<br>Sulphafurazole 75-100mg/kg q6h po<br>or sulfadiazine 75-100mg/kg q6h po | Trimethoprim 960mg q12h IV<br>Sulphamethoxazole 4800mg q12h IV |
| **Rickettsia** | | |
| *Coxiella burnettii* | Tetracycline 2g q6h IV | Chloramphenicol 50mg/kg q6h po |
| **Amoebae** | | |
| *Entamoebae histolytica* | Metronidazole 1600-2800mg q6-8h IV<br>+<br>Diloxanide furoate 1500mg q8h po<br>(after metronidazole completed) | |
| **Viruses** | | |
| Herpes simplex | Acyclovir 15mg/kg q8h IV | |
| Influenza A | Amantadine 200mg q12h po | |
| Cytomegalovirus | No effective therapy | |
| Varicella/zoster | Adenine arabinoside 15mg/kg d IV | |
| **Helminths** | | |
| *Schistosoma* spp. | Praziquantel 40mg/kg stat | |
| Filarioidea nematodes | Diethylcarbamazine 1mg/kg q8h po increasing to 6mg/kg q8h po (over 3 days) | |
| *Leishmania* (kala azar) | Antimony sodium gluconate 6ml d IV | |

q = every. po = oral. IV = intravenous. IM = intramuscular. stat = at once. d = single daily dose.

*Table 9.7* Pneumonia: empirical therapy in the immunocompromised host

| Immune deficiency and disease | Therapy | Infecting organism |
|---|---|---|
| **Cell-mediated Immunity Deficiency** | | |
| AIDS | Trimethoprim-sulphamethoxazole<br>Erythromycin | *Pneumocystis carinii*<br>*Legionella pneumophila*<br>*Mycoplasma pneumoniae*<br>*Chlamydia psittaci* |
| Non-AIDS | As above ± aminoglycoside<br>Beta-lactamase resistant cephalosporin | Aerobic Gram-negative bacilli<br>Aerobic Gram-positive cocci |
| **Humoral Immunity Deficiency** | | |
| Agammaglobulinaemia<br>Hypocomplementaemia<br>Hyposplenism | Penicillin G<br>Beta-lactamase-resistant cephalosporin ± antipseudomonal penicillin with anti-staphylococcal properties | Aerobic Gram-positive cocci<br>and<br>*Haemophilus influenzae* |
| **Granulocyte Deficiency** | | |
| Neutropenia | Aminoglycoside<br>Antipseudomonal penicillin with anti-staphylococcal properties | Aerobic Gram-negative bacilli<br>Aerobic Gram-positive cocci<br>*Pseudomonas aeruginosa*<br>*Staphylococcus aureus* |
| Neutrophil function deficiency | Trimethoprim-sulphamethoxazole<br>Antistaphylococcal penicillin | *Nocardia asteroides*<br>*Staphylococcus aureus* |

*M pneumoniae* should be covered, for example with erythromycin. If the pneumonia develops in a patient with chronic bronchitis and emphysema, there may be coexistent bronchial infection with *H influenzae* or *S pneumoniae* and both of these organisms should be covered, for example with ampicillin. Therapy is then adjusted according to the results of blood and sputum cultures and therapeutic response. In the absence of a firm aetiological diagnosis, and with lack of improvement after 48-72 hours further diagnostic procedures should be undertaken.

Controversy surrounds the best empirical therapy for nosocomial pneumonia. The selection of individual antimicrobial agents will depend highly on the local pattern of antimicrobial sensitivities and the prevalence of problem organisms, such as methicillin-resistant *Staphylococcus aureus* (MRSA). At least 60% of nosocomial pneumonias will be due to Gram-negative bacilli. The incidence of colonisation of the oropharynx with Gram-negative bacilli in seriously ill hospitalised patients approaches 75%. Factors which facilitate this colonisation have been detailed in Table 9.2. The usual regimes combine a broad-spectrum semi-synthetic penicillin plus an aminoglycoside, or a third-generation cephalosporin plus an aminoglycoside, or a broad-spectrum penicillin plus an aminoglycoside. No firm clinical evidence supports the superiority of any one of these regimes. Despite initial excitement at the breadth of cover of the third-generation cephalosporins, monotherapy has proven disappointing in serious infections.

Empirical therapy is vitally important in neutropenic patients and should be commenced promptly once fever is documented unless the febrile episode is obviously related to another cause. The most common pathogens isolated from blood in febrile neutropenic patients are Gram-negative bacilli (*Escherichia coli, Pseudomonas aeruginosa* and *Klebsiella* species) and *S aureus*. Persistent fever in the neutropenic patient with a pulmonary infiltrate despite broad-spectrum antimicrobial cover should provoke attempts to demonstrate invasive aspergillosis, a diagnosis which is frequently missed in this group of patients.[28] The alternative to further invasive procedures is empirical antifungal therapy. Although there is some evidence that the early commencement of antifungal therapy may prevent fatal dissemination, survival usually depends on recovery of the host immune system. Unfortunately, bone marrow recovery may herald the development of gross pulmonary cavitation with subsequent fatal massive haemoptysis.[29]

The growing population of patients suffering from the acquired immune deficiency syndrome (AIDS) has altered the spectrum of pneumonic diseases.[30] Opportunistic infections (Legionnaire's disease and nocardiosis) and the recrudescence of intracellular pathogens (*Pneumocystis carinii* and *Mycobacterium avium-intracellulare)* are the characteristic hallmarks of AIDS. *P carinii* infection occurs in 60 to 85% of patients with AIDS and there are a number of differences compared with other patients with this infection: (i) longer duration of symptoms before diagnosis; (ii) more organisms within the lung, with easier diagnosis with less invasive procedures, such as lung lavage; (iii) longer duration of treatment required; and (iv) longer persistence of organisms in the lung. In a patient with non-proven AIDS empirical therapy should not be given and the specific diagnosis of *P carinii* infection should be sought. If infection is recurrent, empirical treatment, for example trimethoprim-sulphamethoxazole, may be justified.

## Aminoglycosides

The selection of a specific aminoglycoside is dictated by the sensitivity pattern of the organism, relative safety and cost-effectiveness. Aminoglycoside resistance is due to plasmid-mediated aminoglycoside-modifying enzymes which alter the ability of the aminoglycoside to bind to 30S ribosomes within bacterial cell cytoplasm, thereby preventing the induction of a protein which increases the energy-dependent transport of aminoglycoside across the bacterial cell wall.[31] Amikacin is more resistant to these enzymes and therefore is the drug of choice in hospital-acquired Gram-negative bacillary pneumonia where there is a known risk of aminoglycoside resistance (for example, multiresistant *Klebsiella pneumoniae*) or demonstrable resistance on sensitivity testing. Indiscriminate usage outside these limitations is unwise as widespread resistance may occur.

Caution is advised in prescribing aminoglycosides in patients with renal impairment. The dosage should be titrated against renal function and all patients should have careful monitoring of serum levels and renal function. Serum concentrations should be measured half-an-hour after an intravenous dose to demonstrate an adequate peak level, and half-an-hour prior to the next dose so that it may be modified if the trough level shows accumulation of the drug. On serial testing, a rising trough level is a sensitive indicator of a falling glomerular filtration rate, possibly related to aminoglycoside nephrotoxicity. Tobramycin has been shown to cause less nephrotoxicity and marginally less ototoxicity than gentamicin.[32] Gentamicin is the less expensive drug and is more efficacious in *Serratia* infections whereas tobramycin is more effective against *Pseudomonas* strains.[33]

## Cephalosporins

Although second and third generation cephalosporins play an important role in the treatment of pneumonia they are rarely first-line therapy.[34-36] Fortunately, the majority of *S pneumoniae* are exquisitely sensitive to beta-lactam antimicrobial agents; however, a few organisms have developed altered penicillin-binding proteins. If these resistant strains become more widespread it may be necessary to use the aminothiazolyl cephalosporins (cefotaxime and ceftizoxime) as first-line therapy.

*S aureus* produces an inducible and transferable plasmid-mediated beta-lactamase. The second generation cephalosporins, cefuroxime and cefamandole, are more stable against this enzyme than other cephalosporins; however, results of therapy in experimental infection have been contradictory. The mechanism of resistance of *S aureus* to beta-lactamase stable penicillins and cephalosporins is not understood. It is important to realise that strains of *S aureus* resistant to methicillin are also resistant to cephalosporins. Vancomycin is the treatment of choice.[37]

The incidence of beta-lactamase production by *Haemophilus influenzae* varies from 1 to 30% throughout the world. The beta-lactamase stable cephalosporins (cefuroxime, cefotaxime, ceftizoxime, ceftriazone and latamoxef) are effective against both *H influenzae* and most enteric Gram-negative bacilli. *Enterobacter* and *Serratia* pose a serious problem as they contain inducible beta-lactamases which function primarily as cephalosporinases though their mechanism of resistance against beta-lactamase-stable cephalosporins is not fully understood. Ceftazidime and cefoperazone are the only cephalosporins with significant antipseudomonal activity. *Acinetobacter calcoaceticus* may produce a cephalosporinase creating significant resistance to the newer cephalosporins.

## Penicillin

Penicillin G (benzylpenicillin) is the antibiotic of choice for pneumococcal pneumonia; most *S pneumoniae* have a minimum inhibitory concentration of less than 0.1$\mu$g/ml. Local sensitivity patterns will determine whether ampicillin or a beta-lactamase-stable antimicrobial agent is the first choice for *H influenzae*. Amoxycillin has superior enteral absorption to ampicillin. Cloxacillin and azlocillin have superseded methicillin and oxacillin as antistaphylococcal penicillins for intravenous use. Flucloxacillin has the advantage of being taken by the oral route for the latter part of therapy for staphylococcal pneumonia. Piperacillin, ticarcillin, nafcillin, mezlocillin and carbenicillin all have antipseudomonal properties. Monotherapy remains unproven and the preferred therapy for Gram-negative bacillary pneumonia is a combination of an antipseudomonal penicillin plus an aminoglycoside. Inactivation of carbenicillin may occur if it is allowed to remain in solution with an aminoglycoside for 24 hours.[38] This is rarely a practical problem, but may in part explain the difficulty of treating serious Gram-negative bacillary infections with this regime in patients with renal failure who are receiving a single daily dose of an aminoglycoside.

## Anaerobic Infection

Anaerobic infection commonly occurs in conjunction with mixed aerobic Gram-negative bacilli.[39] Therapy should include both aerobic and anaerobic pathogens. Anaerobic infection is often polymicrobial reflecting the diversity of oropharyngeal flora. Sensitivity testing is difficult, but the majority of anaerobes isolated from the oropharynx are sensitive to penicillin; however, some 20% of anaerobic pleuropulmonary infections involve *Bacteroides fragilis* which is more commonly penicillin-resistant. Also, some 20 to 40% of *Bacteroides melaninogenicus* are now penicillin-resistant.[40] Although there is continuing debate as to the pathogenicity of any single anaerobe taken alone, recent reports suggest that penicillin may no longer be the drug of choice in anaerobic lung abscess. Clindamycin appears to offer a superior and quicker cure rate.[41] Unfortunately, reports of clindamycin-resistant *B fragilis* are becoming more frequent. Metronidazole is effective against *B fragilis,* but has not been shown to be superior to penicillin used alone. Cefoxitin and latamoxef are also useful against *B fragilis.* In serious anaerobic pleuropulmonary infections a suitable regime would be two weeks' parenteral therapy with penicillin, cefoxitin and metronidazole, and an aminoglycoside may be required if aerobic Gram-negative bacilli are isolated. Therapy is the continued orally for at least four weeks using amoxycillin and metronidazole.

### Legionnaire's Disease[42]

*Legionella pneumophila* is one of a group of facultative intracellular parasites which require an intact cellular immune system for the containment of infection. Erythromycin and rifampicin, the antimicrobials of choice, are able to penetrate macrophages and inhibit the intracellular growth of *L pneumophila,* but do not kill the bacterium. Hence infection may recrudesce on the cessation of antimicrobial therapy. Erythromycin at a dose of 2 to 4g intravenously per day is the initial therapy of choice. The concomitant administration of rifampicin is advisable in severe cases. Rifampicin should not be used alone due to the potential emergence of resistant strains. Therapy may be changed to the oral route once a clinical response is obtained, but should continue for at least three weeks. Doxycycline is a suitable substitute for erythromycin in the event of intolerable allergy. It has the advantages over other tetracyclines of a long serum half-life allowing single daily dosage, minimal depression of enteral absorption with food, safety in renal insufficiency and lack of vestibular side effects.

The mortality rate for immunosuppressed patients is significantly higher.[43] The use of immunosuppressive agents including corticosteroids should be reduced or ceased where possible. Rarely, strains of *Pseudomonas fluorescens, B fragilis* and other *Pseudomonas* species may cross-react with direct fluorescent antibody testing whereas seroconversion may occur with tularaemia, melioidosis, plague, *B fragilis* infection and leptospirosis.

### Treatment Failure

A poor therapeutic response should prompt an urgent reappraisal of the diagnosis and treatment. Possible explanations include misdiagnosis (non-pneumonic illness, wrong organism(s), significant co-pathogens), the development of resistance during therapy (enzyme induction), complications of pneumonia (abscess or empyema formation, dissemination), drug and oxygen toxicity, and the presence of a hitherto unsuspected immunodeficiency state. It is not too trite to caution that the physician should first ensure that the patient is actually receiving the therapy as prescribed.

## Prophylaxis[44]

Pneumonia commonly complicates chronic bronchial infection. Strategies designed to prevent this are outlined in the subsequent chapters. In principle, they aim to decrease the load of pathogenic organisms via the use of long-term oral antibiotics in usual therapeutic doses or sometimes aerosolised antibiotics. Although nebulised carbenicillin and gentamicin have proved useful in cystic fibrosis,[45] polymixin B used in the intensive care situation did not reduce the mortality of Gram-negative bacillary pneumonia.[46]

A complementary strategy is vaccination of the at-risk population.[47] Anti-pneumococcal vaccine has been shown to reduce the risk of bacteraemic pneumococcal pneumonia but not pneumococcal pneumonia *per se.*[48] Its use is recommended in the splenectomised patient, in multiple myeloma and in chronic granulomatous disease of childhood, at five-year intervals. Antipseudomonal vaccines have not been widely used, but appear to reduce the incidence of invasive pseudomonal infections. Similarly, an anti-*Haemophilus influenzae* vaccine developed for the prevention of childhood meningitis has not been applied to adults with respiratory disease.

Of course most pathogenic bacteria are transferred from patient to patient by medical and nursing staff. Simple hygiene (handwashing) and surveillance procedures (nasal swabs for MRSA) may reduce this. To date, there is no evidence of patient to patient transmission of *L pneumophila*.[49] Although the Centres for Disease Control recommend no isolation procedures for patients with *P carinii* pneumonia[50] it would seem prudent to isolate them from other immunosuppressed patients with negative *P carinii* serology.[51]

## New Antibiotics

The 4-quinolones are potent bacteriocidal agents which act by inhibiting DNA gyrase, an essential enzyme in bacterial metabolism.[52-54] Their spectrum of activity is broad and includes *Pseudomonas aeruginosa* as well as other aerobic Gram-negative organisms, *Staphylococcus aureus,* β-lactamase producing *Haemophilus influenzae* and *Legionella pneumophila,* although there is relative resistance by *Streptococcus pneumoniae*. Clinical studies in pulmonary infection are currently being undertaken with a number of these agents including ciprofloxacin, enoxacin, norfloxacin, ofloxacin and perfloxacin.

Aztreonam, a monobactam, and imipenem, a carbapenem, are two of the more recently developed β-lactams and clinical trials in pulmonary infection are in progress.[55-56] Imipenem has a broad spectrum of activity that includes virtually all clinical isolates apart from *Pseudomonas maltophilia*. Aztreonam has high in-vitro activity against most aerobic Gram-negative organisms, but lacks useful activity against Gram-positive organisms and many anaerobes.

## References


1. Korzeniowski OM. Typical pneumonia syndrome. In: Levison ME, ed. *The pneumonias.* Bristol: John Wright & Sons, 1984: 121.
2. Boscia J, Korzeniowski OM. Atypical pneumonia syndrome. In: Levison ME, ed. *The pneumonias.* Bristol: John Wright & Sons, 1984: 130.
3. Barrett-Connor E. The non-value of sputum culture in the diagnosis of pneumococcal pneumonia. *Am Rev Respir Dis* 1971; 103: 845.
4. Glanville AR, Marlin GE, Hartnett BJS, et al. The use of fibreoptic bronchoscopy with sterile catheter in the diagnosis of pneumonia. *Aust NZ J Med* 1985; 15: 309.
5. Fulkerson WJ. Current concepts. Fibreoptic bronchoscopy. *N Engl J Med* 1984; 311: 511.
6. Wimberley NW, Bass JB, Boyd BW, et al. Use of a bronchoscopic protected catheter brush for the diagnosis of pulmonary infections. *Chest* 1982; 81: 556.
7. Wallace JM, Batra P, Gong H, Ovenfors C. Percutaneous needle aspiration for diagnosing pneumonitis in the patient with acquired immunodeficiency syndrome (AIDS). *Am Rev Respir Dis* 1985; 131: 389.
8. Coonrod JD, Rytel MW. Detection of type-specific pneumococcal antigens by counterimmunoelectrophoresis. Etiologic diagnosis of pneumococcal pneumonia. *J Lab Clin Med* 1973; 81: 778.
9. Young LS. Respiratory infections in the patient at risk: an overview. *Am J Med* 1984; 76(5A): 78.

10. Mufson MA, Manko MA, Kingston JR, Chanock RM. Eaton agent pneumonia — clinical features. *JAMA* 1961; 178: 369.
11. Denny FW, Clyde WA, Glezen WP. *Mycoplasma pneumoniae* disease: clinical spectrum, pathophysiology, epidemiology and control. *J Infect Dis* 1974; 123: 74.
12. Shames JM, George RB, Holliday WB, et al. Comparison of antibiotics in the treatment of *Mycoplasma* pneumonia. *Arch Int Med* 1970; 125: 680.
13. Palmer DL. Microbiology of pneumonia in the patient at risk. *Am J Med* 1984; 76(5A): 53.
14. Hartnett BJS, Marlin GE. Doxycycline in serum and bronchial secretions. *Thorac* 1976; 31: 144.
15. Marlin GE, Davis PR, Rutland J. Berend N. Plasma and sputum erythromycin concentrations in patients with chronic bronchitis. *Thorax* 1980; 35: 441.
16. Marlin GE, Burgess KR, Burgoyne J, et al. Penetration of piperacillin into bronchial mucosa and sputum. *Thorax* 1981; 36: 774.
17. Marlin GE, Nicholls AJ, Funnell GR, Bradbury R. Penetration of cefaclor into bronchial mucosa. *Thorax* 1984; 39: 813.
18. Pennington JE. Penetration of antibiotics into respiratory secretions. *Rev Infect Dis* 1981; 3: 67.
19. Maxwell D. The role of antibiotics given by inhalation in chronic chest disease. *J Antimicrob Chemother* 1983; 11: 203.
20. Marlin GE, Thompson PJ, Jenkins CR, et al. Study of serum levels, venous irritation and gastrointestinal side-effects with intravenous erythromycin lactobionate in patients with bronchopulmonary infection. *Hum Toxicol* 1983; 2: 593.
21. Maddox RR, Rush DR, Rapp RP, et al. Double-blind study to investigate methods to prevent cephalothin-induced phlebitis. *Am J Hosp Pharm* 1977; 34: 29.
22. Huber RC, Riffkin C. In line final filters for removing particles from amphotericin B infusions. *Am J Hosp Pharm* 1975; 32: 173.
23. Masuda JY, Beckerman JH. Particulate matter in commercial antibiotic injectable products. *Am J Hosp Pharm* 1973; 30: 72.
24. Rutland J, Berend N, Marlin GE. The influence of food on the bioavailability of new formulations of erythromycin stearate and base. *Br J Clin Pharmacol* 1979; 8: 343.
25. Shaefer CR, Trincher RC, Rissing JP. Melioidosis: recrudescence with a strain resistant to multiple antimicrobials. *Am Rev Respir Dis* 1983; 128: 173.
26. Donowitz GR, Mandell GL. Empiric therapy for pneumonia. *Rev Infect Dis* 1983; 5: 540.
27. Klastersky J. Empiric treatment of infections in neutropenic patients with cancer. *Rev Infect Dis* 1983; 5: 521.
28. Degregoria MW, Lee WMF, Linker CA, et al. Fungal infections in patients with acute leukemia. *Am J Med* 1982; 73: 543.
29. Albelda SM, Talbot GH, Gerson SL, et al. Pulmonary cavitation and massive haemoptysis in invasive pulmonary aspergillosis. Influence of bone marrow recovery in patients with acute leukemia. *Am Rev Respir Dis* 1985; 131: 115.
30. Stover DE, White DA, Romano PA, et al. Spectrum of pulmonary diseases associated with the acquired immune deficiency syndrome. *Am J Med* 1985; 78: 429.
31. Neu HC. Current mechanisms of resistance to antimicrobial agents in microorganisms causing infection in the patient at risk for infection. *Am J Med* 1984; 76(5A): 11.
32. Smith CR, Lipsky JS, Laskin OL, et al. Double blind comparison of nephrotoxicity and auditory toxicity of gentamicin and tobromycin. *N Engl J Med* 1980; 302: 1106.
33. Bodey GP, Stewart D. In vitro studies of tobramycin. *Antimicrob Agents Chemother* 1972; 2: 109.
34. Perkins RL. Clinical trials of cefotaxime for the treatment of bacterial infections of the lower respiratory tract. *Rev Infect Dis* 1982; 4 (suppl): S421.
35. Kamer RB. Moxalactam: clinical summary of efficacy and safety. *Rev Infect Dis* 1982; 4 (suppl): S721.
36. Gardner WG. Multicentred clinical evaluation of cefoperazone for the treatment of lower respiratory tract infections. *Rev Infect Dis* 1983; 5 (suppl): S137.
37. Sorrell TC, Packham DR, Shanker S, et al. Vancomycin therapy for methicillin-resistant *Staphylococcus aureus. Ann Intern Med* 1983; 97: 344.
38. McLaughlin JE, Reeves DS. Clinical and laboratory evidence for inactivation of gentamicin by carbenicillin. *Lancet* 1971; 1: 261.

39. Bartlett JG. Recent developments in the management of anaerobic infections. *Rev Infect Dis* 1983; 5: 235.
40. Murray PR, Rosenblatt JE. Penicillin resistance and penicillinase production in clinical isolates of *Bacteroides melaninogenicus. Antimicrob Agents Chemother* 1977; 11: 605.
41. Levison ME, Mangura CT, Lorber B, et al. Clindamycin compared with penicillin for the treatment of anaerobic lung abscess. *Ann Intern Med* 1983; 98: 466.
42. Meyer RD. Legionella infections: a review of five years of research. *Rev Infect Dis* 1983; 5: 258.
43. Bock BV, Kirby BD, Edelstein PH, et al. Legionnaire's disease in renal transplant recipients. *Lancet* 1978; 1: 410.
44. Johanson WG. Prevention of respiratory tract infection. *Am J Med* 1984; 76(5A): 69.
45. Hodson ME, Penketh ARL, Batten JC. Aerosol carbenicillin and gentamicin treatment of *Pseudomonas aeruginosa* infection in patients with cystic fibrosis. *Lancet* 1981; 2: 1137.
46. Polk HC, Borden S, Aldrete JA. Prevention of pseudomonas respiratory infection in a surgical intensive care unit. *Ann Surg* 1973; 177: 607.
47. Douglas RM, Riley ID. Pneumococcal disease and its prevention with polyvalent pneumococcal polysaccharide vaccines — a review. *Aust NZ J Med* 1979; 9: 327.
48. Schwartz JS. Pneumococcal vaccine: clinical efficacy and effectiveness. *Ann Intern Med* 1982; 96: 208.
49. Yu, VL, Zuravleff JS, Gavlik L, Magnussen MH. Lack of evidence for person to person transmission of Legionnaire's disease. *J Infect Dis* 1983; 147: 362.
50. Centers for Disease Control. Guideline for isolation precautions in hospitals. *Infect Control* 1983; 4: 245.
51. Hughes WT, Bartley DL, Smith BM. A natural source of infection due to *Pneumocystis carinii. J Infect Dis* 1983; 147: 595.
52. Percival A, ed. Quinolones — their future in clinical practice. International Congress and Symposium Series. London: Royal Society of Medicine Services, Number 104, 1986.
53. Neu HC, Reeves DS, eds. Ciprofloxacin. Pharmacokinetics and clinical experience. *Eur J Clin Microbiol* 1986; 5: 177-261.
54. Wise R, Leigh DA, eds. Perfloxacin — a laboratory and clinical evaluation of a new quinolone. *J Antimicrob Chemother* 1986; 17 (suppl B): 1-118.
55. Remington JS, ed. Carbapenems: a new class of antibiotics. *Am J Med* 1985; 78: 1-159.
56. Scully BE, Neu HC. Use of aztreonam in the treatment of serious infectious due to multiresistant Gram-negative organisms, including *Pseudomonas aeruginosa. Am J Med* 1985; 78: 251-261.

## Further Reading (for material in tables)

57. Abrutyn E. Strategies in the approach to treatment of pneumonia. In: Levison ME, ed. *The pneumonias.* Bristol: John Wright & Sons, 1984: 110.
58. Clarke CW, Marlin GE. Antibiotic treatment of pneumonia. *Aust NZ J Med* 1982; 12: 85.
59. Levison ME. Use of antimicrobial agents. In: Levison ME, ed. *The pneumonias.* Bristol: John Wright & Sons, 1984; 66.
60. Masur H, Shelhamer J, Parrillo JE. The management of pneumonias in immunocompromised patients. *JAMA* 1985; 153: 1769.
61. McLeod DT, Ahmad F, Power JT, et al. Bronchopulmonary infection due to *Branhamella catarrhalis. Br Med J* 1983; 287: 1447.
62. Pennington JE. Respiratory tract infections. Intrinsic risk factors. *Am J Med* 1984; 76(5A): 34.
63. Peterson PK. Host defense abnormalities predisposing the patient to infection. *Am J Med* 1984; 76(5A): 2.
64. Rhame FS, Streiffel AJ, Kersey JH, McGlave PB. Extrinsic risk factors for pneumonia in the patient at high risk of infection. *Am J Med* 1984; 76(5A): 42.
65. Sarosi GA. Management of fungal diseases. *Am Rev Respir Dis* 1983; 127: 250.
66. Young LS. Treatment of respiratory infections in the patient at risk. *Am J Med* 1984; 76(5A): 61.

# Chapter 10

# Chronic Bronchitis and Emphysema

*G.K. Crompton and Andrew P. Greening*

Chronic bronchitis and emphysema may give rise to airflow obstruction, increased work of breathing, impaired gas exchange and, ultimately, disability and death. They are a major world health burden and in the USA alone were said to affect 11 million people in 1982 at a cost of \$26 to \$27 billion.[1] While emphysema is defined anatomically as dilatation of the respiratory air spaces of the lungs with destruction of the interalveolar septa and other pulmonary tissues, chronic bronchitis is defined in clinical terms as chronic cough and sputum production for at least three months for two years.[2]

Following the original observation of Dornhorst[3] patients have been described as 'blue bloaters' or 'pink puffers', the former having hypoxaemia, carbon dioxide retention, secondary polycythaemia and cor pulmonale and the latter, in contrast, being very breathless but with relatively normal arterial gas tensions and no cor pulmonale. In reality, such patients are simply extremes of a continuous spectrum and the well voiced proposition that 'pink puffers' have predominant emphysema and 'blue bloaters' predominant bronchitis is not sustained by clinicopathological studies.[4] Thus, chronic bronchitis and emphysema are best regarded as coexistent diseases and, at the bedside, it is very difficult to say how much bronchitis or emphysema is present in an individual patient.

The disorders are apparently linked by common aetiological factors: cigarette smoking, atmospheric pollutants and occupational dusts. Although cigarette smoking is the most important of the identified causal factors, only a limited proportion of smokers develop hypersecretion and no more than 20% marked airflow obstruction. The mechanisms by which mucus hypersecretion is induced are far from clear, though in animal models there is a marked increase in the rate of multiplication of airway cells and an increase in the size of submucosal glands within a few days of exposure to tobacco smoke. The conventional British view has been that the mucus hypersecretion somehow predisposes the airways to infection, and contributes to airflow obstruction. In contrast Dutch workers have proposed that bronchial hyperreactivity has a central role in the development of permanent airflow obstruction and this may arise from asthmatic-like responses to allergens or other environmental factors.[5]

The pathogenetic mechanisms of emphysema have attracted considerable attention since the recognition of an association between the development of panacinar emphysema at an early age and a genetic deficiency of the major serum anti-elastase, $alpha_1$-antitrypsin ($alpha_1$-proteinase inhibitor),[6] and the observation that papain, a plant enzyme with a broad spectrum of proteolytic activities, was able to produce emphysema-like lesions in rat lung.[7] The present proteinase-antiproteinase hypothesis for the development of emphysema is complex,[8-10] but worthy of summary since it is encouraging new therapeutic developments. Tissue damage in the lung acinus is thought to arise from inadequately inhibited proteolytic activity. Neutrophils and macrophages are the principal cells of origin of the proteinases, of which neutrophil elastase is deemed the most important. The proteinase inhibitors may be derived from serum (eg, $alpha_1$-proteinase inhibitor) or produced locally (eg, antileucoprotease). A much smaller, but perhaps important, contribution is by inhibitors synthesised by macrophages themselves, and includes $alpha_1$-proteinase inhibitor and $alpha_2$-macroglobulin. Oxidants of either cigarette smoke or phagocyte origin can contribute by causing tissue damage directly (lipid peroxidation) or indirectly by inactivating proteinase inhibitors (oxidation of methionine residue(s) at the enzyme's reactive centre).[11] However, oxidant activity in turn is determined by local concentrations of antioxidants.

## Diagnostic Features

To support a diagnosis of chronic bronchitis and emphysema, made on the basis of a clinical history and examination, investigations have traditionally been radiological and physiological. However, since emphysema is defined in pathological terms, diagnosis and quantification in life, by indirect means, must be at best difficult and at worst highly inaccurate.

Three criteria are often accepted for the radiological diagnosis of emphysema from the plain chest X-ray:[12] (i) hyperinflation of the lungs, indicated by low flat diaphragms (maximal curvature of the right diaphragmatic dome less than 1.5cm) and a large retrosternal airspace, with the distance between the anterior margin of the aorta and the posterior border of the sternum, 3cm below the manubrium, being greater than 3 to 4cm on the lateral film;[13] (ii) vascular changes including a prominent pulmonary trunk and large hilar but attenuated peripheral pulmonary vessels, and a narrow, vertical heart; (iii) bullae. However, when these criteria have been applied and the radiological diagnosis of emphysema made, autopsy evidence obtained within six months of the X-ray indicated that only 34% of those actually found to have severe emphysema had been diagnosed radiographically during life.[14] Other authors have recommended the use of whole lung tomography to diagnose and localise emphysema,[15] but this method has not been subjected to the critical analysis of pathological comparisons. The development of computerised tomography (CT) has enabled more accurate estimation of lack of lung tissue (emphysema) and early studies using qualitative assessment of CT scans were encouraging.[16,17] More recently a quantitative analysis of CT scans has been developed and preliminary results using this method indicate a good correlation with pathological evidence obtained on resected lungs.[18]

Patients with chronic bronchitis and emphysema reveal abnormalities on a wide variety of physiological measurements of respiratory function. Airflow obstruction (limitation) is most usefully demonstrated by a reduction in the forced expiratory volume in one second ($FEV_1$) or peak expiratory flow rate (PEFR). In contrast to bronchial asthma the airflow obstruction is persistent with little day-to-day or hour-to-hour variation, either spontaneous or in response to treatment. To determine adequately that patients with chronic asthma are not misdiagnosed as chronic bronchitis and emphysema we would usually recommend that reversibility to an inhaled beta2-adrenoreceptor agonist be checked in the clinic or laboratory, using an adequate (800ug salbutamol, 2mg terbutaline) dose, and at home over a two to four week period monitored by PEFR. Similarly, an outpatient PEFR-monitored steroid trial should be performed, again using adequate doses (prednisolone 40mg per day for two weeks). It is usually accepted that any improvement in $FEV_1$ or PEFR of 15% or more is clinically significant. In those in whom a response of more than 20% is observed a diagnosis of chronic asthma rather than chronic bronchitis should be contemplated. Increases in lung volumes (total lung capacity, functional residual capacity, residual volume), while useful in assessing the severity of lung disease, are not specific for emphysema. Impairment of the carbon monoxide transfer factor ($T_LCO$), or diffusing capacity ($D_LCO$), is frequently observed in emphysema. Indeed, Thurlbeck et al[19] have claimed this as a distinguishing feature. Nevertheless, their data indicate a considerable overlap between patients with severe and mild emphysema. Measurement of the transfer coefficient (kCO, or $T_LCO$ per litre of lung volume) may provide a more sensitive indicator than does $T_LCO$, which is partly volume-dependent.[20]

Ventilation:perfusion (V:Q) lung scanning can provide evidence of extent of pulmonary disease, but the matched V and Q defects are not diagnostic of chronic bronchitis and emphysema, being seen also with bronchial asthma.

## Natural History and Prognosis

The prognosis for patients with chronic bronchitis and emphysema depends upon the severity of their airflow obstruction at the time of presentation and the presence or absence of cor pulmonale. Survival is closely related to the degree of initial impairment of $FEV_1$.[21,22] Thus, in the absence of cor pulmonale, patients with severe airflow obstruction ($FEV_1$ less than 30.5% predicted) have a median survival of 5.1 years, in contrast to 13.5 years for patients with less severe obstruction ($FEV_1$ greater than 42.5% predicted). For patients who also have cor pulmonale the respective median survivals are 2.2 years and 7.0 years.[22]

The progressive decline in $FEV_1$ can be affected by cessation of smoking. Heavy smokers (more than 15 cigarettes per day) have an annual loss of 60 to 80ml $FEV_1$ in contrast to 30 to 40 ml for the normal non-smoker. On stopping smoking the individual's subsequent rate of loss of $FEV_1$ reverts to normal.[23] Exsmokers of more than 10 years have a low death rate from chronic bronchitis and emphysema.[24]

## Goals of Treatment

The ideal is for treatment to prevent the development, or at least the continued deterioration, of the disease process. This requires aggressive antismoking measures and, since it is principally a political decision, the physician will have limited success. However, the 'future developments' discussed below indicate potential therapeutic avenues in disease prevention. In practice, treatment is aimed principally at alleviating bronchoconstriction, eradicating bronchial infections, and giving symptomatic relief from breathlessness.

## Treatment

### General

Although pharmacological interventions provide the mainstay of management of patients with chronic bronchitis and emphysema some general measures are helpful. Cessation of smoking is of major importance. The physician may play an important part in an individual's success or failure at this, since additional support/aids over and above a doctor's verbal advice do not appear to enhance the patient's ability to stop smoking.[25]

Exercise training has been shown to increase exercise performance,[26] though some of the benefit may be indirect, influencing patients' mood and attitudes and beliefs towards their exercise capabilities.[27]

Unless there are individual contraindications, patients should be given an influenza vaccination each autumn. Although the degree of protection conferred will vary with changes in the prevalent influenza strains, this can be a useful preventative measure particularly for those with severe respiratory impairment.

### Bronchodilators

Traditionally ephedrine, alone or in combination with a methylxanthine and a barbiturate, was the standard oral remedy for most patients with chronic obstructive bronchitis. Selective beta2-adrenoreceptor agonists have replaced the indirectly acting sympathomimetic drug ephedrine, and there has been a major change of emphasis in the route of drug administration, inhaled therapy being preferred. Oral methylxanthines are still commonly prescribed, usually as sustained-release formulations but not as combination preparations.

Parasympatholytic remedies have long been used in the treatment of wheezy patients.[28] In early times their benefits were somewhat dubious and the cigarette as an inhalation device would be frowned upon today. Atropine, a naturally occurring plant alkaloid obtained from *A belladonna* and *D stramonium,* was first isolated in 1831.[29] It has unpredictable absorption from the respiratory tract and can give rise to undesirable central nervous system effects since it crosses the blood-brain barrier. Atropine sulphate has fewer unwanted effects and is a more potent bronchodilator, while its quaternary ammonium derivative, atropine methonitrate, is even more potent.[30] Deptropine citrate enjoyed a brief period of popularity in the late 1960s but, although it had been shown that anticholinergic drugs were more likely to be of benefit in chronic obstrucive bronchitis than in chronic asthma,[30,31] widespread use of this type of treatment has only occurred in the last decade following the introduction of ipratropium bromide.[32]

### *Assessment of Bronchodilators*

In emphysema the destruction of interstitial elastic tissue which increases lung compliance and decreases support for the intrathoracic airways may result in airways closure during forced expiratory manoeuvres such as those necessary to record $FEV_1$ and PEFR. Manoeuvres performed at or near functional residual capacity (FRC), as in the body plethysmograph, would be less influenced by loss of lung elastic recoil since intrathoracic pressure variations are much smaller. Hence, significant clinical response to a bronchodilator drug could be missed if objective assessment was confined to a simple ventilatory function reversibility test. Measurements of vital capacity (VC), preferably during a relaxed expiratory manoeuvre, or by helium dilution as part of the measurement of all lung volume compartments, can detect improvement of clinical importance in the absence of appreciable change in $FEV_1$.[33] An individual patient's ability to exercise before and during treatment is also of great value in assessment of bronchodilator responsiveness.[34] Thus lack of significant improvement in $FEV_1$ or PEFR must not be regarded as proof of unresponsiveness. Measurement of VC, lung volumes and exercise tolerance should be made before and during treatment with the drug being assessed.

Patients with chronic bronchitis and emphysema frequently do not respond to conventional doses of inhaled beta2-adrenoreceptor agonists, but can show response to higher doses.[35] It is desirable, therefore, for dose-response assessments to be made in individual cases.

### *Sympathomimetic Bronchodilators*

Selective beta2-adrenoreceptor agonists are now almost exclusively used. Salbutamol[36] and very soon afterwards terbutaline were adopted into clinical practice because of the probably unfounded fears of toxicity of inhaled isoprenaline in the treatment of asthma.[37] After terbutaline came fenoterol, reproterol, and pirbuterol. None of these drugs has any clinically relevant superiority. The equally selective beta2-agonist rimiterol has, however, a shorter duration of action than other drugs and, although it has a more rapid onset of bronchodilator activity, this is probably not of clinical importance.

The argument for inhaled rather than oral administration of these drugs has already been made (Chapter 2) and undoubtedly the inhaled route is superior. The only possible exception is in end-stage disease which has led to hypoxic cor pulmonale when a sympathomimetic agent is being given for its possible effects on the pulmonary vasculature[38] as well as for its bronchodilator properties. For relief of airflow obstruction one of the long-acting selective beta2-preparations for inhalation should be prescribed regularly every four to six hours, and at any other time as required. Ideally a dose-response assessment for each patient should be undertaken (see above). The manufacturer's recommended dose should be ignored, since all are too low and are responsible for irrational undertreatment with beta-agonist drugs. Virtually all patients who get relief from a bronchodilator metered dose inhaler (MDI) will use it more often than instructed and this often leads to unnecessary anxiety for both the patient and his doctor. In chronic obstructive bronchitis and emphysema regular therapy, with extra doses as necessary, is probably a more rational way of using a bronchodilator inhaler than an as necessary basis which is suitable for many patients with asthma.

The dose for each patient should be increased until optimum benefit has been obtained within the dose range which does not give rise to distressing unwanted effects (tremor and/or palpitations). High-dose treatment via a nebuliser has been advocated for patients whose airflow obstruction responds poorly to pressurised aerosol therapy,[39] and there has been a great increase in the domiciliary use of nebulisers for the treatment of chronic bronchitis and emphysema in recent years. However, the apparent benefit of nebulised bronchodilator drugs compared with conventional inhaler therapy is almost certainly simply a reflection of increased dose. Jenkins et al[40] found that salbutamol in doses of 0.2 to 0.6mg delivered via a conventional MDI and 2.5 to 5mg by nebuliser had clinically similar effects in a group of patients with stable chronic airflow limitation. Unwanted effects of high-dose terbutaline can be reduced by using a 750ml plastic spacer device (Nebuhaler), since the spacer system greatly reduces oropharyngeal drug deposition, of which a large proportion is swallowed.[41]

It is likely that spacer systems will be available for salbutamol and other sympathomimetic bronchodilator drugs in the future. Spacer devices overcome the coordination problems many patients have using conventional MDIs[42] and allow more drug to be inhaled,[43] as well as decreasing oropharyngeal drug deposition, and are an important development in the treatment of patients with airways disease.

### *Anticholingeric Bronchodilators*

Several studies have shown anticholinergic agents to be as effective as beta-agonists in chronic bronchitis,[31,44,45] and some have reported evidence of greater improvement with anticholinergics.[46,47] Mann and George,[29] in their review of anticholinergic drugs in the treatment of airways disease, concluded that ipratropium bromide is as effective as beta2-adrenoreceptor agonists in chronic bronchitis, and a subgroup of these patients may respond more favourably to the anticholinergic drug. They also expressed the view that current evidence suggests that concern over possible detrimental effects of ipratropium bromide on airways secretions and clearing is unwarranted.

Ipratropium bromide should be prescribed regularly in a dose of four puffs (0.02mg per value actuation) four times daily. Regular treatment is likely to be more effective than 'as required' use of this inhaler since the onset of bronchodilation is much slower than with inhaled beta-adrenoreceptor agonists.[48] All patients who have been shown to have reversible airways obstruction should have a 'rescue' beta2-agonist bronchodilator inhaler, as well as their MDI containing ipratropium bromide, to be used whenever necessary. It is rarely, if ever, sufficient to prescribe ipratropium bromide alone.

Ipratropium bromide is also available as a nebuliser solution, but the role of this drug via a nebuliser in chronic bronchitis and emphysema has yet to be fully established. Patients who cannot use an MDI, and who cannot be taught how to do so, may be considered for regular domiciliary treatment with ipratropium bromide by nebuliser in a dose of 0.1-0.5mg four times daily. At the time of writing no large-volume spacer system is available specifically for ipratropium bromide, but in the UK at least the canister from the conventional ipratropium MDI fits the Nebuhaler. By using the Nebuhaler and the ipratropium bromide pressurised canister nebuliser systems can be avoided completely.

Older patients may respond better to anticholinergic drugs than to sympathomimetics,[49] and this could be explained by reduced beta-adrenoreceptor responsiveness in the elderly.[50]

*Combination of Ipratropium Bromide and a Selective Beta-adrenoreceptor Agonist*

Combination bronchodilator therapy has been reviewed by Shenfield,[51] who discussed advantages and disadvantages of fixed-dose combinations. Ipratropium bromide is available together with fenoterol hydrobromide in the same MDI. Each dose contains 0.1mg fenoterol hydrobromide and 0.04mg ipratropium bromide. The manufacturer's recommended dose is one or two puffs three or four times daily. We believe there is little or no place for combined bronchodilator preparations. Patients requiring treatment with ipratropium bromide and a beta2-adrenoreceptor agonist, in our experience, obtain more benefit from having two inhalers; ipratropium bromide four puffs six hourly and a beta2-adrenoreceptor agonist MDI used regularly, but not necessarily at the same time as the ipratropium bromide, and at other times as necessary. There is evidence that some patients obtain more relief of airflow obstruction with ipratropium bromide plus a beta2-adrenoreceptor agonist than from either drug alone.[52-54] Therefore, it may be rational for selected patients to have combined anticholinergic plus beta2-adrenoreceptor agonist therapy.

*Methylxanthines*

The evidence that theophylline therapy is of great clinical value in the treatment of chronic bronchitis and emphysema[55-57] is less convincing than that for sympathomimetic and anticholinergic treatment. Aminophylline,[58] like the beta-agonists, increases mucociliary clearance, but this is probably of little clinical importance compared with relief of airflow obstruction. It has also been claimed that aminophylline improves diaphragmatic contractility in normal subjects and in patients with chronic obstructive pulmonary disease,[59,60] but the clinical significance of this has yet to be evaluated. On published evidence presently available it is difficult to give specific guidelines regarding the role of theophyllines in the management of patients with chronic obstructive bronchitis and emphysema. The efficacy of these drugs in the treatment of asthma and in particular in those patients with predominantly nocturnal symptoms is beyond question,[61] and one would expect that methylxanthines should have a beneficial role in the management of reversible airflow obstruction associated with chronic bronchitis. As with other bronchodilator drugs objective evidence of efficacy should be obtained before embarking upon long-term therapy, and with the theophyllines it is important to ensure that adequate serum levels have been achieved before any decision about efficacy is made.[62,63] The presence of cardiac failure, concomitant treatment with erythromycin or smoking may disturb theophylline metabolism and affect serum levels. Sustained-release formulations of aminophylline or theophylline should always be used for oral maintenance therapy. In chronic bronchitis twice daily therapy is probably advisable.

*Corticosteroids*

In recent years there has been considerable controversy about the role of these drugs in the treatment of patients with chronic bronchitis and emphysema. While there is general agreement that short-course systemic therapy should be used in the distressed wheezy patient during exacerbations, providing there are no absolute contraindications, it should be recognised that as a consequence some patients are, thereafter, quite innappropriately labelled 'steroid-responsive' and continued on long-term corticosteroids with all the concomitant unwanted effects.

There is no concensus of opinion about the role of systemic or inhaled corticosteroid drugs in the long-term management of patients with chronic obstructive bronchitis and emphysema. Objective 'steroid assessments' should, of course, be performed before contemplating long-term systemic treatment, but it has been suggested that such an assessment should include a three-month preliminary observation period to prevent an improvement being attributed to corticosteroids when it has, in fact, occurred spontaneously.[64] This is, of course, impracticable in the majority of cases. Curzon et al[65] suggested that corticosteroid responsiveness was unlikely in patients who did not have significant improvement in PEFR after the inhalation of standard doses of ipratropium bromide and/or salbutamol, and Lightbody et al[52] found that the addition of prednisolone to ipratropium bromide and salbutamol did not produce any extra improvement of ventilatory function in patients with chronic bronchitis.

Few patients with chronic bronchitis and emphysema benefit from long-term oral or inhaled corticosteroids. The patients denied beneficial treatment are few compared with those who are given therapy without evidence that it is of any value. Unfortunately, when long-term systemic corticosteroid treatment is started withdrawal is often difficult, and in many cases doses are increased to levels which inevitably lead to unwanted effects which can be life-threatening.

**Antibiotics**

Antibiotic treatment is indicated when bronchial infection is associated with systemic symptoms or deterioration of respiratory symptoms. Some patients are not apparently upset by the presence of purulent sputum, and purulence is often present only in the morning. In these situations it is difficult to know whether antibiotics should be prescribed. These drugs are to be avoided when sputum is obviously mucoid. The general principles of antibiotic treatment have been outlined in Chapter 9. In patients with chronic bronchitis and emphysema macroscopic purulence of sputum is an indication of bronchopulmonary infection. In the vast majority of cases microbiological examination of sputum is not necessary or helpful.[66] Empirical treatment should be given on the assumption that the bacteria responsible are *Haemophilus influenzae* and *Streptococcus pneumoniae.* Treatment must never be delayed until the results of laboratory examination are available.

The majority of exacerbations associated with purulent sputum respond to treatment with oxytetracycline (250mg four times daily), ampicillin or one of its derivatives (250mg three or four times daily), co-trimoxazole (trimethoprim 160mg and sulphamethoxazole 800mg: twice daily), trimethoprim 200mg twice daily, or erythromycin 250mg four times daily. The cephalosporins are effective drugs, but cannot be recommended for routine treatment because they are so much more expensive than ampicillin and other drugs. Patients who have repeated episodes of bronchial infection should be allowed to have a stock supply of a suitable antibiotic to be taken as necessary. Treatment should start as soon as sputum purulence is noticed and be continued for 48 hours after sputum has become mucoid. The traditional 'seven day course' is an anachronism, but a course should probably not be shorter than five days or longer than ten. If sputum remains purulent after five to seven days a change of antibiotic is probably necessary, and at this stage microbiological examination might be helpful.

During influenza epidemics and when bronchial infection has developed in hospital, sputum should be examined in the laboratory at an early stage. In ill patients and in particular those who have evidence of pneumonia, a combination of antibiotics can be given initially to cover *Staphylococcus aureus* and Gram-negative organisms such as *Pseudomonas* and *Proteus* species. Appropriate treatment alterations can be made according to bacteriological investigations and clinical response.

Long-term antibiotic therapy in chronic bronchitis is rarely, if ever, justified. High-dose short-course treatment with ampicillin or one of its derivates (4g daily for three days) is occasionally successful in patients with chronic bronchial infection which has not responded to conventional antibiotic therapy. In some elderly patients with advanced disease and when other treatments have failed we believe it is ethically justifiable to give chloramphenicol 500mg four times daily for five to seven days. This drug may be effective when repeated courses of other antibiotics have not influenced sputum purulence, and in elderly patients with severe chronic airways disease we are of the opinion that the clinical benefits of chloramphenicol treatment far outweigh the exceedingly small risk of bone marrow aplasia.

### Symptomatic Treatment

Distressing breathlessness may be patients' principal complaint. Symptomatic relief may be attempted with a variety of medications. There are conflicting data as to the value of diazepam (25 to 40mg per day) with some authors finding benefit.[67] and others not.[68] In addition, induced drowsiness can be a problem. The antihistamine, promethazine, at a dose of 125mg daily, has been shown to give symptomatic improvement, and objectively increase walking distance.[68] Similarly beneficial results have been reported with dihydrocodeine phosphate (1mg/kg orally).[69] We have also observed useful symptomatic relief, in patients with advanced disease, with other opiate drugs such as diamorphine elixir 5 to 10mg six hourly or pethidine 50 to 100mg six hourly.

### Oxygen Therapy

Acute exacerbations of respiratory failure, in patients with chronic bronchitis and emphysema, require treatment with controlled oxygen therapy.[70,71]

This allows improvement in the degree of hypoxaemia without excessive carbon dioxide retention and resultant respiratory acidosis. On arrival at hospital such patients should have their arterial blood gases determined and be commenced on 24% oxygen via a face mask, such as a Ventimask. After initiation of other therapy (nebulised beta2-agonists, physiotherapy, and diuretics) and equilibration at the new concentration of oxygen (30 minutes) the blood gas measurements should be repeated to ascertain that there is adequate correction of hypoxaemia (arterial $PO_2 > 6.7$kPa, 50mmHg) without an unacceptable rise in arterial $PCO_2$ and hydrogen ion concentration. Under blood gas guidance the inspired oxygen concentration can be increased if required. For patients unable to tolerate a face mask, oxygen can be administered via nasal prongs at a flow rate of one to two litres per minute. Nasal prongs tend to remain in place while the patient is eating, talking and sleeping, but are less accurate in the control of oxygen delivery and at a flow rate of two litres per minute may well deliver 30% oxygen. This can be a disadvantage with patients particularly 'sensitive' to oxygen therapy in whom carbon dioxide retention and acidosis may be induced.

The use of domiciliary oxygen for patients with chronic bronchitis and emphysema raises many questions. Some patients undoubtedly obtain a significant improvement in exercise tolerance from the use of oxygen and this may be a very real benefit for the severely incapacitated who would otherwise be chair-bound or room-bound. Portable oxygen may also allow some house-bound patients to get out. However, there are patients whose use of oxygen at home amounts to that of an expensive placebo, so it behoves doctors advising domiciliary oxygen therapy to prove its benefits for each patient.

The role of long-term domiciliary oxygen therepy is controversial. Two detailed prospective studies have concluded that such treatment can increase patient survival.[72,73] The American trial studied 203 patients, comparing nocturnal oxygen therapy (12h per 24h) with continuous oxygen therapy (19h per 24h). The British trial studied 87 patients, comparing oxygen therapy (15h per 24h) with no oxygen. This study design has been criticised for lack of control therapy (such as compressed air),[74] and it is fair to say that although there was a reduction in mortality for the oxygen-treated group the mechanisms by which this operated were far from clear, since there were no significant differences between patient groups in the rate of change of arterial blood gases, lung function, haematocrit or pulmonary haemodynamics. Patients in these trials had undoubtedly ceased smoking, and the study conclusions should only be applied to exsmokers. Since patients on long-term oxygen therapy often recommence smoking, and in the absence of clear indicators as to which patients may benefit from such therapy, we find it difficult at present to recommend the initiation of such expensive therapy.

The different delivery systems for oxygen, and their advantages and disadvantages are discussed separately in Chapter 3.

## Mucolytics

Mucolytics are often prescribed, to facilitate expectoration by reducing sputum viscosity. These include acetylcysteine, bromhexine, carbocysteine and methylcysteine as oral preparations, and acetylcysteine and tyloxapol for inhalation therapy. Objective tests of mucociliary clearance have failed to demonstrate that such drugs are better than placebo. Oral acetylcysteine has, perhaps, attracted most attention in view of a Swedish report that it can reduce the exacerbation rate in chronic bronchitis.[75] However, the British Thoracic Society trial failed to confirm a beneficial effect.

### Surgery

For a few carefully selected patients surgical removal or collapse of large, localised emphysematous bullae may provide marked relief of breathlessness. Theoretically, there are three reasons why such approaches might benefit dyspnoea. Firstly, if the remaining lung is stretched to develop a greater retractive force it will increase elastic recoil of airways on expiration, and decrease the functional residual capacity and thus the work of breathing.[76] Secondly, although it is rare, the bullous area may have significant 'wasted' ventilation.[77] Thirdly, the bulla(e) may be compressing more normal, adjacent lung tissue causing regions of low ventilation-perfusion ratios. Patients whose emphysema is advanced or generalised are most unlikely to benefit from surgery.

## Future Developments

### Treatment of Hypoxia and Pulmonary Hypertension

Long-term oxygen therapy is discussed separately (page 34). At present there is much interest in the use of almitrine, available in France, but as yet not fully evaluated. It has been shown to increase the arterial $PO_2$ and reduce the arterial $PCO_2$ when given orally, and the improvement is maintained over prolonged periods. However, there is evidence that the drug may actually aggravate pulmonary hypertension. If so, it would be inappropriate to advocate its use simply to improve the arterial $PO_2$ at the expense of increased pulmonary artery pressures. It remains to be seen whether almitrine used in conjunction with calcium antagonists or angiotensin converting enzyme inhibitors would allow improved arterial oxygenation without worsening pulmonary hypertension.

### Proteinase Inhibitor Therapy

Approximately one person per thousand population, of North European origin, has severe $alpha_1$-antitrypsin deficiency. The National Institutes of Health, USA, commenced two long-term studies for the treatment of such individuals. The first, using danazol to increase the biosynthesis of $alpha_1$-antitrypsin,[78] has been discontinued for fear of exacerbating liver disease. The second provides 'replacement therapy' with infused human $alpha_1$-antitrypsin obtained from fractionated pooled serum.[79] Although 4g intravenously once a week appears to boost adequately the antielastase activity of bronchoalveolar lining fluids[80] it may take 10 to 20 years to know whether the development of emphysema can be prevented or even usefully delayed. The logistics and expense of producing sufficient $alpha_1$-antitrypsin for all affected individuals would be formidable. However, genetic engineering has enabled not only expression of the human alpha$_1$-antitrypsin gene in yeast, but also its modification so that an oxidation-resistant alpha$_1$-antitrypsin is synthesised.[81] The gene has also been modified to prevent the protein's glycosylation, since yeast carbohydrate would be antigenically foreign to humans. The resulting antitrypsin has good antielastase activity and does not appear to be unduly antigenic in rabbits. It has, however, a much reduced serum half-life compared with native protein.

Other elastase inhibitors are being explored. Eglin c obtained from the medicinal leech is being produced in commercial quantities from a synthetic gene in *E coli*. Aprotinin has been modified to an elastase inhibitor, rather than a trypsin inhibitor, by substitution of valine for its reactive centre lysine. Both have good in-vitro activity, but will require prolonged clinical trials to determine their efficacy. Less far down the development assembly line are chloromethyl ketones, synthetic active-site inhibitors of neutrophil elastase.[82]

## References


1. Lenfent C. Lung research: government and community. The 1982 Burns Amberson lecture. *Am Rev Respir Dis* 1982; 126: 753.
2. Ciba Guest Symposium. Terminology, definitions and classification of chronic pulmonary emphysema and related conditions. A report of the conclusions of a Ciba guest symposium. *Thorax* 1959; 14: 286.
3. Dornhorst AC. Respiratory insufficiency. *Lancet* 1955; 1: 1185.
4. Thurlbeck WM. Chronic airflow obstruction in lung disease. In: Bennington, ed. *Major problems in pathology;* vol. 5. London: WB Saunders, 1976.
5. Orie NGM, Sluiter HJ, De Vries K, Tammeling GJ, Witkop J. The host factor in bronchitis. In: Orie and Sluiter, eds. *Bronchitis. An international symposium,* 27-29 April, 1960, University of Groningen. Assen: Royal Van Gorcum, 1961: 43.
6. Laurell CB, Ericksson S. The electrophoretic alpha globulin pattern of serum in alpha$_1$-antitrypsin deficiency. *Scand J Clin Lab Invest* 1963; 15: 132.
7. Gross P, Pfitzer EA, Tolker E, Rabyuk MA, Kaschak M. Experimental emphysema: its production with papain in normal and silicotic rats. *Arch Environ Health* 1965; 11: 50.
8. Stockley RA. Proteolytic enzymes, their inhibitors and lung diseases. *Clin Sci* 1983; 64: 119.
9. Idell S, Cohen AB. The protease inhibitor hypothesis of emphysema. In: Flenley and Petty Eds. *Recent advances in respiratory medicine. 3.* Edinburgh: Churchill Livingstone, 1983: 159.
10. Kimbel P. Proteolytic mechanisms of lung injury in the pathogenesis of emphysema. *Chest* 1984; 85 (suppl): 39S.
11. Johnson D, Travis J. The oxidative inactivation of human alpha$_1$-proteinase inhibitor: further evidence for methionine at the reactive center. *J Biol Chem* 1979; 254: 4022.
12. Simon G. Radiology and emphysema. *Clin Radiol* 1964; 15: 293.
13. Simon G, Pride NB, Jones NL, Raimondi AC. Relation between abnormalities in the chest radiograph and changes in pulmonary function in chronic bronchitis and emphysema. *Thorax* 1973; 28: 15.
14. Thurlbeck WM, Simon G. Radiographic appearance of the chest in emphysema. *Am J Roentgenol* 1978; 130: 429.
15. Barter CE, Hugh Jones P, Law JW, Crosbie WA. Radiology compared with xenon 133 scanning and bronchoscopic lobar sampling for assessing regional lung function on patients with emphysema. *Thorax* 1973; 28: 29.
16. Coddington R, Mera SL, Goddard PR, Bradfield JWB. Pathological evaluation of computed tomography images of lungs. *J Clin Path* 1982; 35: 536.
17. Goddard PR, Nicholson EM, Laszlow G, Watt I. Computed tomography in pulmonary emphysema. *Clin Radiol* 1982; 33: 379.

18. Hayhurst MD, Macnee W, Flenley DC, et al. Diagnosis of pulonary emphysema by computerised tomography. *Lancet* 1984; 2: 320.
19. Thurlbeck WM, Dunnill MS, Hartung W, Heard BE, Heppleston AG, Ryder RC. Chronic obstructive lung disease: a comparison between clinical, roentgenologic, functional and morphologic criteria in chronic bronchitis, emphysema, asthma and bronchiectasis. *Medicine (Baltimore)* 1970; 49: 81.
20. Cotes JE. *Lung function: assessment and application in medicine,* 3rd ed. Oxford: Blackwell Scientific Publications, 1975: 416.
21. Boushy SF, Thompson HK, North LB, Beale AR, Snow TR. Prognosis in chronic obstructive pulmonary disease. *Am Rev Respir Dis* 1973; 108: 1373.
22. Traver GA, Cline MG, Burrows B. Predictors of mortality in chronic obstructive pulmonary disease. A 15-year follow-up study. *Am Rev Respir Dis* 1979; 119: 895.
23. Comstock GW, Brownlow WJ, Stone RW, Sartwell PE. Cigarette smoking and changes in respiratory findings. *Arch Environ Health* 1970; 21: 50.
24. Doll R, Peto R. Mortality in relation to smoking: 20 years' observations on male British doctors. *Br Med J* 1976; 2: 1525.
25. British Thoracic Society Research Committee. Comparison of four methods of smoking withdrawal in patients with smoking related diseases. *Br Med J* 1983; 286: 595.
26. Belman MJ, Mittman L. Ventilatory muscle training improves exercise capacity in chronic obstructive pulmonary disease patients. *Am Rev Respir Dis* 1980; 121: 275.
27. Morgan AD, Peck DF, Buchanan DR, McHardy GJR. Effects of attitudes and beliefs on exercise tolerance in chronic bronchitis. *Br Med J* 1983; 286: 171.
28. Christie T. Account of good effects from inhaling the smoke of several species of *Datura,* especially the *Datura fastuosa,* in asthma. *Edinburgh Med Surg J* 1811; 7: 153.
29. Mann JS, George CF. Anticholingeric drugs in the treatment of airways disease. *Br J Dis Chest.* 1985; 79: 209.
30. Altounyan REC. Variation of drug action on airway obstruction in man. *Thorax* 1964; 19: 406.
31. Crompton GK. Comparison of responses to bronchodilator drugs in chronic bronchitis and chronic asthma. *Thorax* 1968; 23: 45.
32. Parkes GE, Brogden RC, Heel TM, Speight TM, Avery GS. Ipratropium bromide: a review of its pharmacological properties and therapeutic efficacy in asthma and chronic bronchitis. *Drugs* 1980; 20: 237.
33. Bellamy D, Hutchison DCS. The effects of salbutamol aerosol on lung function in patients with pulmonary emphysema. *Br J Dis Chest.* 1981; 75: 190.
34. McGavin CR, Artvilini M, Naoe M, McHardy GJR. Dyspnoea disability and distance walked: comparison of estimates of exercise performance in respiratory disease. *Br Med J* 1978; 2: 241.
35. Barclay J, Whiting B, Addis GJ. Salbutamol theophylline interaction. Results of adding maximal effective doses of theophylline to the maximal effects obtainable from salbutamol in chronic bronchitis. *Clin Sci* 1980; 59: 13.
36. Lewis AAG. Salbutamol. *Postgrad Med J* 1971; (suppl 47).
37. Inman WHW, Adelstein AM. Rise and fall of asthma mortality in England and Wales in relation to the use of pressurised aerosols. *Lancet* 1969; 2: 279.
38. Winter RJD, Langford JA, Rudd RM. Effects of oral and inhaled steroids and oral pirbuterol on right and left ventricular function in chronic bronchitis. *Br Med J* 1984; 228: 824.
39. Cochrane GM, Prior JG. The role of bronchodilators in the management of chronic bronchitis and emphysema: In: Clark TJH, ed. *Bronchodilator therapy.* Auckland: ADIS Press, 1984: 188.
40. Jenkins SC, Heaton RW, Moxham J. Comparison of domiciliary salbutamol nebuliser and metered dose inhaler (MDI) in stable chronic airflow limitation. *Thorax* 1985; 40: 232.
41. Lindgren SB, Larsson S. Inhalation of terbutaline sulphate through a conventional actuator or a pear-shaped tube: effects and side-effects. *Eur J Respir Dis* 1982; 63: 504.
42. Crompton GK. Inhalation devices. *Eur J Respir Dis* 1982; 63: 489.
43. Newman SP, Pavia D, Little F, Clarke SW. Deposition of pressurised aerosols inhaled through extension devices. *Am Rev Respir Dis* 1981; 124: 317.
44. Petrie GR, Palmer KNV. Comparison of aerosol ipratropium bromide and salbutamol in chronic bronchitis and asthma. *Br Med J* 1975; 1: 430.

45. Leitch AG, Hopkin JM, Ellis DA, Merchant S, McHardy GJR. The effect of ipratropium bromide and salbutamol on exercise tolerance in chronic bronchitis. *Thorax* 1978; 33: 711.
46. Douglas NJ, Davidson I, Sudlow MF, Flenley DC. Bronchodilatation and the site of airway resistance in severe chronic bronchitis. *Thorax* 1979; 34: 51.
47. Marini JJ, Lakshminarayan S. Atropine and terbutaline aerosols in chronic bronchitis. *Chest* 1981; 80: 285.
48. Shenfield GM, Brogden RN, Ward A. Pharmacology of bronchodilators. In: Clark TJH, ed. *Bronchodilator therapy*. Auckland: ADIS Press, 1984: 17.
49. Ullah MI, Newman GB, Saunders KB. Influence of age on response to ipratropium and salbutamol in asthma. *Thorax* 1981; 36: 523.
50. Marlin GE, Berend N, Harrison AC. Combined cholinergic antagonist and beta-adrenoreceptor agonist bronchodilator therapy by inhalation. *Aust NZ J Med* 1979; 9: 511.
51. Shenfield GM. Combination bronchodilator therapy. *Drugs* 1982; 24: 44.
52. Lightbody IM, Ingram CG, Legge JS, Johnston RN. Ipratropium bromide, salbutamol and prednisolone in bronchial asthma and chronic bronchitis. *Br J Dis Chest* 1978; 72: 181.
53. Brady RE, Easton JG. The value of atropine in the documentation of reversible airways obstruction. *Ann Allergy* 1979; 42: 211.
54. Allen JC, Campbell AH. Dose response of ipratropium bromide assessed by two methods. *Thorax* 1980; 35: 137.
55. Thomas P. The effects of aminophylline and salbutamol in the treatment of 'irreversible' chronic obstructive lung disease: a preliminary report. In Turner Warwick M, Levy J, eds. *New perspectives in theophylline therapy*. Roy Soc Med 1984: 91. (International Congress and Symposium Series No. 78.)
56. Neitrzeba RM, Elliott CG, Adams TD, Yeh MP, Yanowitz FG. Effects of aminophylline upon the exercise performance of patients with stable chronic airflow obstruction. *Bull Eur Physiopathol Respir* 1984; 20: 361.
57. Mahler DA, Matthay RA, Snyder PE, Wells CK, Loke J. Sustained-release theophylline reduces dyspnea in non-reversible obstructive airways disease. *Am Rev Respir Dis* 1985; 131: 22.
58. Sutton PP, Pavia D, Bateman JRM, Clarke SW. The effect of oral aminophylline on lung mucociliary clearance in man. *Chest* 1981; 80 (suppl): 889.
59. Aubier M, De Troyer A, Sampson M,. Macklem PT, Roussos C. Aminophylline improves diaphragmatic contractility. *N Engl J Med* 1981; 305: 249.
60. Murciano D, Aubier M, Lecocguic Y, Pariente R. Effects of aminophylline on diaphragmatic strength and fatigue in patients with chronic obstructive pulmonary disease. *N Engl J Med* 1984; 311: 349.
61. Barnes PJ, Greening AP, Neville L, Timmers J, Poole GW. Single-dose slow-release aminophylline at night prevents nocturnal asthma. *Lancet* 1982; 1: 299.
62. Turner-Warwick M. Study of theophylline plasma levels after oral administration of new theophylline compounds. *Br Med J* 1957; 3: 67.
63. Mitenko PA, Ogilvie RI. Rational intravenous doses of theophylline. *N Engl J Med* 1973; 289: 600.
64. Stokes TC, Shaylor JM, O'Reilly JF, Harrison BDW. Assessment of steroid responsiveness in patients with chronic airflow obstruction. *Lancet* 1982; 2: 345.
65. Curzon PGD, Martin MA, Cooke NJ, Muers MF. Effect of oral prednisolone on response to salbutamol and ipratropium bromide aerosols in patients with chronic airflow obstruction. *Thorax* 1983; 38: 601.
66. Paterson IC, Petrie GR, Robertson JR, Crompton GK. Chronic bronchitis: is bacteriological examination of sputum necessary? *Br Med J* 1978; 2: 537.
67. Mitchell-Heggs P, Murphy K, Minty K, Guz A, Patterson SC, Minty PSB, Rosser RM. Diazepam in the treatment of dyspnoea in the 'pink puffer' syndrome. *Q J Med* 1980; 49: 9.
68. Woodcock AA, Gross EF, Geddes DM, Drug treatment of breathlessness: contrasting effects of diazepam and promethazine in pink puffers. *Br Med J* 1981; 283: 343.
69. Woodcock AA, Gross ER, Gellert A, Shah S, Johnson M, Geddes DM. Effects of dihydrocodeine, alcohol and caffeine on breathlessness and exercise tolerance in patients with chronic obstructive lung disease and normal blood gases. *N Engl J Med* 1981; 305: 1611.
70. Campbell EJW. Respiratory failure. The relation between oxygen concentrations of inspired air and arterial blood. *Lancet* 1960; 2: 10.

71. Hutchison DCS, Flenley DC, Donald KW. Controlled oxygen therapy in respiratory failure. *Br Med J* 1964; 2: 1159.
72. Nocturnal Oxygen Therapy Trial Group. Continuous or nocturnal oxygen therapy in hypoxemic chronic obstructive lung disease: a clinical trial. *Ann Intern Med* 1980; 93: 391.
73. Medical Research Council Working Party. Long-term domiciliary oxygen therapy in chronic hypoxic cor pulmonale complicating chronic bronchitis and emphysema. *Lancet* 1981; 1: 681.
74. Grant IWB. Clinical experience with the oxygen concentrator. *Br Med J* 1983; 287: 685.
75. Boman G, Backer U, Larsson S, Melander B, Wahlander L. Oral acetylcysteine reduces exacerbation rate in chronic bronchitis: report of a trial organised by the Swedish Society for Pulmonary Disease. *Eur J Respir Dis* 1983; 64: 405.
76. Brantigan OC, Mueller E, Kress MB. A surgical approach to emphysema. *Am Rev Respir Dis* 1959; 80: 194.
77. Pride NB, Barter CE, Hugh-Jones P. The ventilation of bullae and the effect of their removal on thoracic gas volumes and tests of overall pulmonary function. *Am Rev Respir Dis* 1973; 107: 83.
78. Gadek JE, Fulmer JD, Gelfand JA, Frank MM. Danazol-induced augmentation of serum $alpha_1$-antitrypsin levels in individuals with marked deficiency of this antiprotease. *J Clin Invest* 1980; 66: 82.
79. Gadek JE, Crystal RG. Experience with replacement therapy in the destructive lung disease associated with severe alpha antitrypsin deficiency. *Am Rev Respir Dis* 1983; 127 (suppl): S45.
80. Gadek JE, Klein HG, Holland PV, Crystal RG. Replacement therapy of alpha antitrypsin deficiency: reversal of proteases antiproteases imbalance within the alveolar structures of PiZ subjects. *J Clin Invest* 1985; 68: 1158.
81. Rosenberg S, Barr PJ, Najarian RC, Hallewell RA. Synthesis in yeast of a functional oxidation-resistant mutant of human $alpha_1$-antitrypsin. *Nature* 1984; 312: 77.
82. Powers JC. Synthetic elastase inhibitors: prospects for use in the treatment of emphysema. *Am Rev Respir Dis* 1983; 127: (suppl): S54.

# Chapter 11

# Respiratory Failure

*John Kolbe*

As the primary function of the lungs is to maintain pulmonary gas exchange one would intuitively define the state of respiratory failure as that state existing when the lungs fail to adequately oxygenate the blood and/or fail to facilitate the removal of carbon dioxide from the blood. For practical purposes respiratory failure is defined as being present whenever the arterial oxygen tension ($PO_2$) is below the normal range for the patient's age, altitude, and posture (a value of less than 60mmHg (8.0kPa) is, however, usually accepted) and/or the arterial carbon dioxide tension ($PCO_2$) is above 45mmHg (6.0kPa). Implicit in this definition is the lack of supplemental oxygen and the exclusion of a state of respiratory compensation for a metabolic alkalosis.

Respiratory failure is not a diagnosis in itself, but a symptom of an underlying condition, either pulmonary or non-pulmonary in origin. Therefore any management of respiratory failure must necessarily include management of the underlying condition. In this chapter I have tried to limit my comments to the management of respiratory failure *per se,* but overlap with, and duplication of, the advice of other authors is sometimes unavoidable. Information on the overall management of respiratory failure is included so that the reader may gain some perspective of the relative roles of drugs and other treatment modalities in this condition.

## Pathophysiological Mechanisms

The derangements in the oxygen and carbon dioxide gas tensions occur via a number of different pathophysiological mechanisms and an understanding of these mechanisms is essential for the rational management of all forms of respiratory failure. These mechanisms, together with clinical examples, are shown in Figure 11.1. Chronic carbon dioxide retention impairs the normal central respiratory control mechanism, which is largely dependent upon a central carbon dioxide drive, and substitutes an increasing dependence upon a peripheral hypoxic drive. Thus the patient is more sensitive to the effects of respiratory depressant drugs and to the effects of supplemental oxygen which eliminates the hypoxic drive.

The symptoms and signs attributable to hypoxia and hypercapnia are shown in Table 11.1. A number of points need to be stressed. The clinical assessment of hypoxia and hypercapnia is notoriously inaccurate and should not be relied upon, therefore measurements of arterial blood gas tensions are essential for diagnosis and assessment of progress of patients with respiratory failure. There is, however, no good correlation between symptoms and signs and the arterial blood gas tensions, and a patient with chronic respiratory failure may demonstrate none of these features. Cyanosis is a very late sign of hypoxia.

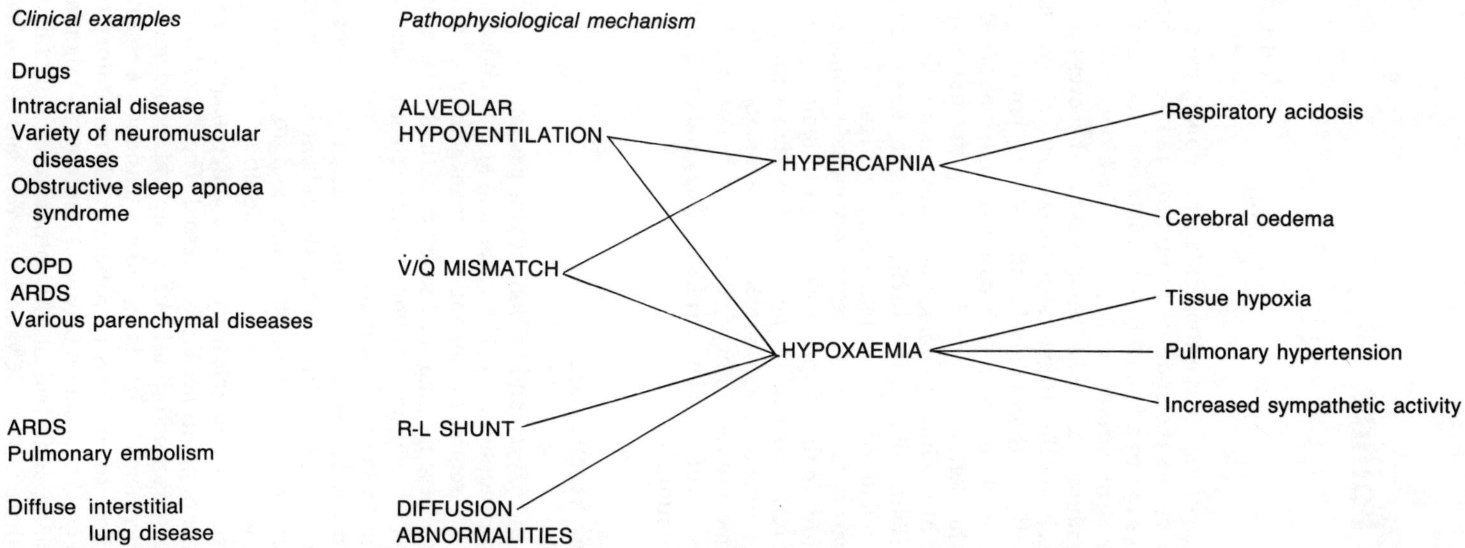


*Figure 11.1* Pathophysiological mechanisms of respiratory failure. COPD = chronic obstructive pulmonary disease. ARDS = adult respiratory distress syndrome. $\dot{V}/\dot{Q}$ = ventilation/perfusion. R-L = right to left.

*Table 11.1* Symptoms and signs of hypoxia and hypercapnia

| Hypoxia | Hypercapnia |
|---|---|
| Confusion | Confusion |
| Restlessness | Somnolence |
| Muscular incoordination | Sweating |
| Tachycardia | Tachycardia |
| Mild hypertension | Mild hypertension |
| Peripheral vasoconstriction | Peripheral vasodilatation |
| Cyanosis | Asterixis |
| | Coma |

Clinical monitoring of the patient's sensorium and cognitive function may be of value in detecting the development of respiratory failure.

## Classification

Respiratory failure is usually due to a generalised condition affecting either the lungs or the respiratory pump mechanism, but may be due to a localised pulmonary abnormality, such as a massive pulmonary embolus. Respiratory failure can be classified in a number of ways; for example, aetiologically, or in terms of the pattern of blood gas abnormality present. For the purpose of this review it will be classified in terms of its rate of onset and the presence or otherwise of severe underlying disease: acute respiratory failure, acute-on-chronic respiratory failure, and chronic respiratory failure.

## Acute Respiratory Failure

In acute respiratory failure, the patient often has no pre-existing pulmonary disease, but develops progressive hypoxaemia following one of a variety of systemic or pulmonary insults. This condition is characterised by marked respiratory distress, hypoxia relatively unresponsive to high concentrations of inspired oxygen, diffuse alveolar shadowing on chest radiograph, and reduced lung compliance in the absence of left ventricular failure. The most satisfactory designation for this non-specific pulmonary disease characterised by increased permeability of the pulmonary vascular endothelium is the 'adult respiratory distress syndrome' (ARDS).

The acute onset of hypoxaemia is poorly tolerated and is often life-threatening. The goals of management in this condition are to treat the underlying cause, reduce pulmonary oedema, maintain oxygen delivery to the tissues and provide general support in order to avoid complications. The management of this condition will be covered in Chapter 15, and will not be therefore discussed further.

## Acute-on-chronic Respiratory Failure

Respiratory failure may develop acutely in patients with underlying disease of the pulmonary parenchyma or chest wall, or in association with neuromuscular diseases causing ventilatory insufficiency. Such acute-on-chronic respiratory failure is often the result of a clearly defined precipitating factor and usually results in both hypoxaemia and hypercapnia. The commonest cause of respiratory failure in this group is an acute exacerbation of chronic obstructive pulmonary disease (COPD). Although respiratory failure does not usually supervene until the underlying condition is severe, most patients survive such exacerbations and an in-hospital mortality rate of less than 5% can be achieved in such patients.[1] However, the long-term prognosis is determined by the nature and severity of the underlying disease.[2]

Common factors that precipitate acute respiratory failure in a patient with chronic disease are intercurrent infection, inappropriate oxygen therapy, inappropriate sedation, an increase in atmospheric pollution, and emergency surgery. The appropriate use of oxygen therapy in this condition is discussed later in this section. Any drug which has a sedative effect is a potential respiratory depressant. Behavioural disorders in patients with respiratory failure are usually due to the effects of hypoxia and/or hypercapnia rather than psychiatric disease. Sedation of such patients is not only inappropriate but hazardous. Instead, management should be directed towards improving the blood gas tensions. The combined effects of anaesthetic agents and abdominal surgery together with analgesic and sedative drugs increase the risk of postoperative respiratory failure, particularly when the severity of the underlying respiratory disease has been underestimated.

The goals of therapy in this condition are the treatment or reversal of the acute precipitating event and support of the patient while this is taking place. Such support of the patient includes maintenance of ventilation and reduction of the work of breathing by the use of bronchodilators, corticosteroids and chest physiotherapy.

## Management

### *Treatment of the Precipitating Event*

Intercurrent infections are the commonest precipitating events and are most common in the winter months and at times when atmospheric pollution is high. They often occur in the absence of fever or a raised white cell count. The initial infection is usually viral in origin, but is shortly followed by a secondary bacterial infection. Any change in colour or volume of the sputum, particularly if microscopy of sputum shows the presence of numerous neutrophils or bacteria, is an indication for antibiotic therapy. The organisms most frequently implicated are *Haemophilus influenzae* and *Streptococcus pneumoniae,* but *Legionella pneumophila* and Gram-negative organisms must also be considered. Parenteral antibiotic therapy should be considered in the first instance and appropriate first-line drugs include ampicillin or amoxycillin (although the emergence of resistant strains of *H influenzae* may reduce the usefulness of these agents), sulphamethoxazole-trimethoprim, cephalosporins (such as cefaclor), tetracycline and erythromycin.

### *General Supportive Measures*

Strict attention to fluid and electrolyte balance is important in correcting the frequently associated dehydration, hyponatraemia and hypokalaemia. Patients with acute-on-chronic respiratory failure are frequently dehydrated due to increased losses from the respiratory tract, the presence of fever, and the lack of fluid intake, and to obtain adequate rehydration intravenous fluids are usually necessary. Although inadequate hydration causes secretions to be difficult to mobilise and impairs mucociliary function, overhydration has no role in making secretions less viscous.

### *Controlled Oxygen Therapy*

Inevitably the patient with acute-on-chronic respiratory failure has hypoxaemia and thus oxygen therapy is indicated. Oxygen, like any other drug, must be ordered and administered in a specific dose (concentration or flow rate), the means of administration must be specified, and the response must be carefully monitored both clinically and with serial blood gas analyses. Like other drugs oxygen has well recognised side effects and in high concentrations definite toxicity. It must therefore be used judiciously. The principles of oxygen therapy and its hazards are fully discussed in Chapter 3.

### *Bronchodilator Therapy*

The rationale for the use of bronchodilators in respiratory failure is that there is usually a variable degree of reversible airflow obstruction present in these patients, and reversal of such obstruction would provide benefits in terms of gas exchange, removal of excessive secretions and reduction in the work of breathing.

Some patients have an acute fall in arterial oxygen tension after the administration of bronchodilators as a result of worsening ventilation-perfusion mismatch. This is due to an increased blood flow to poorly ventilated areas in association with an increased cardiac output, reversal of hypoxic vasoconstriction, and selective deposition of aerosol in better ventilated areas of the lung. This is particularly important in these acutely ill patients who are on the steep portion of the oxyhaemoglobin dissociation curve where a fall in arterial $PO_2$ will be accompanied by a significant fall in oxygen saturation. Although recent studies suggest that this phenomenon may not be as significant as previously thought, bronchodilator therapy should probably always be given with supplemental oxygen.

Details of available bronchodilator drugs are given in Chapter 6 and 10. Even in severely ill patients, adequate administration of beta2-sympathomimetic agents has been reported with the use of metered dose inhalers. In practice patients with acute-on-chronic respiratory failure often cannot use their metered dose inhalers effectively because they are too dyspnoeic or confused, and for more reliable drug administration nebulised aerosols are recommended. Intravenous (IV) administration is usually not necessary and is restricted to those patients who are too ill to manage a nebuliser. The higher doses used and the systemic administration lead to increased side effects.

Gas-driven or ultrasonic nebulisers are preferred for the supply of the aerosol. Arguments for the use of intermittent positive pressure breathing (IPPB) to deliver aerosols are based on the premise that the large breaths taken with IPPB decrease airway obstruction, prevent atelectasis and help the removal of secretions. There is little evidence to support such contentions and the same effects can be achieved without the use of IPPB.[3]

### *Corticosteroids*

The pharmacology of corticosteroids is discussed in Chapter 8, and their use in chronic bronchitis and emphysema in Chapter 10.

### *Respiratory Stimulants*

The efficacy of these drugs in patients with respiratory failure is still debated. Details of their actions are given in Chapter 4.

### *Mobilisation of Tracheobronchial Secretions*

Many patients with acute-on-chronic respiratory failure have problems with increased volumes of tenacious secretions, and removal of such secretions would improve gas exchange and reduce the work of breathing. A number of methods have been used in this endeavour. These include nebulised mists, mucolytic agents and physiotherapy.

**Nebulised mists.** Aerosols of water or saline have been used in an attempt to liquify tracheobronchial secretions in order to aid their removal by mucociliary transport and/or by cough. Only a very small proportion of the aerosol produced by air jets or ultrasonic nebulisers is deposited in the lung,[4] and this is therefore unlikely to significantly alter the visco-elastic characteristics of the tracheobronchial secretions. Humidification of inspired air and inhalation of bland aerosols does not increase mucociliary clearance in experimental animals or normal humans, but stimulation of mucociliary clearance has been observed in patients with COPD after inhalation of saline aerosols.[5,6]

Caution must be observed regarding the use of water aerosols particularly in that subgroup of patients with bronchial hyper-responsiveness. Aerosols of hypotonic as well as hypertonic solutions are well recognised precipitants of bronchoconstriction in such patients,[7] and may thus lead to aggravation of the gas exchange abnormalities in an already severely compromised patient. Aerosol generators and nebulisers may also serve as sources of nosocomial infection. Although dry air may have an adverse effect on mucociliary clearance and increase the osmolality of tracheal secretions, there seems to be insufficient justification for the administration of water or saline aerosols to improve clearance of tracheobronchial secretions, particularly in view of the potentially adverse effects of such aerosols.

Much of the evidence for the efficacy of mist therapy in pulmonary disease is based on studies of children with cystic fibrosis.[8,9] Recent evidence suggests that the underlying defect in cystic fibrosis may be a disorder of ion and water transport at a number of sites such as the sweat glands, nasal epithelium and tracheobronchial epithelium.[10-14] In the tracheobronchial epithelium, the primary defect appears to be an impermeability of the apical cell membrane to chloride ions in the presence of a normal absorptive sodium pump. This leads to the net absorption of ions and water and to relative dehydration of secretions. Hence in this condition there is at least a theoretical basis for a beneficial effect of saline aerosols. Whether amiloride, which inhibits sodium absorption from the apical cell membrane but has little effect on the submucosal gland secretion of sodium and chloride, is beneficial requires definitive study.

Basal ion and water transport in airways is mainly under cholinergic control, probably via effects on submucosal gland output.[15] In vitro such transport can be influenced by numerous drugs, such as frusemide, ouabain, amiloride and terbutaline, as well as various autacoids such as histamine, acetylcholine, adrenaline, $PGE_2$, $PGF_{2a}$, vasoactive intestinal peptide and substance P.[16] Whether pharmacologically induced changes in water and ion transport across the respiratory epithelim can favourably influence the properties of secretions and aid their removal in patients with various forms of respiratory failure awaits the results of future studies.

**Mucolytic agents.** Mucolytic agents are used in an attempt to reduce the viscosity of tracheobronchial secretions and thus make them easier to mobilise and remove. Although studies confirm acetylcysteine as an effective agent to liquify both mucoid and purulent bronchial secretions *in vitro* no mucolytic agent has established itself as being of benefit in the management of patients with respiratory failure.[17] Mucolytic agents can cause oedema of the bronchial wall and bronchospasm and, although pretreatment with a bronchodilator has been recommended, the safest course of action would seem to be avoidance of such agents altogether.

Detergents such as propylene glycol 5% and glycerin 5% have no significant mucolytic effects, but are used in an attempt to improve the hydration of the secretions. There is no evidence that these agents increase mucociliary clearance or improve pulmonary function,[17] and in vitro they have little more sputum-thinning activity than water or saline.

**Physiotherapy.** The goal of chest physiotherapy is to clear excessive tracheobronchial secretions and in doing so support the defence mechanisms of the lung, reduce the work of breathing, improve gas exchange and reduce the risk of additional pulmonary infection and alveolar collapse.

Despite its widespread use, the benefits of physiotherapy in patients with acute-on-chronic respiratory failure remain controversial. There are a number of studies demonstrating a lack of benefit from physiotherapy in acute exacerbations of COPD,[18-20] and others showing an acute detrimental effect in terms of lung volumes and arterial oxygenation.[21,22]

However, the volume of the sputum appears to be an important factor in determining whether chest physiotherapy is effective. Physiotherapy is without benefit and potentially hazardous in acutely ill patients without sputum production. Its usefulness is restricted to those patients producing moderate or large quantities of sputum,[22,23] even if such patients require mechanical ventilation.[22]

### *Mechanical Ventilation*

Some patients will be so ill at presentation, or will rapidly and progressively deteriorate in spite of the above measures, that they will require mechanical ventilation. A detailed description of the various forms of mechanical ventilation and the use of other associated treatment modalities is beyond the scope of this text and will not be discussed further. Circumstances vary greatly and the type of ventilatory support must be tailored to the patient's individual needs. Management of the patient with respiratory failure requiring mechanical ventilation should be undertaken in an intensive care unit by physicians familiar with the techniques required for intubation and mechanical ventilation and aware and capable of dealing with any complications that may arise.

*Avoidance of Complications*

Arrhythmias, especially atrial arrhythmias, are common in acute-on-chronic respiratory failure and may be aggravated by hypoxia, acidosis and certain drugs such as sympathomimetics and theophylline. Anti-arrhythmic drugs are relatively ineffective in the control of such arrhythmias and correction of hypoxaemia, acid-base balance and electrolyte abnormalities are most important.

Pulmonary embolism may complicate the course of respiratory failure in a significant proportion of patients,[24] and there is evidence that this proportion can be reduced, without significant complications, by the use of low-dose heparin prophylaxis.[25]

Gastrointestinal bleeding from superficial gastric ulceration occurs frequently in patients with acute respiratory failure. Rates of 18 to 25% have been reported, but this frequency can be significantly reduced by the prophylactic administration of antacids via a nasogastric tube.[26,27]

## Chronic Respiratory Failure

Some patients because of severe underlying disease have permanent severe derangement of arterial blood gas tensions so that, by the definition given earlier, they remain in a state of chronic respiratory failure. The prognosis of such patients depends on the severity and nature of the underlying disease and in the vast majority the long-term outlook is poor. The commonest cause of chronic respiratory failure is severe COPD, but it may also be the result of diffuse interstitial lung disease, chest wall disorders and a variety of neuromuscular disorders.

### Management

*Bronchodilator Therapy*

The rationale for the use of bronchodilators in chronic respiratory failure, particularly those with COPD, is that most patients have some degree of reversibility of their airflow obstruction,[28,29] and thus marginal benefit will be gained by many and substantial benefit by some. The use of such drugs should not necessarily be restricted only to those patients who demonstrate an acute response on spirometric testing because of the relative insensitivity of these tests and the potential for long-term versus short-term benefit. Also 'non-responders' to a single bronchodilator may respond to another class of bronchodilator.

Such therapy includes beta2-sympathomimetics, oral methylxanthines (theophylline), anticholinergic drugs and calcium antagonist drugs. The use of these agents has been fully discussed in the chapter dealing with chronic bronchitis and emphysema (Chapter 10).

## *Corticosteroids*

There are no well documented studies proving the efficacy of long-term corticosteroid therapy in the majority of patients with respiratory failure. The published reports give conflicting results, and many are uncontrolled, not double-blind, and depend on subjective end-points.[30] However, a proportion of patients has a substantial improvement in symptoms and/or lung function tests after steroids. Therefore each case in this heterogeneous group must be considered individually with respect to the efficacy of steroid therapy. There are no clinical or laboratory markers which reliably identify the steroid-responsive group. If the patient's response to maximal bronchodilator therapy is less than satisfactory, a trial of steroids for two to four weeks is justified. In those patients in whom there has not been an objective improvement in serial lung function tests, steroids should be slowly withdrawn. Clinical judgement must be used in those patients who give a convincing history of improved exercise tolerance without an objective improvement in lung function tests. The situation in which the patient is placed on long-term steroid therapy without objective benefit and subsequently develops severe steroid side effects must be avoided. Between 11 and 28% of such patients may be expected to have a substantial improvement in lung function tests,[31-33] and in this group the steroid therapy is altered to an alternate-day regimen employing the lowest dose of steroid that will maintain the level of improvement.

## *Pulmonary Vasodilators*

In many patients with chronic respiratory failure, the disease process is complicated by the development of pulmonary hypertension and cor pulmonale. (The term cor pulmonale denotes right ventricular enlargement, hypertrophy and/or dilation, secondary to an abnormality of the lungs, ventilatory pump or control of breathing and does not necessarily imply overt clinical right ventricular failure.) Chronic hypoxia is the major aetiological mechanism in the development and progression of pulmonary hypertension and the sequence of pathophysiological changes occurring as a result of chronic hypoxia is shown in Figure 11.2. Destruction of pulmonary capillaries is not the major mechanism in the development of pulmonary hypertension as two-thirds to three-quarters of the capillaries need to be destroyed before pulmonary hypertension develops. Cor pulmonale is not the only serious consequence of pulmonary hypertension: these patients are at an increased risk of pulmonary embolism and sudden death. Fourteen per cent of the deaths in the Nocturnal Oxygen Therapy Trial (NOTT) study were sudden and presumably the result of arrhythmias.[34]

The mechanism of hypoxic vasoconstriction is not known but two theories predominate. The first states that hypoxia may cause release of mediators which cause vasoconstriction. A number of mediators such as serotonin, histamine, various prostaglandins ($PGD_2$, $PGI_2$, $PGF_{2\alpha}$) and leukotrienes are able to modulate pulmonary arterial tone, but a definite role for any single mediator or group of mediators is not proven. Leukotrienes seem to play a central role in hypoxic vasoconstriction in the isolated perfused adult rat and ferret lungs, in intact sheep and in awake rats. The second theory states

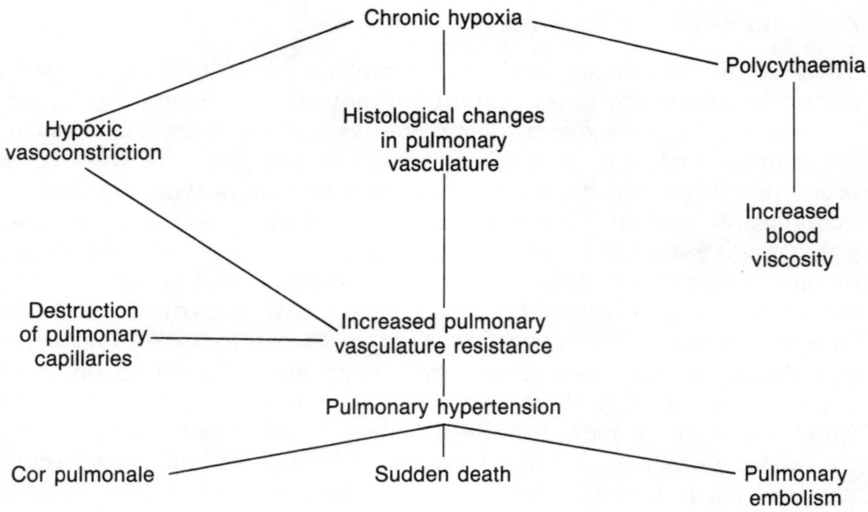


*Figure 11.2* Pathophysiological consequences of chronic hypoxia.

that hypoxia may alter the membrane potential in vascular smooth muscle cells, interfere with the ability of these cells to maintain transmembrane concentration gradients, and thus allow entry of extracellular calcium into the smooth muscle cell which leads to vasoconstriction.

In patients with COPD complicated by hypoxic cor pulmonale and carbon dioxide retention, the reported three-year mortality varies from 32 to 100%.[35-42] Therefore, in recent years therapy has been directed at reducing the elevated pulmonary artery pressure in patients with severe underlying disease.

Two broad therapeutic approaches may be taken to the problem of secondary pulmonary hypertension. The first approach is the early identification and treatment of patients with mild pulmonary hypertension in the hope of preventing progression of the disease and perhaps reversing changes which have taken place. Such early identification of patients is limited by an inability to measure pulmonary artery pressure non-invasively and the insensitivity of clinical criteria. Although cor pulmonale is found at autopsy in about 45% of patients with COPD, only about 30% of these will have had electrocardiographic or chest radiographic evidence of this complication. The arterial $PO_2$ is probably the best single indicator; 80% of patients with an arterial $PO_2$ of less than 60mmHg (8.0kPa) have right ventricular hypertrophy. The assessment of these patients is further complicated by the fact that pulmonary artery pressure is not a stable parameter, and patients with a normal pressure at rest may develop pulmonary hypertension during exercise, sleep or periods of acute respiratory failure. It is not known at what level pulmonary hypertension *per se* becomes harmful, nor at what level of pulmonary artery pressure intervention should take place.

The other therapeutic approach and the most common form of pharmacological intervention is treatment of the patient with established pulmonary hypertension and cor pulmonale in the hope of reducing the pulmonary artery pressure, increasing the cardiac output, reducing symptoms, improving exercise tolerance and increasing longevity. Because of the complex relationship between pressure and blood flow, estimation of the degree of reversibility of the vasoconstriction and the response to drug therapy is often very difficult.[43] Also there are no suitable non-invasive methods of assessing the degree of reversibility of pulmonary hypertension.

The use of vasodilators in patients with chronic respiratory failure complicated by pulmonary hypertension is based on the following premises: (i) that an increased afterload is the major insult to the right ventricle in cor pulmonale; (ii) that active and hence reversible pulmonary vasoconstriction makes a significant contribution to the increased pulmonary vascular resistance; (iii) that prolonged relief of the vasoconstriction will lead to reversal of the histological changes in the pulmonary arterioles; (iv) that if the pulmonary vascular resistance can be reduced, there must be sufficient residual right ventricular function to pump blood through the lungs — right ventricular dysfunction has been demonstrated in most patients with hypoxic COPD,[44,45,46] and in patients with cor pulmonale there is relative endocardial ischaemia during exercise; and (v) that drugs active as vasodilators in the systemic circuit are likely to be active also in the pulmonary circuit.

Some of the drugs which have been used as pulmonary vasodilators are shown in Table 11.2. However, oxygen is the most effective pulmonary vasodilator and its long-term domiciliary use will be discussed later in this chapter. In normal subjects most drugs that dilate the pulmonary vascular bed also dilate the systemic vascular bed, but it is not possible to predict the relative effects of the drugs in the two vascular beds. If the pulmonary vascular bed is hyporesponsive, the isolated systemic vasodilatation would lead to systemic hypotension and reduced cardiac output. The other major side effect of these agents is worsening of hypoxaemia by the selective reversal of hypoxic vasoconstriction and worsening of ventilation-perfusion mismatch. These risks can be minimised by initially using low intravenous doses of a short-acting vasodilator whilst carefully monitoring haemodynamic parameters.

*Table 11.2* Agents which have pulmonary vasodilating properties

| | |
|---|---|
| *Alpha-adrenergic Blockers* | *Smooth Muscle Relaxants* |
| Tolazoline | Hydrallazine |
| Phentolamine | Minoxidil |
| | Prazosin |
| *Beta-adrenergic Agonists* | Diazoxide |
| Isoprenaline | Nitroprusside |
| | Nitrates |
| *Parasympathomimetics* | *Calcium Channel Blockers* |
| Acetylcholine | Diltiazem |
| | Nifedipine |
| *Eicosanoids* | Verapamil |
| Prostacyclin | *Converting Enzyme Inhibitors* |
| $PGE_1$ analogues | Captopril |
| *Leukotriene Synthetase and Receptor Blockers* | |

There is no agreement as to the best vasodilator drug, apart from oxygen, for the treatment of hypoxic pulmonary hypertension. Such therapy should be reserved until more conventional treatment with bronchodilators and controlled supplemental oxygen has failed to alleviate the pulmonary hypertension and cor pulmonale. At our present state of knowledge, any vasodilator therapy should be part of an appropriately controlled trial, and institution of treatment should take place under intensive haemodynamic monitoring. In chronic respiratory failure short-term haemodynamic benefit has been demonstrated with a number of agents including glyceryl trinitrate (nitroglycerin), $PGE_1$, hydrallazine and nifedipine, but short-term haemodynamic efficacy does not necessarily indicate long-term haemodynamic benefit, and a haemodynamic effect does not necessarily translate into improved exercise tolerance or increased longevity.[47]

Early reports of the short-term success of these agents ushered in a phase of great enthusiasm. However, more recent reports of therapeutic failures and unwanted, even dangerous, side effects have tempered this initial enthusiasm. Hydrallazine has been most studied as a pulmonary vasodilator in chronic respiratory failure. Results of studies of the haemodynamic effects of this agent have ranged from those showing significant improvement,[48-50] to those showing little or no haemodynamic improvement,[51] and those showing detrimental effects.[52] At present there is insufficient evidence to support the widespread use of hydrallazine as a pulmonary vasodilator.

As pulmonary vasoconstriction is dependent on the availability of calcium to the effector cell, drugs which inhibit the voltage-dependent entry of calcium into smooth muscle cells may theoretically be useful in the management of hypoxic pulmonary vasoconstriction. Such agents may also prevent the release of mediators which are important in vasoconstriction. Nifedipine is approximately one hundred times more active in inhibiting voltage-dependent calcium entry into vascular smooth muscle cells than diltiazem or verapamil, and is thus the most potent drug in its effects on the pulmonary vasculature. Nifedipine inhibits hypoxic vasoconstriction in laboratory animals[53] and in patients with acute respiratory failure.[54] In a controlled double-blind study of COPD patients with pulmonary hypertension, nifedipine acutely reduced both pulmonary artery pressure and pulmonary vasculature resistance at rest and during exercise under hypoxic conditions. Nifedipine, when added to low-flow oxygen therapy, further reduced pulmonary vasculature resistance at rest and during exercise.[55] However, in some patients with severe COPD and pulmonary hypertension, nifedipine causes a significant fall in the arterial $PO_2$ due to inhibition of hypoxic pulmonary vasoconstriction,[55,56] although because of the increased cardiac output, oxygen delivery to the tissues may be increased.

In rats, nifedipine inhibited the development of right ventricular hypertrophy and muscularisation of the pulmonary arterioles of animals exposed to intermittent hypoxia. Nifedipine, when used in established pulmonary hypertension, caused partial regression of right ventricular hypertrophy and muscularisation of the pulmonary arterioles.[57] Whether long-term nifedipine therapy prevents or reverses the pathological changes of cor pulmonale in humans is not known.

As a pulmonary vasodilator, $PGE_1$, which has the beneficial feature of being metabolised and largely inactivated in the lung, has been useful on a short-term basis.[58] More recently, OP-1206, an orally active $PGE_1$ derivative, has produced acute beneficial haemodynamic effects in patients with COPD or pulmonary fibrosis.[59]

Leukotrienes, specifically leukotriene $C_4$, have been suggested as mediators involved in the production of hypoxic vasoconstriction, and various structurally dissimilar inhibitors of leukotriene synthesis and/or action have been shown to inhibit hypoxic pulmonary vasoconstriction in the isolated rat[60] and ferret lung,[61] in intact sheep,[62] and in awake rats.[63] Whether such agents are useful in patients with chronic respiratory failure and pulmonary hypertension is not yet known.

Pulmonary hypertension and cor pulmonale may also complicate the course of cystic fibrosis and indicate a poor prognosis. Although extensive studies of vasodilator therapy have not been undertaken initial work suggests that, while oxygen therapy may have beneficial haemodynamic effects in such patients, there is no evidence that supports the use of vasodilator drugs.[64]

Hence the role of vasodilator drugs is still not clear and a number of major questions remain unanswered. Which drug or drugs are most effective and is there a selective pulmonary vasodilator? What are the effects of long-term therapy with vasodilators and do these agents reverse histological changes, improve exercise tolerance or increase longevity? How can patients most likely to benefit from vasodilator therapy and those most likely to suffer adverse effects be identified non-invasively?

### *Long-term Oxygen Therapy*

Hypoxia is the most effective and consistent stimulus to the development of pulmonary hypertension[65] and resting levels of pulmonary artery pressure are inversely correlated with resting arterial oxygen pressure, pre-sleep oxygen saturation and mean sleep oxygen saturation.[66] Thus the reversal of hypoxia may be expected to have haemodynamic benefit. Indeed, oxygen therapy is the only therapy proven to improve survival of patients with chronic respiratory failure.

The present use of long-term domiciliary oxygen is based primarily on the results of two hallmark studies performed in the late 1970s: the British Medical Research Council (MRC) Working Party study (1981)[67] and the Nocturnal Oxygen Therapy Trial (NOTT) Group study (1980).[34] In the MRC trial of patients with COPD complicated by cor pulmonale and carbon dioxide retention, mortality was reduced in the nocturnal oxygen group (15 hours a day) compared with the no-oxygen group (45.2% compared with 66.7%), although the survival advantage which occurred only for the men did not emerge until after 500 days. In the long-term survivors, although the pulmonary artery pressure was not consistently lower, it appeared that oxygen therapy prevented the progression of hypoxia and pulmonary hypertension. There was no associated rise in the arterial $PCO_2$.

In the NOTT trial the overall mortality of hypoxic COPD patients in the nocturnal oxygen therapy group (12 hours a day) was 1.94 times that of the continuous oxygen therapy group (17.7 hours a day). Continuous oxygen therapy appeared most beneficial to those with poor pulmonary function, hypoventilation, mental disturbances, and least disturbed pulmonary haemodynamics. Neither oxygen programme resulted in correction or near-correction of the baseline haemodynamic abnormality although the continuous oxygen group did show improvements in pulmonary artery pressure, pulmonary vascular resistance, and stroke volume index, while the nocturnal oxygen group showed stable haemodynamic parameters. For both groups the changes in mean pulmonary artery pressure during the first six months were associated with subsequent survival suggesting that the haemodynamic response to oxygen therapy is predictive of survival.[66]

Hence oxygen therapy sufficient to abolish severe hypoxaemia improved mortality in patients with COPD, and the longer the period of oxygen therapy (and hence reversal of hypoxia) the greater the benefits. Periods of therapy less than 12 hours a day do not produce significant benefit. Although data obtained on long-term oxygen therapy have come from studies of patients with COPD most believe that such data are applicable to other forms of hypoxic lung disease.

The precise mechanism by which long-term oxygen therapy improves mortality is not known, but the potential beneficial effects are shown in Figure 11.3. Oxygen acutely reverses hypoxic vasoconstriction and it has been suggested that those patients with cor pulmonale due to COPD who show a fall in mean pulmonary artery pressure greater than 5mmHg (0.7kPa) when breathing 28% inspired oxygen for 24 hours have a better two-year survival rate than those who do not have a fall in pulmonary artery pressure.[68] In many patients, however, administration causes little acute change in

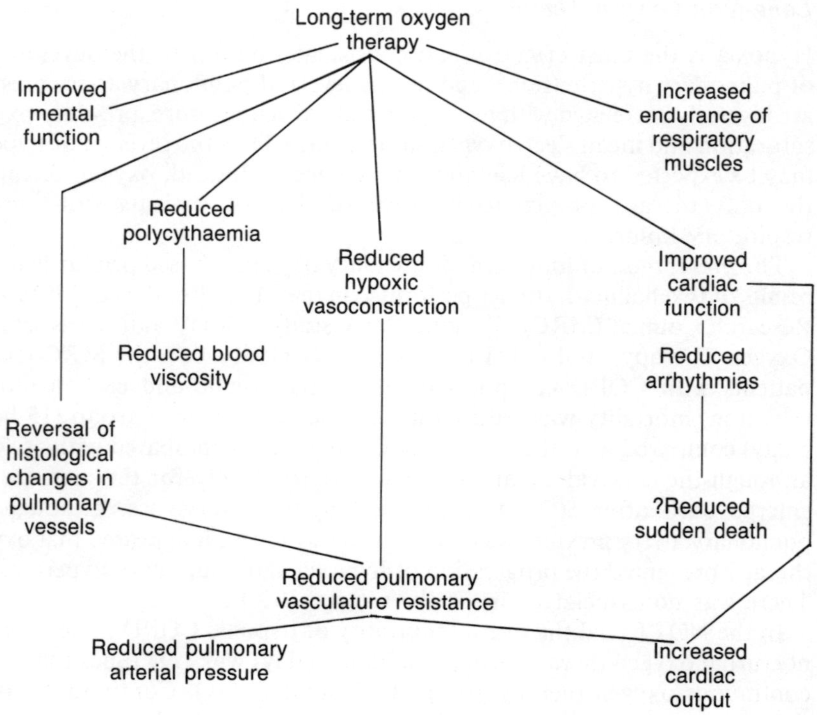


*Figure 11.3* Beneficial effects of long-term oxygen therapy.

pulmonary artery pressure[66] suggesting that this may not be the major mechanism of action of oxygen therapy. In animal studies, increasing duration of normal oxygenation caused a progressive reversal of the physiological and pathological consequences of hypoxia.[69,70] Similarly, brief administration of oxygen to a patient with COPD complicated by pulmonary hypertension or to a high-altitude dweller causes only slight temporary relief of pulmonary hypertension. However, prolonged reflief of hypoxia by oxygen administration in patients with COPD[71,72] or permanent descent to sea level of high-altitude dwellers[73] leads to gradual reversal of pulmonary hypertension, suggesting that reversal of the histological changes in the pulmonary blood vessels may have taken place.

The arterial oxygen saturation falls transiently in sleep, particularly REM sleep, in many patients with respiratory failure. The mechanism by which this occurs is complex, but is likely to be due to periods of hypoventilation rather than to associated obstructive sleep apnoea.[74] The awake arterial $PO_2$ correlates with the severity of the nocturnal hypoxaemia[74-76] and a causal relationship has been postulated between these episodes of nocturnal transient worsening of hypoxaemia, which are associated with transient elevations of pulmonary artery pressure, and the development of sustained pulmonary hypertension and cor pulmonale.[77,78] Nocturnal supplemental oxygen can alleviate these episodes of desaturation without causing important rises in arterial $PCO_2$, and prevent the associated rise in pulmonary artery pressure[79,80] and the associated cardiac arrhythmias.[81,82] Long-term therapy with nocturnal oxygen leads to a lower mean pulmonary artery pressure, lower pulmonary vascular resistance and increased cardiac output in a significant proportion of patients.[83] The unproven implication is that in patients with COPD and nocturnal hypoxaemia, nocturnal oxygen therapy may prevent the development of sustained pulmonary hypertension and cor pulmonale. At present it is not known when low-flow nocturnal therapy should be instituted and which patients are likely to benefit most. Routine pulmonary function tests correlate poorly with nocturnal events, but the high degree of correlation between arterial $PO_2$ during wakefulness and the lowest level of arterial $PO_2$ during sleep suggests that this parameter may be a useful indicator.

Most studies indicate that hypoxaemic COPD patients whose arterial $PO_2$ worsens with exercise will improve their exercise endurance and capacity when given supplemental oxygen. Menkes et al[84] suggest that patients with exercise-induced dyspnoea whose $PO_2$ is between 60 and 65mmHg (8.0-8.6kPa) should be evaluated with an exercise test. If the $PO_2$ falls significantly and oxygen improves exercise tolerance, the patient should receive domiciliary oxygen. Limited data are available in patients with restrictive lung disease, but it is suggested that supplemental oxygen during exercise improves exercise endurance but not work capacity.

The fundamental mechanism of dyspnoea is incompletely understood, but it is clear that it may or may not be associated with hypoxaemia severe enough to affect tissue oxygenation. Oxygen therapy should be limited to the treatment of hypoxaemia and its consequences rather than the subjective relief of dyspnoea *per se*. There is, however, at least one well designed and controlled study of 'normoxic' at-rest patients with marked dyspnoea that clearly shows that oxygen therapy relieves dyspnoea and improves exercise tolerance.[85] These patients did not desaturate during exercise and there was no means of predicting those patients more likely to benefit.

The ACCP-NHL BI National Conference on Oxygen Therapy[86] suggested that before the initiation of long-term oxygen therapy all four following conditions should be met: (i) an accurate, current diagnosis must have been established; (ii) an optimal medical regimen prescribed by a physician knowledgeable in chest disease must have been in effect; (iii) the patient's condition must have been stable for at least one month and have recovered from any acute exacerbation; (iv) oxygen therapy must have been shown to, or can reasonably be predicted to, improve the hypoxaemia or tissue hypoxia, or provide overall clinical benefit. Such circumstances would include an arterial $PO_2$ of less than 55mmHg (7.3kPa), secondary polycythaemia, and evidence of pulmonary hypertension and/or cor pulmonale.

Continued cigarette smoking by patients receiving oxygen therapy is contraindicated because it reduces the physiological benefit of the therapy, and for safety reasons. Also there is a reluctance to offer relatively scarce public resources to patients who will not help themselves by giving up smoking.[87]

Long-term oxygen therapy is given at a concentration to alleviate hypoxaemia, that is, to maintain the arterial $PO_2$ above 60mmHg (8.0kPa). There are three main sources of oxygen for domiciliary use: compressed gas oxygen cylinders, liquid oxygen and oxygen concentrators, and the choice between these depends upon patient requirements and mobility, initial and long-term costs, and local availability and services. Supplementation is usually accomplished by administration of a low concentration of oxygen via a nasal cannula or mask for at least 15 hours a day. Patients with intermittent hypoxaemia may benefit from oxygen therapy during these periods; for example, during sleep, air travel or exercise. Like all other forms of therapy there must be an assessment of the clinical and physiological effects of therapy, and the continued need for oxygen therapy should be evaluated on several occasions during the first year and then on a yearly basis.

### *Treatment of Respiratory Muscle Fatigue*

Over recent years it has become clear that respiratory muscle fatigue contributes to the pathogenesis of both acute and chronic hypercapnic respiratory failure.[88] There are a number of factors present in patients with underlying lung disease which contribute to the development of respiratory muscle fatigue. These include: (i) increased work and energy cost of breathing; (ii) reduced efficiency of the respiratory muscles; (iii) abnormal patterns of breathing with increased use of intercostal and accessory muscles; (iv) reduced inspiratory muscle strength due to the mechanical disadvantage of the diaphragm in patients with hyperinflation; (v) compromise of inspiratory muscle strength by malnutrition, hypoxia and acidosis; and (vi) atrophy of the diaphragm and intercostal muscles particularly in patients with severe airflow obstruction.[89] Inspiratory muscle fatigue leads to dyspnoea, tachypnoea, reduced exercise tolerance, paradoxical abdominal movements, and finally respiratory acidosis and failure.

Management of respiratory muscle fatigue may include rest, use of pharmacological agents, or respiratory muscle training. Rest of the respiratory muscles is achieved by the introduction of mechanical ventilation while the work of breathing is reduced with the use of bronchodilators and corticosteroids. Daily intermittent rest of the respiratory muscles by means of mechanical ventilation has been shown to improve respiratory muscle strength, ventilatory performance and function in a group of COPD patients with respiratory failure. It is not clear what duration of rest is required to permit recovery of the respiratory muscles from acute fatigue, nor the effects of intermittent rest combined with other treatment modalities.

Theophylline has a beneficial effect on respiratory function in experimental animals,[90-92] normal subjects,[93] and in patients with severe airway disease.[94] In a study of patients with severe COPD, hypoxaemia and hypercapnia, oral doses of theophylline sufficient to produce serum levels in the therapeutic range increased diaphragmatic strength and suppressed diaphragmatic fatigue in all patients who received it, and this effect persisted for at least 30 days. All subjects who received theophylline were reported to have experienced subjective relief.[94] Although in some trials oral theophylline produced relief of dyspnoea in patients with COPD and chronic respiratory failure,[95,96] in other studies this drug did not reduce dyspnoea either acutely[97] or with longer term treatment,[98] whether or not improvements in lung volumes occurred.[96,98] Although Leitch et al[99] reported a slight increase in exercise capacity in patients with COPD, this was associated with a significant increase in $FEV_1$, and a similar but slightly greater improvement in exercise capacity occurred with the use of oral salbutamol. This improvement was of the order seen with placebo in other studies.[100] Hence on the basis of present information there is insufficient evidence to recommend the use of oral theophylline in respiratory failure on the basis of its effect on dyspnoea or exercise tolerance, particularly in view of the drug's potentially toxic side effects.

The major limiting factor to exercise in many patients with chronic respiratory failure is an impaired ventilatory capacity, and therefore improvement of maximum sustained ventilatory capacity through respiratory muscle training might be expected to increase exercise tolerance. Indeed, a number of investigators have reported that respiratory muscle training improves respiratory muscle function and exercise tolerance in patients with severe COPD.[101-103] However, the results of the study by Pardy et al[103] suggested that respiratory muscle training may benefit only that group of patients whose exercise tolerance is limited specifically by the development of respiratory muscle fatigue.

Various exercise training programmes have had variable effects on the exercise performance of patients with severe COPD, some showing no effects and others showing only minor effects.[104-107] With some exceptions,[108] most studies which have compared a somatic exercise programme with specific respiratory muscle training programmes have demonstrated greater increases in exercise performance with the respiratory muscle training programme or a combination of the programmes.[103,109]

Of concern is evidence that some patients with severe respiratory failure who are required to inspire through resistive devices during respiratory muscle training may acutely develop hypoventilation and arterial desaturation when simple clinical tolerance for a specified time is used in selecting a suitable training load.[103,110] Hence, prior to the institution of an inspiratory muscle training programme it is important to determine whether respiratory muscle fatigue develops during exercise, and is therefore likely to be a limiting factor, and to ensure that the training load is appropriate and does not lead to acute hypoventilation and an associated derangement in arterial blood gas tensions.

*Physiotherapy*

Many patients with respiratory failure have excessive tracheobronchial secretions due to a number of factors: excessive production of secretions by increased numbers of goblet cells and hypertrophied submucous glands, impaired mucociliary clearance, and decreased cough efficiency. Chest physiotherapy is undertaken in an effort to clear these excessive secretions and, although its use is widespread, Jones[111] in his review of this subject found little objective data to support its use in chronic respiratory failure.

The essential prerequisite for effectiveness of chest physiotherapy is that the volume of tracheobronchial secretions be large and able to be loosened by percussion and/or vibration and carried to the pharynx by gravity, aided by postural drainage, or by coughing. Those studies which show a beneficial effect of physiotherapy in chronic respiratory failure are those performed on patients producing large volumes of sputum.[112,113] However, if the patient is producing little or no sputum, then physiotherapy is unlikely to be beneficial.[114-116]

When cough is prohibited, postural drainage increases the clearance of central airway secretions and the amount of sputum production in patients with excessive tracheobronchial secretions.[117] Physiotherapy is more effective than cough alone in clearing secretions from the peripheral lung, but may be no more effective than cough alone in removing secretions from the central airways.[118] Whether therapy such as external vibration improves clearance of excessive tracheobronchial secretions is not yet clear,[119] but animal studies suggest that chest wall vibrations at frequencies which are near the natural ciliary beat frequency produce enhanced tracheal mucus transport.[120]

Hence physiotherapy may benefit those patients with chronic respiratory failure who produce large volumes of sputum (more than 30ml per day). Physiotherapy should be performed after the administration of bronchodilator drugs, and supplemental oxygen should be given to severely hypoxaemic patients. The long-term effects of physiotherapy on sputum production and removal, pulmonary function, prevention of complications, and the natural history of the underlying disease are unknown.

*Digoxin and Diuretics*

Digoxin has not been shown to improve right heart function in chronic respiratory failure patients without left heart failure,[121] and should not be used for isolated cor pulmonale. Although acute digitalisation may enhance the ionotropic state of the right ventricle, it also increases pulmonary artery pressure and pulmonary vascular resistance, thus offsetting any beneficial effects.[122] The increased susceptibility to digoxin toxicity of patients with chronic respiratory failure is associated with an increased sensitivity to the drug rather than to an alteration in its metabolism.[122]

In chronic respiratory failure the accepted indication for digoxin is left ventricular failure unresponsive to diuretic therapy alone. There is a high rate of left ventricular dysfunction in patients with cor pulmonale and the cause of this remains controversial. With the advent of potent more specific antiarrhythmic drugs digoxin is no longer the drug of choice for supraventricular arrhythmias with rapid ventricular response.

Diuretic therapy may be useful in those patients with chronic respiratory failure who have fluid retention, but often such oedema is resistant to diuretics. Usually an improvement in oxygenation will promote a brisk diuresis even in the absence of diuretics by decreasing pulmonary vascular resistance and increasing cardiac output.[123] Cautious use of diuretics is recommended as they can cause hypokalaemia, hypochloraemia and a metabolic alkalosis which can reduce alveolar ventilation and increase the affinity of haemoglobin for oxygen, leading to tissue hypoxia. Also the liberal use of diuretics reduces right ventricular preload and, if right ventricular filling pressure (or volume) is reduced below a critical level, the cardiac output falls. Diuretics should be reserved for patients with overt right ventricular failure in whom the markedly increased preload is a significant contribution to the impaired cardiac output.

*Other Therapies*

Continuous antibiotic therapy reduces the number of exacerbations in patients who have frequent relapses, but does not influence the rate of decline of pulmonary function or increase longevity. In most patients with chronic respiratory failure antibiotics are reserved until the first sign of an intercurrent infection.

Rehabilitation is an essential part of the comprehensive management of patients with chronic respiratory failure as their condition almost invariably requires social, psychological and possibly vocational adjustments. A rehabilitation programme consists of physical therapy, psychological counselling and patient education. Such programmes are best performed on an outpatient basis by a team consisting of the physician, nurse, physiotherapist, social worker and others, such as a psychologist. After a period of intensive therapy and instruction, the patients continue their therapy at home with frequent follow-up visits for reinforcement and evaluation.

The use of mechanical ventilation in chronic respiratory failure is usually restricted to certain types of respiratory failure: those patients with neuromuscular disorders who are chronically ill and in whom more conservative measures have not succeeded in maintaining alveolar ventilation at an acceptable level. When the work of breathing is normal and secretions are controllable intubation and subsequent tracheostomy are unnecessary and ventilation can be satisfactorily maintained using devices such as the whole-body respirator or 'iron lung', the flexible cuirass body respirator, the rocking bed, the chest-shell respirator, and the abdominal pneumobelt. Mechanical ventilation may be used in selected patients, again mainly those with neuromuscular disorders, to prevent severe hypoxaemia as a result of sleep-induced hypoventilation.

From the above discussion it should be clear that much of the drug therapy used in respiratory failure is directed towards the underlying condition rather than the respiratory failure *per se*. It is anticipated that in the future drug therapy will be more specifically directed towards prevention and/or reversal of the pathophysiological manifestations of respiratory failure such as pulmonary hypertension, cor pulmonale and respiratory muscle fatigue. As a result of these focused therapeutic interventions, it is expected that patients will benefit in terms of reduction of dyspnoea, improved exercise tolerance and increased longevity.

## References


1. Bone RC, Pierce AK, Johnson RL Jr. Controlled oxygen administration in acute respiratory failure in chronic obstructive pulmonary disease: a reappraisal. *Am J Med* 1978; 65: 896.
2. Martin LVH, Marshall RL. Survival of chronic bronchitics after intermittent positive pressure ventilation. *Anaesthesia* 1973; 28: 10.
3. Murray JF. Review of the state of the art in intermittent positive pressure breathing therapy. *Am Rev Respir Dis* 1974; 110 (suppl): 193.
4. Asmundsson T, Johnson RF, Kilburn KH, Goodrich JK. Efficiency of nebulisers for depositing saline in human lung. *Am Rev Respir Dis* 1973; 108: 506.
5. Pavia D, Thompson ML, Clarke SW. Enhanced clearance of secretions from the human lung after administration of hypertonic saline aerosol. *Am Rev Respir Dis* 1978; 117: 199.
6. Clarke SW, Lopez-Vidriero MT, Pavia D, Thompson ML. The effect of sodium 2-mercapto-ethane sulphonate and hypertonic saline aerosols on bronchial clearance in chronic bronchitis. *Br J Clin Pharmacol* 1979; 7: 39.
7. Eschenbacher WL, Boushey HA, Sheppard D. Alteration in osmolarity of inhaled aerosols causes bronchoconstriction and cough but absence of a permeant ion causes cough alone. *Am Rev Respir Dis* 1984; 129: 211.
8. Matthews LW, Doershuk CF, Spector S. Mist tent therapy of obstructive pulmonary lesion of cystic fibrosis. *Pediatrics* 1967; 39: 176.
9. Doershuk CF, Matthews LW, Gillespie CT, Lough MD, Spector S. Evaluation of jet type and ultrasonic nebulisers in mist therapy for cystic fibrosis. *Pediatrics* 1968; 41: 723.
10. Quinton PM. Chloride impermeability in cystic fibrosis. *Nature* 1983; 301: 421.
11. Quinton PM, Byman J. Higher bioelectric potentials due to decreased chloride absorption in the sweat glands of patients with cystic fibrosis. *N Engl J Med* 1983; 308: 1185.
12. Knowles M, Gatzy J, Boucher R. Increased bioelectric potential difference across respiratory epithelia in cystic fibrosis. *N Engl J Med* 1981; 305: 1489.
13. Knowles MR, Stutts MJ, Spock A, Fisher N, Gatzy JT, Boucher RC. Abnormal ion permeation through cystic fibrosis respiratory epithelium. *Science* 1983; 221: 1067.
14. Knowles M, Gatzy J, Boucher R. Relative ion permeability of normal and cystic fibrosis nasal epithelium. *J Clin Invest* 1983; 71: 1410.
15. Knowles M, Murray M, Shullal J, et al. Bioelectric properties and ion flow across excised human bronchi. *J Appl Physiol* 1984; 56: 868.
16. Widdicombe JH, Welsh MJ. Ion transport in the dog tracheal epithelium. *Fed Proc* 1980; 39: 3062.
17. Barton AD. Aerosolised detergents and mucolytic agents in the treatment of stable chronic obstructive pulmonary disease. *Am Rev Respir Dis* 1974; 110 (suppl): 104.
18. Anthonisen P, Riis P, Sogaard-Andersen T. The value of lung physiotherapy in the treatment of acute exacerbations of chronic bronchitis. *Acta Med Scand* 1964; 175: 715.
19. Petersen SE, Esmann V, Honcke P, Munker C. A controlled study of the effect of treatment in chronic bronchitis. An evaluation using pulmonary function tests. *Acta Med Scand* 1967; 182: 293.
20. Newton DAG, Stephenson A. Effect of physiotherapy on pulmonary function. *Lancet* 1978; 2: 228.
21. Campbell AH, O'Connell JM, Wilson F. The effect of chest physiotherapy upon the $FEV_1$ in chronic bronchitis. *Med J Aust* 1975; 1: 33.
22. Connors AF, Hammon WE, Martin WJ, Rogers RM. Chest physical therapy. The immediate effect on oxygenation in acutely ill patients. *Chest* 1980; 78: 559.

23. Holody B, Goldberg HS. The effect of mechanical vibration physiotherapy on arterial oxygenation in acutely ill patients with atelectasis and pneumonia. *Am Rev Respir Dis* 1981; 124: 372.
24. Neuhaus A, Bentz RR, Weg JG. Pulmonary embolism in respiratory failure. *Chest* 1978; 73: 460.
25. Harris SK, Bone RL, Ruth WE. The efficacy of low-dose heparin for prevention of pulmonary embolism in a respiratory intensive care unit. *Am Rev Respir Dis* 1977; 115: 118.
26. Harris SK, Bone RL, Ruth WE. Gastrointestinal haemorrhage in a respiratory intensive care unit. *Chest* 1977; 72: 301.
27. Hastings PR, Skillman JJ, Bushnell S, Silen W. Antacid titration in the prevention of acute gastrointestinal bleeding: a controlled, randomized trial in 100 acutely ill patients. *N Engl J Med* 1978; 298: 1041.
28. Payne CB, Chester EH, Hsi BP. Airway responsiveness in chronic obstructive pulmonary disease. *Am J Med* 1967; 42: 554.
29. Connellan SJ, Gough SE. The effects of nebulised salbutamol on lung function and exercise tolerance in patients with severe airflow obstruction. *Br J Dis Chest* 1982; 76: 135.
30. Sahn SA. Corticosteroids in chronic bronchitis and pulmonary emphysema. *Chest* 1978; 73: 789.
31. Shim C, Stover DE, Williams MH Jr. Response to corticosteroids in chronic bronchitis. *J Allergy Clin Immunol* 1978; 62: 363.
32. Mendella LA, Manfrida J, Warren CPW, Anthonisen NR. Steroid response in stable chronic obstructive pulmonary disease. *Ann Intern Med* 1982; 96: 17.
33. Blair GP, Light RW. Treatment of chronic obstructive pulmonary disease with corticosteroids. Comparison of daily vs alternate day therapy. *Chest* 1984; 86 524.
34. Nocturnal Oxygen Therapy Trial Group. Continuous or nocturnal oxygen therapy in hypoxemic chronic obstructive lung disease. *Ann Intern Med* 1980; 93: 391.
35. Boushey SR, Coates EO. The prognostic value of pulmonary function tests in emphysema. *Am Rev Respir Dis* 1964; 90: 553.
36. Renzetti AD, McClement JH, Litt BD. The Veterans Administration co-operative study of pulmonary function III: mortality in relation to respiratory function in chronic obstructive lung disease. *Am J Med* 1966; 41: 115.
37. Jones NL, Burrows B, Fletcher CM. Serial studies of 100 patients with chronic airway obstruction in London and Chicago. *Thorax* 1967; 22: 327.
38. Ude AC, Howard P. Controlled oxygen therapy and pulmonary heart failure. *Thorax* 1971; 26: 572.
39. Burrows B, Kettel LJ, Niden AH, Rabinowitz M, Diener CF. Patterns of cardiovascular dysfunction in chronic obstructive pulmonary disease. *N Engl J Med* 1972; 286: 912.
40. Boushey SF, Thompson HK, North LB, Beale AR, Snow TR. Prognosis in chronic obstructive pulmonary disease. *Am Rev Respir Dis* 1973; 108: 1373.
41. Diener CF. Burrows B. Further observations on the course and prognosis of chronic obstructive lung disease. *Am Rev Respir Dis* 1973; 111: 719.
42. Damsgaard T, Kok-Jensen A. Prognosis in severe chronic obstructive lung disease. *Acta Med Scand* 1974; 196: 103.
43. Hyman AL, Kadowitz PJ. Vasodilator therapy for pulmonary hypertensive disorders. *Chest* 1984; 85: 145.
44. Ellis JH Jr, Kirch D, Steele PP. Right ventricular ejection fraction in severe chronic airway obstruction. *Chest* 1977; 71 (suppl): 281.
45. Matthay RA, Berger HJ, Davis RA, et al. Right and left ventricular exercise performance in chronic obstructive pulmonary disease: radionuclide assessment. *Ann Intern Med* 1980; 93: 234.
46. Mahler DA, Brent BN, Loke J, Zaret BJ, Matthay RA. Right ventricular performance and central circulatory hemodynamics during upright exercise in patients with chronic obstructive pulmonary disease. *Am Rev Respir Dis* 1984; 130: 722.
47. Rubin LJ. Cardiovascular effects of vasodilator therapy for pulmonary artery hypertension. *Clin Chest Med* 1983; 4: 309.
48. Rubin L, Peter R. Hemodynamics at rest and during exercise after oral hydralazine in patients with cor pulmonale. *Am J Cardiol* 1981; 47: 116.

49. Rubin LJ, Handel F, Peter RH. The effects of oral hydralazine on right ventricular end diastolic pressure in patients with right ventricular failure. *Circulation* 1982; 65: 1369.
50. Keller CA, Shepard JW, Chun DS, Dolan GF, Vasquez P, Minh V-D. Effects of hydralazine on hemodynamics, ventilation and gas exchange in patients with chronic obstructive pulmonary disease and pulmonary hypertension. *Am Rev Respir Dis* 1984; 130: 606.
51. Lupi-Herrera E, Seoane M, Verdejo J. Hemodynamic effect of hydralazine in advanced stable chronic obstructive pulmonary disease with cor pulmonale. *Chest* 1984; 85: 156.
52. Tuxen DV, Powles AC, Mathur PN, Pugsley SO, Campbell FJ. Detrimental effects of hydralazine in patients with chronic airflow obstruction and pulmonary hypertension. *Am Rev Respir Dis* 1984; 129: 388.
53. Kennedy T, Summer W. Inhibition of hypoxic pulmonary vasoconstriction by nifedipine. *Am J Cardiol* 1982; 50: 864.
54. Simonneau G, Escourrou P, Duroux P, Lochhart A. Inhibition of hypoxic pulmonary vasoconstriction by nifedipine. *N Engl J Med* 1981; 304: 1582.
55. Kennedy TP, Michael JR, Huang C-K, et al. Nifedipine inhibits hypoxic pulmonary vasoconstriction during rest and exercise in patients with chronic obstructive pulmonary disease. *Am Rev Respir Dis* 1984; 129: 544.
56. Melot C, Hallemans R, Naeije R, Mols P, Lejeune P. Deleterious effects of nifedipine on pulmonary gas exchange in chronic obstructive pulmonary disease. *Am Rev Respir Dis* 1984; 130: 612.
57. Stanbrook HS, Morris KG, McMurtry IF. Prevention and reversal of hypoxic pulmonary hypertension by calcium antagonists. *Am Rev Respir Dis* 1984; 130: 81.
58. Naeije R, Melot C, Mols P, Hallemans R. Reduction in pulmonary hypertension in decompensated chronic obstructive pulmonary disease. *Am Rev Respir Dis* 1982; 125: 1.
59. Ishizaki T, Miyabo S, Mifune J, et al. OP-126, a prostaglandin $E_1$ derivative. Effects of oral administration to patients with chronic lung disease. *Chest* 1984; 85: 382.
60. Morganroth ML, Reeves JT, Murphy RC, Voelkel NF. Leukotriene synthesis and receptor blockers block hypoxic pulmonary vasoconstriction. *J Appl Physiol* 1984; 56: 1340.
61. Gottlieb J, McGeady M, Adkinson NF, Hayes E, Sylvester JF. Inhibition of hypoxic pulmonary vasoconstriction in ferret lungs by nordihydroguaiuretic acid (NDGA). *Am Rev Respir Dis* 1984; 129: A343.
62. Ahmed T, Oliver W. Does slow reacting substance of anaphylaxis mediate hypoxic pulmonary vasoconstriction? *Am Rev Respir Dis* 1983; 127: 566.
63. Morganroth ML, Stenmark KR, Morris KG, et al. Diethylcarbamazine inhibits acute and chronic hypoxic pulonary vasoconstriction in awake rats. *Am Rev Respir Dis* 1985; 131: 488.
64. Geggel RL, Dazar AL, Fyler DC, Reid LM. Effect of vasodilators at rest and during exercise in young adults with cystic fibrosis and chronic cor pulmonale. *Am Rev Respir Dis* 1985; 131: 531.
65. Fishman AP. Hypoxia on the pulmonary circulation: how and where it acts. *Circ Res* 1976; 38: 221.
66. Timms RM, Khaja FU, Williams GW, and the NOTT Group. Hemodynamic response to oxygen therapy in chronic obstructive pulmonary disease. *Ann Intern Med* 1985; 102: 29.
67. Report of the Medical Research Council Working Party. Long term domiciliary oxygen therapy in chronic hypoxic cor pulmonale complicating chronic bronchitis and emphysema. *Lancet* 1981; 1: 681.
68. Ashutosh K, Mead G, Dunsky M. Early effects of oxygen administration and prognosis in chronic obstructive pulmonary disease and cor pulmonale. *Am Rev Respir Dis* 1983; 127: 399.
69. Kay JM. Effects of continuous and intermittent normoxia on chronic hypoxic pulmonary hypertension, right ventricular hypertrophy and polycythemia in rats. *Am Rev Respir Dis* 1980; 121: 993.
70. Kay JM, Suyama KL, Keane PM. Effect of intermittent normoxia on muscularisation of pulmonary arterioles induced by chronic hypoxia in rats. *Am Rev Respir Dis* 1981; 123: 454.
71. Abraham AS, Cole RB, Bishop JM. Reversal of pulmonary hypertension by prolonged oxygen administration to patients with chronic bronchitis. *Circ Res* 1968; 23: 147.
72. Weitzenblum E, Sautegeau A, Ehrhart M, Mammosser M, Pelletier A. Long-term oxygen therapy can reverse the progression of pulmonary hypertension in patients with chronic obstructive pulmonary disease. *Am Rev Respir Dis* 1985; 131: 493.

73. Sime F, Penaloza D, Ruiz L. Bradycardia, increased cardiac output and reversal of pulmonary hypertension in altitude natives living at sea level. *Br Heart J* 1971; 33: 647.
74. Catterall JR, Douglas NJ, Calverley PMA, et al. Transient hypoxaemia during sleep in chronic obstructive pulmonary disease is not a sleep apnea syndrome. *Am Rev Respir Dis* 1983; 128: 24.
75. Koo KW, Sax DS, Snider GL. Arterial blood gases and pH during sleep in chronic obstructive pulmonary disease. *Am J Med* 1975; 58: 663.
76. Bye PTP, Issa F, Berthon-Jones M, Sullivan CE. Studies of oxygenation during sleep in patients with interstitial lung disease. *Am Rev Respir Dis* 1984; 129: 27.
77. Flenley DC. Clinical hypoxia: causes, consequences and correction. *Lancet* 1978; 1: 542.
78. Block AJ, Boysen PG, Wynne JW. The origins of cor pulmonale. A hypothesis. *Chest* 1979; 75: 109.
79. Boysen PG, Block AJ, Wynne JW, Hunt LA, Flick MR. Nocturnal pulmonary hypertension in patients with chronic obstructive pulmonary disease. *Chest* 1976; 76: 536.
80. Goldstein RS, Ramcharan V, Bowes G, McNicholas WT, Bradley D, Phillipson EA. Effect of supplemental nocturnal oxygen on gas exchange in patients with severe obstructive lung disease. *N Engl J Med* 1984; 310: 425.
81. Flick MR, Block AJ. Nocturnal versus diurnal cardiac arrhythmias in patients with chronic obstructive pulmonary disease. *Chest* 1979; 75: 8.
82. Tirlapur VG, Mir MA. Nocturnal hypoxemia and associated electrocardiographic changes in patients with chronic obstructive airway disease. *N Engl J Med* 1982; 306: 125.
83. Fletcher EC, Levin DC. Cardiopulmonary hemodynamics during sleep in subjects with chronic obstructive pulmonary disease. *Chest* 1984; 85: 6.
84. Menkes HA, Bleeker ER, Smith PL. Obstructive pulmonary disease. In: Harvey AM, Jones RL, McKusic VA, et al, eds. *The principles and practice of medicine,* 21st ed. Norwalk: Appleton-Century Crofts, 1984.
85. Woodcock AA, Gross ER, Geddes DM. Oxygen relieves breathlessness in 'pink puffers'. *Lancet* 1981; 1: 907.
86. Neff TA, Conway WA, Lakshiminarayan S, Petty TL, Solliday NH. Indications for oxygen therapy. *Chest* 1984; 86: 239.
87. Flenley DC. Long-term home oxygen therapy. *Chest* 1985; 87: 99.
88. Grassino A, Gross D, Macklem PT, Roussos Ch, Zagelbaum G. Inspiratory muscle fatigue is a factor that limits exercise. *Bull Eur Physiopathol Respir* 1979; 15: 105.
89. Rochester DF. The respiratory muscles in COPD. State of the art. *Chest* 1984; 85 (suppl): 47S.
90. Sigrist S, Thomas D, Howell S, Roussos Ch. The effect of aminophylline on inspiratory muscle contractility. *Am Rev Respir Dis* 1982; 126: 46.
91. Aubier M, Murciano D, Viires N, Lecocguic Y, Palacios S, Pariente R. Increased ventilation caused by improved diaphragmatic efficiency during aminophylline infusion. *Am Rev Respir Dis* 1983; 127: 148.
92. Howell S, Roussos Ch. Isoproternol and aminophylline improve contractility of fatigued canine diaphragm. *Am Rev Respir Dis* 1984; 129: 118.
93. Aubier M, De Troyer A, Sampson M, Macklem P, Roussos Ch. Aminophylline improves diaphragmatic contractility. *N Engl J Med* 1981; 305: 249.
94. Murciano D, Aubier M, Lecocguic Y, Pariente R. Effects of theophylline on diaphragmatic strength and fatigue in patients with chronic obstructive pulmonary disease. *N Engl J Med* 1984; 311: 349.
95. Jenne JW, Siever JR, Druz WS, Solana JV, Cohen SM, Sharp JT. The effect of maintenance theophylline therapy on lung work in severe chronic obstructive pulmonary disease while standing and walking. *Am Rev Respir Dis* 1984; 130: 600.
96. Mahler DA, Matthay RA, Snyder PE, Wells CK, Loke J. Sustained-release theophylline reduces dyspnea in nonreversible obstructive airways disease. *Am Rev Respir Dis* 1985; 131: 22.
97. Eaton ML, Green BA, Church TR, McGowan T, Niewoehner DE. Efficacy of theophylline in irreversible airflow obstruction. *Ann Intern Med* 1980; 92: 758.
98. Eaton ML, MacDonald FM, Church TR, Niewoehner DE. Effects of theophylline on breathlessness and exercise tolerance in patients with chronic airflow obstruction. *Chest* 1982; 82: 538.

99. Leitch AG, Morgan A, Ellis DA, Bell G, Haslett C, McHardy GJR. Effect of oral salbutamol and slow release aminophylline on exercise tolerance in chronic bronchitis. *Thorax* 1981; 36: 787.

100. Evans WV. Plasma theophylline concentrations, six minute walking distances, and breathlessness in patients with chronic airflow obstruction. *Br Med J* 1984; 289: 1649.

101. Andersen JB, Dragsted L, Kann T, et al. Resistive breathing training in severe chronic obstructive pulmonary disease patients. A pilot study. *Scand J Respir Dis* 1979; 60: 151.

102. Belman MJ, Mittman C. Ventilatory muscle training improves exercise capacity in chronic obstructive pulmonary disease patients. *Am Rev Respir Dis* 1980; 121: 273.

103. Pardy RL, Rivington RN, Despas PJ, Macklem PT. The effects of inspiratory muscle training on exercise performance in chronic airflow limitation. *Am Rev Respir Dis* 1981; 123: 426.

104. Pierce AK, Taylor HF. Archer RK, Miller WF. Response to exercise training in patients with emphysema. *Arch Intern Med* 1964; 113: 28.

105. Nicholas JJ, Gilbert R, Gabe R, Auchincloss JH. Evaluation of an exercise therapy program for patients with chronic obstructive pulmonary disease. *Am Rev Respir Dis* 1970; 102: 1.

106. Bass H. Whitcomb JF, Forman R. Exercise training: therapy for patients with chronic obstructive pulmonary disease. *Chest* 1970; 57: 116.

107. Vyas MN, Bannister EW, Morton JW, Grzybowski S. Response to exercise in patients with chronic airway obstruction. *Am Rev Respir Dis* 1971; 103: 390.

108. Belman M, Sieck G, Mazar A. Ventilatory muscle training and pulmonary rehabilitation. *Chest* 1984; 85 (suppl): 83S.

109. Geiger MJ. Katzoff MN. A comparison of inspiratory muscle training and exercise training in a COPD population. *Am Rev Respir Dis* 1984; 129 (suppl): A35.

110. Jenderlinic P, Muspratt JA, Miller MJ. Inspiratory muscle training in clinical practice. Physiologic conditioning or habituation to suffocation? *Chest* 1984; 86: 870.

111. Jones NL. Physical therapy: present state of the art. *Am Rev Respir Dis* 1974; 110: 132.

112. Cochrane GM, Webber BA, Clarke SW. Effects of sputum on pulmonary function. *Br Med J* 1977; 2: 1181.

113. Feldman J, Traver GA, Taussig LM. Maximal expiratory flows after postural drainage. *Am Rev Respir Dis* 1979; 119: 239.

114. May DB, Munt PW. Physiological effects of chest percussion and postural drainage in patients with stable chronic bronchitis. *Chest* 1979; 75: 29.

115. Murray JF. The ketchup bottle method. *N Engl J Med* 1979; 300: 1155.

116. Mohsenifar Z, Rosenberg N, Goldberg HS, Koerner SK. Mechanical vibration and conventional chest physiotherapy in outpatients with stable chronic obstructive lung disease. *Chest* 1985; 87: 483.

117. Oldenberg FA, Dolovich MB, Mongomery J, Newhouse M. Effects of postural drainage, exercise and cough on mucus clearance in chronic bronchitis. *Am Rev Respir Dis* 1979; 120: 739.

118. Bateman JRM, Newman SP, Daunt KM, Sheahan NF, Pavia D, Clarke SW. Is cough as effective as chest physiotherapy in the removal of excessive tracheobronchial secretions? *Thorax* 1981; 36: 683.

119. Pavia D, Thomson ML, Phillapakos D. A preliminary study of the effect of a vibrating pad on bronchial clearance. *Am Rev Respir Dis* 1976; 113: 92.

120. King M, Phillips DM, Gross M, Vartain V, Chang HK, Zidulka A. Enhanced tracheal mucus clearance with high frequency chest wall compression. *Am Rev Respir Dis* 1983; 128: 511.

121. Mathur PN, Powles ACP, Pugsley SO, McEwan MP, Campbell EJM. Effect of digoxin on right ventricular function in severe chronic airflow obstruction. A controlled clinical trial. *Ann Intern Med* 1981; 95: 283.

122. Green LH, Smith TW. The use of digitalis in patients with pulmonary disease. *Ann Intern Med* 1977; 87: 459.

123. Kilburn KH, Powell AR. Renal function in respiratory failure. *Arch Intern Med* 1971; 127: 754.

# Chapter 12

# Tuberculosis

*N. W. Horne*

Tuberculosis remains a major problem in many areas of the world. In economically developing countries the disease is one of the principal causes of suffering and death. It has been estimated that there are 15 to 20 million infectious cases worldwide and about three million deaths annually, 80% of which occur in developing countries. By contrast the disease may well be virtually eradicated from large areas of the developed countries — North America, Australasia and Europe — within 25 years. The problems associated with the decline of tuberculosis have been discussed by Horne.[1]

The clinical features of respiratory tuberculosis are well known, and most are non-specific. Cough, sputum and haemoptysis are the main respiratory symptoms but vague chest pain, wheeze, pleuritic pain and breathlessness also occur. The disease may present as a pleural effusion or spontaneous pneumothorax and may be discovered in the course of investigation of some other disease. Constitutional symptoms are often lacking but fever, loss of weight, loss of appetite and fatigue may be present.

## Diagnostic Features

The definitive diagnosis of tuberculosis is made by the identification of *Mycobacterium tuberculosis* from sputum, laryngeal swab or gastric washings. Characteristic histological features with or without the presence of tubercle bacilli may be identified from bronchial washings or biopsy, needle lung biopsy, resected lung or lymph nodes. Radiographic examination including, where appropriate, tomography is mandatory but there are no radiographic appearances which cannot be mimicked by other diseases, and vice versa. The tuberculin test is of limited diagnostic value, except in young children.

## Natural History and Prognosis

This can be expressed quite simply. Prior to the introduction of chemotherapy, 75% of patients with sputum smear-positive disease would die within five years. Current chemotherapy offers the possibility of cure in all patients with drug-sensitive infections, and in the vast majority of drug-resistant infections, providing there is compliance with treatment.

## Goals of Treatment

The main aim of treatment is cure. Modern chemotherapy is so effective that if proper drug regimens are prescribed and the patient is wholly cooperative with treatment then cure takes place in 100% of patients with drug-sensitive tubercle bacilli and in the vast majority of patients who have drug-resistant organisms. A subsidiary, but nevertheless important, aim is to render the patient non-infectious and thus prevent spread of disease. These aims are elaborated below.

## Rationale of Chemotherapy of Tuberculosis

In earlier 'standard' chemotherapy using streptomycin, para-amino salicylic acid (PAS) and isoniazid, drug combinations were selected with a view to preventing drug resistance. The organisms were eventually killed or died out after many months of treatment. The new concept of short-term chemotherapy is different, the object being to select combinations of drugs that are rapidly sterilising.

The population of mycobacteria within lesions in man consists of several identifiable groups.[2] One group consists of metabolically active, continuously growing bacilli, for example, in cavity walls; some bacilli are found mainly inside cells in which the environment is acid, an environment in which pyrazinamide is especially effective; some organisms are mostly dormant but have occasional spurts of metabolism, and others are fully dormant and appear to die off gradually. The importance of individual drugs in this context has been evaluated by Fox.[3]

In short-course chemotherapy two drug actions are involved, bactericidal activity and sterilisation. From studies of sputum in the early days of treatment it was found that isoniazid is particularly bactericidal, rifampicin is less so, and pyrazinamide and streptomycin have very low activity.[4] The sterilizing role has been described by Grosset.[5] Rifampicin and pyrazinamide are very potent sterilisers in the mouse, the most potent sterilising combinations being isoniazid plus pyrazinamide and isoniazid plus rifampicin. The addition of streptomycin or ethambutol makes no contribution to the sterilising capacity or the capacity of either of these combinations to eliminate 'persisters'.

It is of crucial importance, especially for patients harbouring large bacterial populations, to prevent further bacterial multiplication so that the disease is brought under control as soon as possible. This not only saves the lives of some patients and prevents disastrous gross lung destruction in others, but it also limits the dissemination of infection in the community. Treatment with three or four drugs in the initial phase will almost always prevent the emergence of drug-resistant mutants and will with few exceptions secure a successful outcome in patients with initially drug-resistant infection[6] preventing the emergence of 'persisters'. A good regimen is one that largely overcomes the influence of initial drug resistance. The employment of drugs with a high sterilising effect in the continuation phase is designed to eliminate relapse.

The practical application of these principles is discussed below.

## Drugs and Regimens

The chemotherapy of pulmonary tuberculosis demands a detailed knowledge not only of the individual drugs which are effective, but also of the regimens which are essential to a successful outcome of treatment.

It is almost 25 years since it was established that with appropriate combinations of drugs administered for a sufficiently long period of treatment and given strict compliance by the patient, treatment would be 100% effective in patients with initially sensitive organisms,[7] and relapse would be rare.[8] Earlier effective regimens have, however, been superseded by short-term chemotherapy. The short-term regimens now recommended have the advantages of reducing chronic toxicity, of making compliance by the patient easier, of being highly effective even in the presence of initial infection with drug-resistant organisms, and of making relapse highly unlikely even in patients complying with treatment for periods as brief as four months.[9]

The realisation that short-course chemotherapy could produce highly effective results emerged in the early 1970s and studies in Britain[10] and in France[11] consolidated the accumulating evidence. Treatment with rifampicin and isoniazid for nine months, supplemented in an initial two-month period of intensive therapy by *either* ethambutol or streptomycin, produced excellent results and the so-called nine-month regimen became the established recommendation, ethambutol being more commonly prescribed than streptomycin because of the more frequent toxicity associated with the latter drug. Subsequent studies[12] demonstrated that six-month regimens were capable of producing similar excellent results provided that four drugs were used in the intensive initial period which must include pyrazinamide.

The current recommended treatment for smear-positive disease is as follows: *initial intensive phase* (two months) isoniazid, rifampicin, pyrazinamide and *either* ethambutol or streptomycin; *continuation phase* (four months) isoniazid plus rifampicin.

The initial reluctance to use pyrazinamide should now have been overcome following its reappraisal which showed low toxicity provided it is prescribed strictly in the recommended dose (Table 12.1).

It is often asked whether the duration of treatment can be reduced in smear-negative but culture-positive disease. Current evidence suggests that it is inadvisable to give less than six months' treatment in these circumstances. Recent studies have shown that there is a 15% relapse rate in three-month, and a 9% relapse rate in four-month daily regimens.[13]

The cost of drugs is important in developing countries. Intermittency reduces the cost and there are effective regimens which are either intermittent throughout or contain an initial period of daily treatment. If initial resistance is common there are advantages in choosing the longer dose regimens containing rifampicin and those which contain pyrazinamide in the initial intensive phase. The choice of regimen is becoming increasingly complex. Intermittent regimens are reviewed in detail by Fox[3] and Horne.[6] The most commonly used supervised regimen in developed countries is streptomycin and isoniazid daily for 12 weeks followed by streptomycin plus isoniazid twice weekly to a total period of 12 months. An initial period of four weeks' daily treatment gives 98% success.

*Table 12.1* Dosage and adverse effects of antituberculosis drugs:1*

| | Dosage | | | Adverse effects | |
|---|---|---|---|---|---|
| Drug | Adult | Children | Intermittent | More common | Rare |
| Isoniazid | 300mg<br>In chemoprophylaxis, 5mg/kg<br>In miliary TB, 12mg/kg | 10mg/kg | 15mg/kg | Hypersensitivity, hepatitis | Peripheral neuropathy, toxic psychosis, pellagra, haemolytic anaemia, agranulocytosis |
| Rifampicin | Less than 50kg, 450mg<br>Over 50kg, 600mg | 10-20mg/kg | 600-900mg<br>600-900mg | Gastrointestinal, hypersensitivity, hepatitis<br>Induction of liver enzymes<br>Toxicity of intermittent therapy | Thrombocytopenic purpura, pseudomembranous colitis, pseudo-adrenal crisis |
| Ethambutol | 25mg/kg for 2 months; then 15mg/kg. Renal disease (see text) | See text | 3 times weekly, 30mg/kg<br>Twice weekly, 45 mg/kg | Retrobulbar neuritis | Hypersensitivity, hepatitis |
| Pyrazinamide | Less than 50kg, 1.5g<br>50-74kg, 2.0 g<br>More than 75kg, 2.5g | 40mg/kg (max 2g) | 3 times weekly, 2.0g<br>Twice weekly, 3.0g<br>3 times weekly, 2.5g<br>Twice weekly, 3.5g | Arthralgia, hepatitis | Gastrointestinal, photosensitivity of skin, sideroblastic anaemia |
| Streptomycin | Less than 30kg, 750mg<br>More than 30kg, 1g (750mg if over 40 years)<br>Renal disease, see text<br>Intrathecal 50-100mg | 20mg/kg (max 1g)<br>Intrathecal 1mg/kg (max 50mg) | 1g | Ototoxicity (vestibular disturbance) | Ototoxicity (deafness), hypersensitivity, renal damage, blood dyscrasias, lupoid reaction |

*This table should be read in conjunction with the text.

## Individual Agents

The dosage of antituberculosis drugs is shown in Tables 12.1 and 12.2 and recommendations regarding adjustment of dose in special circumstances, such as liver or renal disease, are described below. *All these drugs should be given in a single daily dose.* Isoniazid/rifampicin and isoniazid/ethambutol should be given in a combined formulation. A single preparation including rifampicin, isoniazid and pyrazinamide has been formulated. Because of its relatively low dose of pyrazinamide, its efficacy must await the results of clinical trials. Research into the activity of long-acting rifampicins is in progress.

Adverse effects from antituberculosis drugs are not frequent, but they are diverse and some are potentially serious. The following paragraphs amplify Tables 12.1 and 12.2. The reader is referred for more detailed information to reviews of adverse reactions[14] and practical drug management.[15]

All the main drugs can cause cutaneous and general reactions and hepatitis. The most common causative agents of hypersensitivity reactions are streptomycin, para-aminosalicylic acid (PAS) and thiacetazone. They usually occur in the first four weeks of treatment and if treatment is not stopped the reactions may become severe. The drug or drugs responsible for the reaction should be identified by giving small test doses and resuming adequate chemotherapy as soon as possible, using not less than two drugs to which the patient is not hypersensitive. Desensitisation to the offending drug or drugs should then be carried out. Girling[14] describes the practical techniques of desensitisation in detail.

Hepatitis may be caused by all the antituberculosis drugs: it may be due to a single drug or to combinations.[14] Hepatitis is an indication for stopping treatment. Treatment with the same drugs can often be resumed uneventfully, but liver function should be carefully monitored.

### *Rifampicin (Rifampin)*

Rifampicin is normally administered orally. An intravenous preparation is available (300mg in 10ml). The drug is almost completely absorbed from the gastrointestinal tract after an oral dose and it is partly deacetylated in the liver by an enzyme which is induced in the first few days of treatment. It is excreted almost completely by the bile, but is to some extent excreted in the urine, there being an enterohepatic circulation.

Rifampicin is well tolerated and rarely causes serious toxicity. It should be administered with caution to patients with chronic liver disease and alcoholics, as it may cause hepatitis, and also to elderly patients. Liver function should be monitored in these patients, but is not normally required. Because it induces microsomal enzymes it reduces the clinical efficacy of concomitantly administered corticosteroids, oral contraceptives, oral diabetic agents, some narcotics and analgesics, digoxin and coumarin anticoagulants. Subtherapeutic serum concentrations and poor clinical response to treatment have been reported when rifampicin and ketoconazole are given together.[16] Pseudomembranous colitis, pseudo-adrenal crisis and osteomalacia have also been described as toxic effects.

The following reactions are commoner with intermittent therapy, but may occur rarely with daily treatment: cutaneous reactions, gastrointestinal symptoms, thrombocytopenic purpura. Intermittent therapy may also cause shock and shortness of breath, the 'flu' syndrome, acute haemolytic anaemia and acute renal failure. These reactions are fully described by Girling.[14] Patients should be warned that the urine, and occasionally other body secretions, will turn red. If the drug is reintroduced after a short interval, it should be started in small, gradually increasing doses to prevent the possibility of severe reactions.

*Isoniazid*

Isoniazid is extremely well tolerated and rarely causes adverse reactions, hepatitis and peripheral neuropathy being the most important. Pyridoxine 10mg daily should be given in conjunction when the dosage exceeds 400mg. Nausea and anorexia are rare.

There is a genetically determined variation between different subjects in the rate of acetylation. In certain ethnic groups — the Japanese, Koreans and particularly the Eskimos — the prevalence of rapid inactivators is high (50 to 95%) whereas it is only 5% in South India.

*Ethambutol*

The most important adverse effect is retrobulbar neuritis causing reduced visual acuity, central scotomata and disturbances of red-green perception and, rarely, peripheral field defects. These effects are dose-related and are very rarely seen in dosages of 15mg/kg or below. Successful litigation, with the award of substantial damages, has been undertaken in circumstances where routine eye examinations have not been undertaken. The serum urea or creatinine and visual acuity using the Snellen test chart should be recorded in the notes prior to starting treatment. Patients who normally wear spectacles for distant vision should be tested wearing them. The drug should not be given to patients with greatly reduced visual acuity. The patient should be told to stop the drug immediately if impairment of vision is noted, and to report this occurrence at once. This fact should also be recorded in the notes. Patients observing impairment of visual acuity should be referred immediately for specialist ophthalmological examination. Routine tests of visual acuity during treatment are not recommended. The drug should be avoided in young children who may not be able to give early warning of failing vision.

Ethambutol is well tolerated. Mild hyperuricaemia occurs; cutaneous reactions and hepatitis are extremely rare. The dosage schedule for patients with impaired renal function is described below.

*Streptomycin*

The main adverse effect is ototoxicity, chiefly vestibular damage, though deafness may occur. It occurs more commonly in the elderly. Attention to the correct dose is essential. The trough plasma concentrations should not exceed 2μg/ml. Patients must be warned to stop treatment at once if vestibular or auditory symptoms occur.

Hypersensitivity reactions are not common and anaphylaxis occurs very rarely. The drug should not be given in myasthenia gravis, because it is a weak neuromuscular blocker. It should be avoided in pregnancy if possible. Dermatitis may occur in streptomycin handlers.

### *Pyrazinamide*

Hepatotoxicity was common when pyrazinamide was first used, but occurs very rarely in the dose now recommended.[12] Arthralgia occurs in about 5% of patients and is associated with a rise in serum uric acid concentration. It usually responds to symptomatic treatment.

### *Other Anti-tuberculosis Drugs*

Thiacetazone and PAS are commonly used as companion drugs to isoniazid in regimens recommended in developing countries because of their relative cheapness. The other drugs are used in the management of drug-resistance or hypersensitivity problems. The following notes amplify Table 12.2.

*Thiacetazone* is well tolerated in some communities but not in others particularly those of Mongolian ethnic origin. It is important to determine its acceptability in a community before it is widely used. Cross-resistance can occur with ethionamide and prothionamide. It is usually given in a combined preparation (*Thiazina*). *PAS* has been largely replaced by other drugs in technically advanced countries. Aqueous solutions are unstable and should not be used if they are darker than freshly prepared solutions. The drug should not be given when a restricted sodium intake is necessary. *Ethionamide* and *prothionamide* diffuse readily into the cerebrospinal fluid (CSF). They are teratogenic and must be avoided in pregnancy. *Cycloserine* has low potency. Suicide has been recorded as an adverse effect and the drug should be avoided in patients with a history of epilepsy or psychiatric illness.

## Drugs in Special Situations

### *Acute Miliary Tuberculosis*

It should be borne in mind that meningitis is a potential complication of miliary tuberculosis. In order to ensure a higher level of isoniazid in the cerebrospinal fluid the dose should be increased to 10 to 12mg/kg. Pyridoxine 10mg daily should also be given as prophylaxis against peripheral neuropathy. Pyrazinamide should always be included in the treatment regimen as it has been shown to achieve highly effective levels in the cerebrospinal fluid both in the presence of inflamed meninges and in the healing stage. There is debate as to whether steroids should be used in miliary tuberculosis, but this form of the disease is occasionally the cause of the adult respiratory distress syndrome,[17] and should such occur, high-dose steroids, commencing with 40mg prednisolone daily, should be given.

### *Pregnancy*

Tuberculosis should be treated without delay even if the patient is pregnant.

Isoniazid, rifampicin and ethambutol all cross the placental barrier, but all are safe in pregnancy. Isolated cases of psychomotor retardation and convulsions due to isoniazid have been reported, but the evidence is incon-

*Table 12.2* Dosage and adverse effects of antituberculosis drugs: 2*

| Drug | Dosage | | Adverse effects | |
|---|---|---|---|---|
| | Adult | Children | More common | Rare |
| Thiacetazone | 150mg | 4mg/kg | Gastrointestinal | Hepatitis, agranulocytosis, haemolytic anaemia |
| PAS (sodium salt) | 10-15g† | 300mg/kg | Gastrointestinal, febrile cutaneous reactions | Hypokalaemia, blood dyscrasias |
| Ethionamide, Prothionamide | Less than 50kg,‡, 750mg<br>50kg or more, 1g | | Gastrointestinal, metallic taste in mouth<br>Teratogenic | Hepatitis, cutaneous reactions |
| Cycloserine | 500mg | | Confusion, slurred speech, convulsions | Psychosis, suicide |
| Kanamycin, Capreomycin, Viomycin | As streptomycin (Table 12.1). Monitor serum electrolyte concentrations | | | |

*This table should be read in conjunction with the text.
†In two divided doses.
‡Administer at night to avoid daytime nausea.

clusive. The concurrent administration of pyridoxine 10mg daily is a sensible precaution if high-dose isoniazid is being given. Rifampicin was shown to be teratogenic to rodents when given in a dose much in excess of that used in routine practice in humans. Some clinicians automatically recommend abortion if rifampicin has been taken early in pregnancy, but this is a viewpoint which must be difficult to defend.

Streptomycin is potentially ototoxic and there are some reports which have shown that audiograms in children born to mothers who have been given streptomycin in pregnancy have demonstrated a perceptible hearing loss in the higher frequencies. Therefore, with other drugs readily available, streptomycin should be avoided if at all possible. The same advice relates to capreomycin and kanamycin. There is insufficient evidence regarding the use of pyrazinamide, PAS, thiacetazone and cycloserine, but they appear to be safe. Ethionamide and prothionamide have been shown to be teratogenic and must be avoided in pregnancy.

I agree with the statement made by the Committee on Chemotherapy of Tuberculosis[18] that 'Tuberculosis and the administration of these drugs [isoniazid, ethambutol and rifampicin] are not indications for therapeutic abortion'.

*Hepatic Disease*

Many of the antituberculosis drugs are hepatotoxic. In mild hepatic dysfunction, such as alcoholism, there may not be any need for special care, but it is an indication for regular monitoring of hepatic function. Elevation of the concentration of serum aspartate aminotransferase (AST) or alanine aminotransferase (ALT) above four times normal, or of serum bilirubin above 50μmol/L are indications for a review of treatment. Patients with established hepatic failure may be treated with streptomycin and ethambutol, a third drug in the form of isoniazid or rifampicin being introduced cautiously. Drug level monitoring is essential in these circumstances.

*Renal Disease*

Because of its method of clearance, rifampicin may be given in normal dose.

Isoniazid requires no adjustment unless creatinine clearance is less than 10ml/min. If it is reduced below this level, isoniazid should be given at a dose of 150 to 200mg daily, though serum levels should not exceed 1μg/ml before the next dose or dialysis. Pyridoxine 10mg daily should also be administered prophylactically.

The aminoglycosides are excreted exclusively and ethambutol predominantly by the kidneys, and should be avoided if possible in renal failure. If they must be given streptomycin should be given at such intervals that the trough serum levels do not exceed 4μg/ml. For patients on regular dialysis 0.75g of streptomycin should be given four to six hours before dialysis.

Ethambutol should be given in a dose of 25mg/kg three times a week to patients with a creatinine clearance of 50 to 100ml/min, and twice a week if the clearance lies between 30 and 50ml/min. For patients on dialysis 25mg/kg should be given four to six hours before dialysis for thrice-weekly programmes, increased to 45mg/kg for twice-weekly and to 90mg/kg for once-weekly dialysis.

Thiacetazone and PAS should be avoided.

### Management of Drug-Resistant Tuberculosis

This is a complex problem requiring specialist skill. Adherence to a few straightforward rules should prevent the emergence of drug resistance. However, some patients may relapse because of bad chemotherapy in the past, and others are unsuspectedly infected with drug-resistant organisms. The subject can be dealt with only briefly here, but detailed practical advice is given in a review by Crofton.[19]

In patients suspected of having acquired resistance, the following appraisal should be made. A detailed history of chemotherapy should be written down, reference to case records being made if possible. If the clinical state permits it, treatment should be delayed until the results of drug-sensitivity testing are known. The following rules should then be observed. At least three antituberculous drugs which have not previously been received and to which organisms are or are likely to be sensitive should be used. The possibility of cross-resistance between drugs should be borne in mind. It is not unusual for five or six drugs to be given initially. Fully supervised treatment is essential. Because of the toxicity of 'reserve' drugs, frequent changes of regimen may be necessary. Never give monotherapy at any stage. Monitor very closely the bacteriological status. Where there is multiple resistance to the main drugs consider surgical resection in localised disease.

## Disease due to Mycobacteria other than *Mycobacterium tuberculosis*

Particularly in certain areas infections of this nature are presenting an increasing problem. Such infections can be extremely difficult to treat because these organisms are commonly resistant to several, and in some instances to all, antituberculosis drugs. There are excellent reviews of the general subject,[20] and of disease due to *M avium-intracellulare*.[21] The main groups of mycobacteria encountered, and recommended forms of treatment are shown in Table 12.3. Specialists in respiratory medicine may encounter mycobacterial infections in other systems and these are included for completeness. Surgical resection in some cases of pulmonary disease may well prove to be the only certain method of cure.

## Extrapulmonary Tuberculosis

There has been no evaluation of short-course chemotherapy in extrapulmonary disease for a variety of reasons, mainly the inability to assemble enough patients in one location and the variety of anatomical sites involved. There are also some difficulties in accurate assessment of response. There are a number of good studies which demonstrate that short-course chemotherapy gives excellent clinical results with freedom from relapse.

*Table 12.3* Summary of recommended treatment of mycobacterial infections other than *M tuberculosis*

| Mycobacterial species | Commonest clinical features* | Recommended treatment |
|---|---|---|
| *Kansasii* | Pulmonary disease | Streptomycin (first three months), rifampicin, isoniazid and ethambutol for at least two years; consider resection surgery |
| *Marinum* | Swimming pool and fish tank granuloma | Usually heal spontaneously ? trimethoprim and sulphamethoxazole |
| *Scrofulaceum* | Cervical lymph nodes in children | ? as for *avium* |
| *Avium* | Lymph nodes, pulmonary disease (disseminated disease) | At least four drugs, including rifampicin and streptomycin, intensively for two years; consider resection surgery |
| *Xenopi* | Pulmonary diseae | As for *avium* but may be possible to modify as some strains are sensitive to a number of drugs |
| *Ulcerans* | Skin ulcers (Buruli ulcer) | Surgical excision and skin graft: rifampicin; (clofazimine) |
| *Fortuitum* | Injection abscess, pulmonary disease, post-cardiac surgery | Four drugs from gentamicin, amikacin, streptomycin, erythromycin and ethionamide according to sensitivity tests |
| *Chelonei* | Injection abscess, post-cardiac surgery, (rarely mycobacterial septicaemia), dissemination after renal homografts | |

*Diseases of meninges, genitourinary tract and skeleton are rare manifestations of infection by rapid growers in particular.

Among these can be cited genitourinary[22,23] and lymph node[24] tuberculosis. On theoretical grounds and in view of the data from published studies it seems that the duration of treatment in extrapulmonary disease should be similar to that in pulmonary tuberculosis.

## Compliance

For over 25 years, chemotherapy regimens have been available which are capable of ensuring 100% rates of cure.[7,8] Why is it that all treated patients are not cured? The reasons for failure lie partly with physicians and partly with patients; the reasons have been described by Fox.[9]

Death still occurs far too frequently partly from failure to diagnose the disease and sometimes from failure to institute early treatment. Physicians continue to prescribe regimens which are manifestly inadequate; they fail to recognise that many patients from other countries may have an important degree of initial resistance — for example, 25% to isoniazid and 4.6% to rifampicin in Korea, 12.6% of Hispanics in the United States of America, and 16.3% in Hong Kong;[1] and they tinker about with monotherapy during the management of toxic reactions. Neglect of adequate explanation to patients is sometimes responsible.

The patient may fail to comply because of ignorance, lack of intelligence, or indifference and these may be difficult to overcome. Complex social problems, the stigma of disease, psychiatric illness and alcoholism are other factors. Enlisting the aid of relatives in supervising treatment and regular checks of drug consumption and urine tests to determine the presence of drug metabolites also lessen failure.

## Chemoprophylaxis of Tuberculosis

By using the tuberculin skin test and additional epidemiological criteria one can identify persons who are at a higher risk of developing tuberculosis.

### Primary Chemoprophylaxis

Primary (infection) chemoprophylaxis refers to the use of antituberculosis drugs in uninfected persons who are tuberculin-negative in order to prevent infection. The only indication in this context is to prevent infection of infants by sputum smear-positive mothers. There is no indication for the use of mass prophylaxis.

### Secondary Chemoprophylaxis

There is considerable disagreement regarding the degree of use of secondary (disease) chemoprophylaxis; that is, the use of drugs in infected individuals with no clinical evidence of tuberculosis in order to prevent the development of disease. In several large-scale well-designed clinical trials, isoniazid reduced the incidence of tuberculosis during the year of medication by 70 to 80%,[25] and in those who took most of the drug may have afforded 90% protection.[26] There is evidence that a high level of protection was afforded for up to 20 years. Isoniazid in a dose of 300mg (10mg/kg in children, maximum 300mg) given in a single dose for 12 months is recommended. Research into the possible role of rifampicin in prophylaxis is being conducted. Reluctance to use isoniazid more frequently is due to the small risk of hepatitis. The risk is age-related with an overall occurrence of slightly greater than 1%.[27] Under 20 years of age the risk is extremely small, but it rises to 1.2% from 35 to 49 years and to about 2% over 50 years of age. Patients should be seen at monthly intervals, but routine liver function tests are not recommended.

The decision to recommend chemoprophylaxis should be based on an estimation of the risk of developing the disease, the risk of isoniazid-induced hepatitis, the likelihood of compliance, and the epidemiological background.

In technically advanced countries, prophylaxis is generally advised in the following groups: (i) recently infected persons — all tuberculin convertors and all close contacts under 35 years of age of infectious persons; (ii) tuberculin-positive children under five years of age because of the risk of meningitis; (iii) strongly positive tuberculin reactors known to be at special risk, such as recent immigrants from countries with a high prevalence of tuberculosis; and (iv) immunosuppressed patients, those with chronic renal insufficiency, renal transplantation, or conditions associated with substantial weight loss (gastrectomy, intestinal bypass). Patients with radiographic abnormalities should be given treatment with at least two antituberculosis drugs.

## Surgical Treatment

Chemotherapy is now so effective that the indications for surgical treatment are few in number.

Surgical treatment for an uncomplicated residual open cavity would have been invariably employed in past years. This is no longer an indication, but if the cavity has been colonised by *Aspergillus fumigatus* with formation of a mycetoma, resection should be considered in the absence of specific contraindications.

Surgical resection requires consideration and may be desirable in the following circumstances: (i) as a diagnostic measure when all other methods of investigation have failed to resolve the problem; (ii) when, after careful appraisal of all the circumstances, it is considered that the patient is unlikely to cooperate throughout the whole period of treatment; (iii) when drug-resistant infection is present and there is intolerance to reserve drugs; (iv) when there are recurrent intractable non-tuberculous infections, often accompanied by haemoptysis, and for removal of a mycetoma; (v) very rarely, in primary tuberculosis, for the removal of mediastinal glands which are life-threatening; and (vi) tuberculous empyema.

It must be emphasised that surgical resection does not render unnecessary a proper course of chemotherapy, for there may be other lesions present which are the potential seeds of relapse.

Surgical treatment may be necessary in selected patients suffering from skeletal tuberculosis, and extremely rarely in the management of lymph node or renal disease.

## Corticosteroid Treatment

Corticosteroids have no place in the routine treatment of pulmonary tuberculosis.[28] However, their use is mandatory in the treatment of the adult respiratory distress syndrome which sometimes complicates acute miliary tuberculosis and, less commonly, acute extensive pulmonary tuberculosis.

Corticosteroids (prednisolone 5mg four times daily for two to three weeks, followed by decreasing dosage over a further two to four weeks according to severity) aid absorption of pleural fluid and may avoid the need for further aspiration.[29]

Severe drug reactions may require steroid treatment and desensitisation is sometimes necessary under steroid cover.

## Hospitalisation and Isolation

The majority of patients should be treated wholly as outpatients. The general advice given in the code of practice of the Joint Tuberculosis Committee of the British Thoracic Society (1983) is as follows: 'For practical purposes patients with pulmonary tuberculosis in whose sputum tubercle bacilli were seen on direct examination should be regarded as non-infectious after two weeks of chemotherapy including rifampicin but may not remain so unless regular and adequate chemotherapy is continued thereafter.'[30] More prolonged isolation may be advisable for teachers and others in close contact with young people, and for patients in contact with immunosuppressed persons. Longer isolation may be considered for irresponsible people and patients excreting drug-resistant mycobacteria. Infectious patients should be accommodated in a well-ventilated single room or in a ward specifically set aside for patients with infectious tuberculosis. They should be advised to cover the mouth when coughing. Barrier nursing and special care of fomites are unnecessary. Patients in whom three or more sputum smears give negative results on direct examination, and those who have extrapulmonary tuberculosis, do not require isolation. It is not uncommon for tuberculosis to be diagnosed in patients already in hospital, but their retention is justifiable only in the following circumstances: (i) infectivity as defined above; (ii) severe constitutional illness, adult respiratory distress syndrome, potentially life-threatening forms of the disease such as miliary or meningeal disease, or haemoptysis; (iii) the management of severe manifestations of drug toxicity including hypersensitivity reactions; and (iv) coexisting disease such as renal or hepatic disease requiring specialist management.

## Patient Education

It is important to emphasise the possibilities for cure which now exist, and that cure depends wholly on the patients taking chemotherapy faithfully throughout the recommended period even though they are feeling entirely well. Written instructions detailing the regimen are helpful. Specific indications should be spelled out for stopping treatment and seeking immediate advice: for example, impairment of vision (ethambutol), dizziness (streptomycin) and febrile cutaneous reactions (all drugs). Enlisting the help of relatives is valuable in the elderly and in potentially uncoperative patients.

## References

1. Horne NW. Some problems of tuberculosis in decline. *Br Med J* 1984; 288: 1249.
2. Mitchison DA. Treatment of tuberculosis. *J R Coll Physicians* 1980; 14: 91.
3. Fox W. Short course chemotherapy for tuberculosis. In: Flenley DC, ed. *Recent advances in respiratory disease 2.* Edinburgh, London, Melbourne, New York: Churchill Livingstone, 1980: 183.
4. Jindani A, Aber VR, Edwards A, Mitchison DA. The early bactericidal activity of drugs in patients with pulmonary tuberculosis. *Am Rev Respir Dis* 1980; 121: 939.
5. Grosset J. The sterilising value of rifampicin and pyrazinamide in experimental short course chemotherapy. *Tubercle* 1958; 59: 287.

6. Horne NW. Short-course chemotherapy for tuberculosis. In: Flenley DC, Petty TL, eds. *Recent advances in respiratory disease 3*. Edinburgh, London, Melbourne, New York: Churchill Livingstone, 1983: 226.
7. Crofton J. 'Sputum conversion' and the metabolism of isoniazid. *Am Rev Tuberc Respir Dis* 1958; 77: 869.
8. Ross JD, Horne NW, Grant IWB, Crofton JW. Hospital treatment of pulmonary tuberculosis. A follow-up study of patients admitted to Edinburgh hospitals in 1953. *Br Med J* 1958; 1: 237.
9. Fox W. Compliance of patients and physicians: experience and lessons from tuberculosis. *Br Med J* 1983; 287: 33: 101.
10. British Thoracic and Tuberculosis Association. Short course chemotherapy in pulmonary tuberculosis. *Lancet* 1976; 2: 1102.
11. Brouet G, Roussel G. Trial 6.9.12. Overall methods and results. *Rev Fr Mal Respir* 1977; 5 (suppl 1): 5.
12. British Thoracic Society. A controlled trial of 6 months' chemotherapy in pulmonary tuberculosis. Final report: results during the 36 months after the end of chemotherapy and beyond. *Br J Dis Chest* 1984; 78: 330.
13. Hong Kong Chest Service/Tuberculosis Research Centre, Madras/British Medical Research Council. A controlled trial of 2-month, 3-month and 12-month regimens of chemotherapy for sputum smear-negative pulmonary tuberculosis. *Am Rev Respir Dis* 1981; 115: 138.
14. Girling DJ. Adverse effects of anti-tuberculosis drugs. *Drugs* 1982; 23: 56.
15. Ross JD, Horne NW. *Modern drug treatment in tuberculosis*. 6th ed. London: Chest, Heart and Stroke Association, 1983.
16. Doble N, Hykin P, Shaw R, Keale EE. Pulmonary *Mycobacterium tuberculosis* in acquired immune deficiency syndrome. *Br Med J* 1985; 291: 849.
17. So SY, Yu D. The adult respiratory distress syndrome in miliary tuberculosis. *Tubercle* 1981; 62: 49.
18. Committee on Chemotherapy of Tuberculosis. Standard therapy for tuberculosis 1985. *Chest* 1985; 87 (supplement): 117S.
19. Crofton J. The prevention and management of drug-resistant tuberculosis. *Ann Med (Barc)* 1984; 70: 205.
20. Wolinsky E. Non-tuberculous mycobacteria and associated diseases. *Am Rev Respir Dis* 1979; 119: 107.
21. Committee on *M. intracellulare* Disease. Disease due to *Mycobacterium avium intracellulare. Chest* 1985; 87: 139S.
22. Skutil S, Varga J, Obsitnik M, Moro I. Six months chemotherapy of urogenital tuberculosis. *Bull Int Union Tuberc* 1982; 57: 46.
23. Wong SH, Lau WY, Ho KK, Fan ST, Yiu TF, Chan SL. The management of urinary tuberculosis — a logical approach. *Br J Urol* 1984; 56: 349.
24. British Thoracic Society Research Committee. Short course chemotherapy for tuberculosis of lymph nodes: a controlled trial. *Br Med J* 1985; 290: 1106.
25. Ferebee SH. Controlled chemoprophylaxis trials in tuberculosis: a general review. *Adv Tuberc Res* 1970; 17: 28.
26. Comstock GW, Baum C, Snider DE. Isoniazid prophylaxis among Alaskan Eskimos: a final report of the Bethel isoniazid studies. *Am Rev Respir Dis* 1979; 119: 827.
27. Kopanoff DE, Snider DE, Caras GJ. Isoniazid-related hepatitis. *Am Rev Respir Dis* 1978; 117: 991.
28. Horne NW. A critical evaluation of corticosteroids in tuberculosis. *Adv Tuberc Res* 1966; 15: 1.
29. Menon NK. Steroid therapy in tuberculous pleural effusion. *Tubercle* 1964; 45: 17.
30. Joint Tuberculosis Committee of the British Thoracic Society. Control and prevention of tuberculosis: a code of practice. *Br Med J* 1983; 287: 1118.

# Chapter 13

# Primary Pulmonary Hypertension

*D.N. Sharpe*

Numerous pathological processes can result in pulmonary hypertension. In many cases, the cause will be apparent from clinical assessment. In such conditions as mitral valve disease, intracardiac left-to-right shunting, parenchymal lung disease or thromboembolism, treatment will be directed towards the underlying cause. The outcome of treatment will be determined by the potential reversibility of the causative condition and the concomitant changes which have occurred in the pulmonary vasculature.

In some cases, however, there is no clinically identifiable cause, in which case the pulmonary hypertension may be designated primary, idiopathic or, perhaps most appropriately, unexplained. The syndrome of primary pulmonary hypertension occurs most commonly in young women, although presentation in childhood is well known.[1] Occasionally a familial pattern of presentation may occur.[2,3] Apart from genetic susceptibility possibly related to vascular hyper-reactivity, various agents have been linked with pulmonary hypertension including the drugs aminorex[4] and fenfluramine[5] and the alkaloid crotaline.[6] Progressive pulmonary vascular disease has also been associated with the use of oral contraceptives.[7,8]

## Diagnostic Features

Clinical presentation is generally at a late stage in the disease when pulmonary hypertension is severe. The commonest initial symptoms are dyspnoea on exertion and tiredness. At a late stage, chest pain, haemoptysis, oedema or syncope may occur. The clinical signs are those of increased pressure in the pulmonary arterial circulation and right heart, and signs of right heart failure may occur at a late stage.

The chest X-ray characteristically shows cardiac enlargement, proximal dilatation and peripheral 'pruning' of pulmonary arteries. The electrocardiographic changes reflect right heart dilatation and hypertrophy. Echocardiography is helpful in confirming the presence of right heart dilatation and hypertrophy and typically the M mode pulmonary valve echo will show a flattened diastolic slope, a loss of the 'a' wave and systolic notching, which are relatively specific for pulmonary hypertension. An estimate of pulmonary arterial pressure can be obtained using Doppler techniques.[9,10] Echo-Doppler techniques will assist in ruling out valvular and left ventricular disease, and radionuclide ventilation-perfusion lung scanning can exclude major pulmonary embolism. Haematological and other investigations will be directed towards excluding treatable causes of secondary pulmonary hypertension particularly the connective tissue diseases, systemic lupus erythematosus, scleroderma and rheumatoid disease.

The place of lung biopsy in management is not clearly established and remains controversial. Open lung biopsy is generally preferred to other methods which are more hazardous and may not provide an adequate sample.

A variety of histological appearances is encountered, emphasising the heterogeneous pathological nature of the condition.[11,12] The finding of medial hypertrophy alone implies an early stage of disease and potential reversibility. This appears to be followed by the development of fixed obstructive disease with intimal proliferation, fibrosis and necrosis, and characteristic arterial plexiform lesions. Commonly, in-situ thrombosis is found which may be either primary or secondary. Other diagnostic possibilities include pulmonary arteritis, thromboembolism and veno-occlusive disease which may be difficult to distinguish clinically from primary pulmonary hypertension without lung biopsy.

## Natural History and Prognosis

The prognosis of primary pulmonary hypertension is extremely poor, with approximately 50% of patients dying within two years of diagnosis and 75% within five years.[13,14] However, there is considerable individual variation and a proportion of patients remains stable for many years. It is important that every patient presenting with pulmonary hypertension be fully investigated to ensure that no possible treatable cause of secondary hypertension is present.

Medical treatment is generally only palliative and in most cases clearly has little if any effect on disease progression. The response to vasodilator treatment depends to some extent on the histological characteristics and stage of the disease. Diagnosis in the early stages of the disease and the demonstration of medial hypertrophy without irreversible obstructive changes would appear to increase the likelihood of a beneficial response to treatment. The variable responses reported to different vasodilator drugs reflect to some extent the spectrum of histological characteristics and potential reversibility. While treatment options are limited and may not affect prognosis, the variable nature of the disease and response to treatment justify full investigation and a trial of treatment with careful monitoring. Recently heart-lung transplantation has been employed in a few selected terminal cases.

## Goals of Treatment

There is no effective treatment for the basic underlying disease process which remains ill-understood. Therapeutic options which may be considered are aimed at preventing or reversing thrombosis in the pulmonary vasculature, lowering the elevated arterial resistance and pressure, and treating right heart failure and associated systemic venous congestion.

## Treatment

### Anticoagulants

Long-term oral anticoagulation is generally recommended in view of the finding of arterial thrombosis in a high proportion of patients on lung biopsy or at autopsy, and also to prevent secondary thromboembolism. Although there is no definite evidence of benefit from this approach from a controlled prospective trial, a large retrospective study has demonstrated improved survival in patients with primary pulmonary hypertension receiving oral anticoagulants compared with those who did not.[13]

## Vasodilator Drugs

A wide range of vasodilator agents has been employed in the treatment of primary pulmonary hypertension. None has been shown more effective than others although there are numerous reports of haemodynamic and symptomatic improvement with many of these drugs in individual cases and small groups of patients.

The rationale for the administration of vasodilator drugs in primary pulmonary hypertension compares with that related to their administration in chronic left ventricular failure. However, whereas in left ventricular failure the elevated systemic vascular resistance is generally reversible and provides the basis for beneficial afterload reduction, in primary pulmonary hypertension the elevated pulmonary vascular resistance may be fixed. Furthermore, vasodilator therapy cannot be applied selectively to the pulmonary circulation. Thus in primary pulmonary hypertension where elevated pulmonary vascular resistance is related to obstructive irreversible structural changes, selective systemic vasodilatation with no reduction in pulmonary vascular resistance may result in systemic hypotension and possibly coronary and cerebral hypoperfusion. Right ventricular output and hence left ventricular filling and cardiac output may be further compromised as a result of systemic venodilatation and reduction in right ventricular filling. Negative inotropic effects of some vasodilator drugs may also contribute to haemodynamic deterioration.

Thus vasodilator drugs should be given carefully on a trial basis with haemodynamic monitoring to compare the response to different agents and avoid adverse effects. Although most vasodilator agents act predominantly on the systemic circulation and also produce a fall in pulmonary vascular resistance to some extent, significant reduction in pulmonary artery pressure is much more difficult to achieve. Changes in pulmonary vascular resistance alone are not necessarily a reliable guide to response which is best judged by comparing the percentage fall in pulmonary vascular resistance with the percentage fall in systemic vascular resistance.[15] A beneficial pulmonary vasodilator response is characterised by a fall in pulmonary resistance greater than the fall in systemic resistance, accompanied by a significant fall in pulmonary artery pressure without a significant change in systemic pressure.

Of the beta-adrenoreceptor agonists, isoprenaline (isoproterenol) has been most widely used. Sustained clinical improvement with sublingual isoprenaline over a period of years has been reported in an individual in whom reduction in moderately elevated pulmonary artery pressure was demonstrated on several separate occasions during this time.[16] While other studies have demonstrated haemodynamic improvement with isoprenaline,[17,18] unfavourable effects have also been reported due to the inotropic effect exceeding the pulmonary vasodilator effect and causing a further increase in pulmonary artery pressure.[19] Experience has also been reported with alpha-adrenoreceptor antagonists such as tolazoline intravenously,[20] and phentolamine intravenously and orally[21,22] with varying results.

Direct-acting vasodilators, particularly diazoxide[23-25] and hydrallazine[26-28] have been used in primary pulmonary hypertension, again with mixed results. The variable haemodynamic response to vasodilator treatment that can occur in primary pulmonary hypertension is well exemplified by the disparate response to hydrallazine.[26-28] In one study hydrallazine was effective in markedly reducing pulmonary vascular resistance and increasing cardiac output in four patients without causing changes in systemic arterial pressure or oxygen saturation.[26] These changes were demonstrated at rest and during exercise and continued after long-term treatment. Therapy was well tolerated and exercise tolerance and symptoms improved.

In contrast, in another study which included six patients with primary pulmonary hypertension,[28] hydrallazine produced only moderate pulmonary vasodilatation with the decrease in resistance in the systemic circulation exceeding that in the pulmonary circuit, no significant decrease in pulmonary artery and right heart pressures but substantial reduction in systemic arterial pressure and an increase in heart rate. The conclusion from this study was that careful invasive haemodynamic verification of a beneficial drug response is necessary before long-term treatment is contemplated, and that empirical hydrallazine therapy in patients with pulmonary hypertension can cause adverse reactions and should not be undertaken.

Calcium channel antagonists offer a further therapeutic option in the treatment of pulmonary hypertension.[29] Experimental studies in dogs in whom pulmonary hypertension was produced by hypoxia or infusion of prostaglandin $F_{2\alpha}$ suggest that nifedipine may be a more effective pulmonary vasodilator than verapamil or diltiazem.[30] A number of case reports claim short and long term haemodynamic and symptomatic improvement with calcium channel antagonists in pulmonary hypertension.[31-36] A favourable haemodynamic and symptomatic response to nifedipine sublingually and orally both short and long term has also been reported in a larger series of patients.[37] However, adverse effects were noted in this study. One patient who experienced systemic vasodilatation in the absence of a pulmonary vasodilator response had a marked increase in pulmonary artery pressure, probably due to reflex sympathetic stimulation causing an increased heart rate and cardiac output. The negative inotropic effect of calcium channel antagonists, particularly verapamil, may also be detrimental to patients with primary pulmonary hypertension who have pre-existing right ventricular dysfunction.[38] Thus the overall haemodynamic response to calcium channel antagonists, as with other vasodilators, will depend on the extent to which selective pulmonary vasodilatation is achieved with the additional factor of possible negative inotropic effect.

Other vasodilators of potential benefit include the serotoninergic antagonist ketanserin, the angiotensin converting enzyme inhibitor captopril[39] and prostacyclin.[40-41] Although beneficial in some cases, none of these appears to provide a particular advantage over other vasodilators. Prostacyclin may be helpful in identifying patients with reversible pulmonary hypertension who may respond to conventional vasodilators. While it is a potent vasodilator, it can only be given parenterally and has a relatively high incidence of side effects including headache, nausea and vomiting, flushing and systemic hypotension. Oxygen inhalation in hospital or at home may attenuate pulmonary vasoconstriction and increase blood oxygen saturation and is commonly used.[42]

In conclusion, although a variety of vasodilator agents has been investigated in the treatment of primary pulmonary hypertension, none has been proven particularly effective. Although the syndrome remains unexplained and treatment palliative, full investigation and a trial of treatment with careful monitoring is justifiable in all cases to rule out possible remediable causes and achieve optimal treatment of any component of reversible pulmonary vasoconstriction. While selective pulmonary vasodilating agents with minimal side effects may yet be developed, prognosis is likely to remain very poor with such a high proportion of patients presenting at a late stage when pulmonary hypertension is severe and irreversible. In the future, heart-lung transplantation may provide long-term benefit for advanced disease, although its role in treatment has yet to be defined clearly.

## References


1. Farrar JF, Reye RDK, Stucker D. Primary pulmonary hypertension in childhood. *Br Heart J* 1961; 23: 605-615.
2. Melmon KL, Braunwald E. Familial pulmonary hypertension. *N Engl J Med* 1963; 269: 770-775.
3. Loyd JE, Primm RK, Newman JH. Familial primary pulmonary hypertension: clinical patterns. *Am Rev Respir Dis* 1984; 129: 194-197.
4. Kay JM, Smith P, Heath D. Aminorex and pulmonary circulation. *Thorax* 1971; 26: 262-270.
5. Douglas JG, Munro JF, Kitchin AH, Muir AL, Proudfoot AT. Pulmonary hypertension and fenfluramine. *Br Med J* 1981; 283: 881-883.
6. Meyrick B, Reid L. Development of pulmonary arterial changes in rats fed *Crotalaria spectabilis*. *Am J Pathol* 1979; 94: 37-48.
7. Oakley CM, Somerville J. Oral contraceptives and progressive pulmonary vascular disease. *Lancet* 1968; 1: 890-893.
8. Kleiger RE, Boxer M, Ingham R, Harrison DC. Pulmonary hypertension in patients using oral contraceptives. *Chest* 1976; 69: 143-147.
9. Yock PG, Popp RL. Noninvasive estimation of right ventricular systolic pressure by Doppler ultrasound in patients with tricuspid regurgitation. *Circulation* 1984; 70: 657-662.
10. Kitabatake A, Inoue M, Asao M, et al. Noninvasive evaluation of pulmonary hypertension by a pulsed Doppler technique. *Circulation* 1983; 68: 302-309.
11. Wagenvoort CA, Wagenvoort N. Primary pulmonary hypertension: a pathologic study of the lung vessels in 156 clinically diagnosed cases. *Circulation* 1970; 42: 1163-1184.
12. Bjornsson J, Edwards WD. Primary pulmonary hypertension: a histopathologic study of 80 cases. *Mayo Clin Proc* 1985; 60: 16-25.
13. Fuster V, Steele PM, Edwards WD, Gersh BJ, McGoon MD, Frye RL. Primary pulmonary hypertension: natural history and the importance of thrombosis. *Circulation* 1984; 70: 580-587.
14. Suarez LD, Sciandro EE, Llera JJ, Perosio AM. Long term follow-up in primary pulmonary hypertension. *Br Heart J* 1979; 41: 702-708.
15. Rich S, Martinez J, Lam W, Levy PS, Rosen KM. Reassessment of the effects of vasodilator drugs in primary pulmonary hypertension: guidelines for determining a pulmonary vasodilator response. *Am Heart J* 1983; 105: 119-127.
16. Pietro DA, La Bresh KA, Shulman RM, Folland ED, Parisi AF, Sasahara AA. Sustained improvement in primary pulmonary hypertension during six years of treatment with sublingual isoproterenol. *N Engl J Med* 1984; 310: 1032-1034.
17. Shettigar UR, Hultgren HN, Specter M, Martin R, Davies DH. Primary pulmonary hypertension: favourable effect of isoproterenol. *N Engl J Med* 1976; 295: 1414-1415.
18. Daoud FS, Reeves JT, Kely DB. Isoproterenol as a potential pulmonary vasodilator in primary pulmonary hypertension. *Am J Cardiol* 1978; 42: 817-822.

19. Elkayam U, Frishman WH, Yoran C, Strom J, Sonnenblick EH, Cohen MN. Unfavourable haemodynamic and clinical effects of isoproterenol in primary pulmonary hypertension. *Cardiovasc Med* 1977; 3: 1177-1180.
20. Rudolph AM, Paul MH, Sommer LS, Nadas AS. Effects of tolazoline hydrochloride (priscoline) on circulatory dynamics of patients with pulmonary hypertension. *Am Heart J* 1958; 55: 424-432.
21. Ruskin JN, Hutter AM Jr. Primary pulmonary hypertension treated with oral phentolamine. *Ann Intern Med* 1979; 90: 772-774.
22. Cohen ML, Krozon I. Adverse hemodynamic effects of phentolamine in primary pulmonary hypertension. *Ann Intern Med* 1981; 95: 591-592.
23. Wang SWS, Pohl JEF, Rowlands DJ, Wade EG. Diazoxide in treatment of primary pulmonary hypertension. *Br Heart J* 1978; 40: 572-574.
24. Klinke WP, Gilbert JAL. Diazoxide in primary pulmonary hypertension. *N Engl J Med* 1980; 302: 91-92.
25. Honey M, Cotter L, Davies N, Denison D. Clinical and haemodynamic effects of diazoxide in primary pulmonary hypertension. *Thorax* 1980; 35: 269-276.
26. Rubin LJ, Peter RH. Oral hydralazine therapy for primary pulmonary hypertension. *N Engl J Med* 1980; 302: 69-73.
27. Lupi-Herrera E, Sandoval J, Seoane M, Bialostozky D. The role of hydralazine therapy for pulmonary arterial hypertension of unknown cause. *Circulation* 1982; 65: 645-650.
28. Packer M, Greenberg B, Massie B, Dash H. Deleterious effects of hydralazine in patients with pulmonary hypertension. *N Engl J Med* 1982; 306: 1326-1331.
29. Packer M. Therapeutic application of calcium-channel antagonists for pulmonary hypertension. *Am J Cardiol* 1985; 55: 196B-201B.
30. Young TE, Lundquist LJ, Chesler E, Weir EK. Comparative effects of nifedipine, verapamil, and diltiazem on experimental pulmonary hypertension. *Am J Cardiol* 1983; 51: 195-200.
31. Landmark K, Refsum AM, Simonsen S, Storstein O. Verapamil and pulmonary hypertension. *Acta Med Scand* 1978; 204: 299-302.
32. Camerini F, Alberti E, Klugmann S, Silvi A. Primary pulmonary hypertension: effects of nifedipine. *Br Heart J* 1980; 44: 352-356.
33. Kambara H, Fujimoto K, Wakabayasi A, Kawai C. Primary pulmonary hypertension: beneficial therapy with diltiazem. *Am Heart J* 1981; 101: 230-231.
34. De Feyter PJ, Kerkkamp HJJ, de Jone JP. Sustained beneficial effect of nifedipine in primary pulmonary hypertension. *Am Heart J* 1983; 105: 333-334.
35. Wise JR. Nifedipine in the treatment of primary pulmonary hypertension. *Am Heart J* 1983; 105: 693-694.
36. Saito D, Haraoka S, Yoshida H, et al. Primary pulmonary hypertension improved by long-term oral administration of nifedipine. *Am Heart J* 1983; 105: 1041-1042.
37. Rubin LJ, Nicod P, Hillis LD, Firth BG. Treatment of primary pulmonary hypertension with nifedipine. A hemodynamic and scintigraphic evaluation. *Ann Intern Med* 1983; 99: 433-438.
38. Packer M, Medina N, Yushak M, Wiener I. Detrimental effects of verapamil in patients with primary pulmonary hypertension. *Br Heart J* 1984; 52: 106-111.
39. Ikram H, Maslowski AH, Nicholls MG, Espiner EA, Hull FTL. Haemodynamic and hormonal effects of captopril in primary pulmonary hypertension. *Br Heart J* 1982; 48: 541-545.
40. Guadagni DN, Ikram H, Maslowski AH. Haemodynamic effects of prostacyclin ($PGI_2$) in pulmonary hypertension. *Br Heart J* 1981; 45: 385-388.
41. Rubin LJ, Groves BM, Reeves JT, Frosolono M, Handel F. Prostacyclin-induced acute pulmonary vasodilation in primary pulmonary hypertension. *Circulation* 1982; 65: 334-338.
42. Nagasaka Y, Akutsu H, Lee YS, Fujimoto S, Chikamori J. Long term favourable effect of oxygen administration on a patient with primary pulmonary hypertension. *Chest* 1978; 74: 299-300.

# Chapter 14

# Cystic Fibrosis

*Margaret E. Hodson*

Cystic fibrosis is a disease characterised by chronic bronchopulmonary infection, malabsorption and a high sweat sodium concentration. It is a multisystem disease and its features are fully described in basic textbooks.[1-4] The first clinical and pathological description of this condition was published in 1938.[5] At that time, 80% of babies born with cystic fibrosis died within one year of birth, but now many are surviving into adult life. The best survival figures come from 'specialised cystic fibrosis centres'[6,7] indicating that 80% of patients should reach 19 or 20 years of age. In the UK a recent study by the British Paediatric Association suggests that in the next five years we can expect 200 patients to reach 15 years of age.[8] The improved survival is probably due to better paediatrics and improvements in physiotherapy and chemotherapeutic agents particularly antibiotics. The increasing number of new patients presents an exciting therapeutic challenge.

## Diagnostic Tests

The diagnosis of cystic fibrosis depends on a careful history and examination and is confirmed by the sweat test.[9] The method used is that of Gibson and Cooke.[10] A sweat sodium of above 60mmol/L in childhood is considered to be diagnostic. Sweating is induced by pilocarpine iontophoresis, the secretions are collected and then analysed chemically for the chloride and sodium concentration. The pad under the positive electrode is soaked with 0.4% pilocarpine nitrate solution, and the pad under the negative electrode in N/10 magnesium sulphate solution. The iontophoresis enhances the penetration of the pilocarpine into the sweat glands and so stimulates sweating.

Unfortunately the sweat test is less discriminating after puberty as the normal person's sweat electrolytes rise with age and the sweat sodium may easily reach 60 to 90 mmol/L. When making a diagnosis of cystic fibrosis in an adult, at least two sweat sodium values of over 70mmol/L should be obtained on separate occasions.[11] Pretreatment with fludrocortisone increases the usefulness of the sweat test in adults.[12] After baseline tests have been performed a daily dose of $3mg/m^2$ (5mg for the average adult) of fludrocortisone acetate is given for two days and the sweat test is repeated. In cystic fibrosis patients the sodium values do not fall below 70mmol/L, contrasting with normal adults.

## Pancreatic Enzymes

About 85% of patients with cystic fibrosis have symptomatic steatorrhoea,[13] and abnormalities of pancreatic exocrine secretion can be detected in almost all patients. Patients pass frequent, bulky, pale, offensive, greasy, semi-formed stools. This is socially embarrassing and causes malnutrition. The pancreatic enzymes which are deficient include amylase, trypsin and lipase which are important for the digestion of carbohydrate, protein and fat respectively. Absorption of the fat soluble vitamins A, D, E and K and some minerals may also be affected.

The majority of patients are deficient in pancreatic enzymes and require replacement enzyme therapy. The enzymes used are usually derived from the hog pancreas, but some preparations contain enzymes of plant origin and some bile salts. A variety of preparations is available (Table 14.1); these vary from country to country.

*Table 14.1* Some pancreatin preparations in units BP

| Preparation | Lipase | Protease | Amylase |
|---|---|---|---|
| **Powder** | | | |
| Pancreatin BP | 20 000/g | 1400/g | 24 000/g |
| *Pancrex V* (Paines & Byrne) | 25 000/g | 1400/g | 30 000/g |
| **Enteric-coated Granules** | | | |
| *Pancrex* (Paines & Byrne) | 5000/g | 300/g | 4000/g |
| **Capsules** | | | |
| *Cotazym* (Organon) | 14 000 | 500 | 10 000 |
| *Pancrex V* (Paines & Byrne) | 8000 | 430 | 9000 |
| **Tablets, Enteric-coated** | | | |
| *Nutrizym* (Merck) | 10 000 | 560 | 10 000 |
| *Pancrex V forte* (Paines & Byrne) | 5600 | 330 | 5000 |
| **Enteric-coated Granules in Capsules** | | | |
| *Creon* (Duphar) | 8000 | 210 | 9000 |
| Pancrease (Ortho-Cilag) | 5000 | 330 | 2900 |

1. Powders are suitable for infants and young children, but are rapidly inactivated by the acid of the stomach. These uncoated preparations are unpleasant to taste.
2. Enteric-coated preparations protect the enzyme until the alkaline medium of the duodenum is reached. However, as there is defective production of bicarbonate from most cystic fibrosis pancreases[14] and also increased acid production in the stomach, a strong enteric coating may not be fully digested.
3. Enteric-coated granules which are in gelatine capsules. These are relatively new on the market and are still being fully evaluated. However, it appears that they may give better protein and fat absorption and the patient may need to take fewer of these capsules per meal than with other forms of enzyme replacement therapy.

Pancreatic enzyme preparations should be taken just before or during each meal and with snacks. Powder for an infant can be mixed in a little milk and given on a teaspoon. It should not be mixed in the feeding bottle or sprinkled on food as this makes it unpalatable. The dose of enzyme is chosen to reduce the frequency and consistency of the stool to that which is optimal for the patient, and the dose that ensures that the child thrives and the adult maintains an adequate body weight.

In young children large doses of enzymes may cause perioral or perianal irritation. This is improved by a reduction in the dose. Occasionally patients may become allergic to hog pancreatin preparations in powder form.

Excessive pancreatic enzymes can cause abdominal pain and constipation. Increased levels of urinary uric acid have been found in some patients on large doses of pancreatic extracts. A reduction in the amount of enzyme taken returns the level of uric acid excreted to normal.

## $H_2$-Receptor Antagonists

Pancreatic enzymes are most effective at an alkaline pH. There is evidence of jejunal hyperacidity in cystic fibrosis. The giving of sodium bicarbonate in high doses with food is unpalatable. However, in some patients agents which reduce gastric acid secretion, such as cimetidine or ranitidine, may improve absorption.[15] If cimetidine is used it should be given in a dose of 400mg forty minutes before each meal. An enzyme, as an uncoated preparation, should then be given at the beginning and during the meal.

## Vitamins

It is the fat-soluble vitamins which particularly need supplementation in cystic fibrosis.

### Vitamin A

Serum levels are low in cystic fibrosis[16] although clinical deficiency is rare. Supplementation with 5000-10 000IU/day is recommended.

### Vitamins B and C

These water-soluble vitamins are present in most standard multivitamin preparations and deficiency is not recorded in cystic fibrosis. Reduced absorption of vitamin B12 is present, but the serum level is usually normal.

### Vitamin D

Rickets do not occur in cystic fibrosis except where there is severe coexisting liver disease. All patients, however, have low serum levels unless given supplements.[17] Supplementation with 400 to 800IU/day is recommended.

### Vitamin E

Vitamin E levels are generally low.[18] Severe vitamin E deficiency has resulted in spinocerebellar degeneration.[19] Vitamin E is an antioxidant and helps to protect unsaturated fatty acids from breakdown. It has been suggested that a combination of low serum vitamin E and low serum selenium may predispose to neoplasia.[20] Two hundred milligrams of a water-soluble preparation daily are recommended.

### Vitamin K

Deficiency may occur, especially in infants, causing bleeding due to hypoprothrombinaemia. Absorption of vitamin K is less, due to the steatorrhoea, and synthesis of vitamin $K_2$ by intestinal bacteria is less if antibiotics are being taken. If the prothrombin time is prolonged vitamin K, 10mg daily as a water-soluble preparation, is indicated.

## Minerals

### Iron

Iron absorption appears normal in cystic fibrosis, but deficiency may occur probably due to an inadequate intake. Supplementation by standard iron preparations is adequate if intake is low.

### Zinc

Low plasma zinc levels have been reported in a few cases of cystic fibrosis and may be associated with growth retardation.[21] If indicated, 61.8mg of zinc sulphate as a monohydrate may be given one to three times daily.

### Selenium

Serum levels in cystic fibrosis are usually low.[20] Selenium is contained in human red cell glutathione peroxidase which protects cells from oxidation and is in this way similar to vitamin E. Selenium toxicity is easily induced and therefore routine supplementation is not advised. It is more important to ensure adequate levels of vitamin E.

## Nutritional Supplements

Poor nutrition is present in the majority of patients with cystic fibrosis. It is due to maldigestion, malabsorption, chronic pulmonary infection and poor nutritional intake. The malabsorption may be partly counteracted by pancreatic enzymes. Chronic pulmonary infection is treated energetically, but attention to nutritional intake is also vital. The caloric requirements in cystic fibrosis are often above normal due to the chronic infection, and the excess caloric loss in the stools is not fully counteracted by pancreatic enzymes. A patient who has chronic infection may not feel like eating and so becomes accustomed to eating small meals. Children often have a ravenous appetite,[22] but older patients frequently eat less than their requirements.[23] It is essential to monitor the child's weight and height, and the older patient's weight. Regular assessment of dietary intake is also recommended. All patients with malabsorption are encouraged to take a high calorie, high protein diet, with a normal fat content and are given sufficient enzymes to control the frequency of the bowel action. If enzymes alone do not achieve this, then the addition of an $H_2$-receptor blocker may be helpful. In only a few patients is fat restriction required. However, when advanced respiratory disease is present it is usually necessary to give nutritional supplements to maintain caloric intake.

Simple measures such as encouraging the patient to eat three meals daily with snacks mid-morning, mid-afternoon and before retiring are helpful. Some patients need extra supplements such as medium chain triglycerides (MCT) as an oil or incorporated in special milks, *Pregestimil* or *Portagen* (Mead Johnson). Older patients may use glucose polymers such as *Caloreen*

(Roussell), *Polycal* (Cow & Gate) or *Maxijul* (Scientific Hospital Supplies) added to food or drinks. Skimmed milk based products such as *Build-up* (Carnation) are available in several flavours and may be made up with milk or water. Raw eggs and ice cream can also be used to fortify milks or custards.

Other methods of supplementary nutrition have been used. Nasogastric or nasojejunal feeding have been used and an increase in body weight has been reported.[24] Older patients resent having a tube passed each night and if the tube is left down it is socially embarrassing and impedes the vitally important chest physiotherapy. Parenteral intravenous nutrition has been shown to be beneficial.[25,26] Some work has been done on gastrostomy and jejunostomy feeding, but this requires further evaluation. These invasive methods of supplementary nutrition may be useful in the short term, but are not a long-term solution to the nutritional problems of the cystic fibrosis patient. Whenever possible, oral supplementation should be used.

## Antibiotics

The major cause of morbidity and mortality in cystic fibrosis is pulmonary infection.[27,28] The major bacterial pathogens are *Staphylococcus aureus, Haemophilus influenzae* and *Pseudomonas aeruginosa;*[29] viruses may also act as important triggers to acute episodes of pulmonary infection in patients already colonised with these bacteria.[30]

Regular physiotherapy[31] is an essential part of treatment.

Infection with *Staphylococcus aureus* should be treated with flucloxacillin or erythromycin. Fusidic acid may be added in cases of severe infection. *H influenzae* infection may be treated with amoxycillin, tetracycline (not in children), erythromycin, co-trimoxazole or oral cephalosporins. In severe infection chloramphenicol may be very effective. Amoxycillin with clavulanic acid (*Augmentin*) may have a limited role in the treatment of *H influenzae* infection where beta-lactamases are also present in the sputum. Some of these oral antibiotics are used at higher doses than are conventionally given in an attempt to achieve higher levels in the sputum.

There is currently no generally available oral antibiotic effective against *Ps aeruginosa.* However, pilot studies on a quinolone, ciprofloxacin, are encouraging.[32] Present practice in a few centres is to treat patients with intravenous antibiotics every three months irrespective of symptoms,[33] but the most common practice is to treat patients chronically infected with *Ps aeruginosa* with antibiotics when there is an acute deterioration as indicated by an increase in cough, sputum or breathlessness, together with a deterioration in chest radiograph, peak expiratory flow rate, forced expiratory volume in one second or forced vital capacity. Patients are treated for a minimum of 10 days, or until maximum improvement is obtained. Drugs are usually given in hospital by intravenous cannula, such as a Venflon cannula with heparin-saline lock, but some patients may learn to give their own antibiotics at home. A few patients requiring frequent treatment may have a Portacath implanted in the chest wall to provide easy venous access. Two antibiotics are commonly given to take advantage of synergy and perhaps reduce the emergence of drug-resistant strains. The currently available preparations are carboxypenicillins (carbenicillin, ticarcillin), ureidopenicillins (azlocillin, mezlocillin, piperacillin), third generation cephalosporins (ceftazidime, cefsulodin), and aminoglycosides (gentamicin, tobramycin, netilmicin and amikacin).

Piperacillin is best avoided in the treatment of cystic fibrosis patients as febrile reactions have been seen following its use. There is no clinical evidence of superiority of one or other of these drugs. Ticarcillin has been compared with carbenicillin,[34] azlocillin with carbenicillin,[35] tobramycin with gentamicin,[36] and ceftazidime with azlocillin and gentamicin,[37] and no difference in clinical response has been demonstrated.

### Aerosol Antibiotics

These are mainly used for the treatment of *Pseudomonas* infection. It has been shown that the use of aerosol carbenicillin and gentamicin improves lung function and reduces the frequency of hospital admissions.[38] Azlocillin[39] and ceftazidime[40] have also been shown to be similarly effective. These preparations are given twice daily after physiotherapy. They are used as maintenance treatment and not to treat acute exacerbations of infection. The doses used are shown in Table 14.2. If two antibiotics are used these should not be mixed but given sequentially. It is vital that a nebuliser and high flow compressor (8 to 12 litres/minute) are used which will deliver small particles. The majority of particles should be less than five microns in diameter to ensure good penetration of the bronchopulmonary tree.[41] Arrangements should also be made to discharge exhaled antibiotics to the outside air. An Ambu-valve and a length of corrugated tubing are satisfactory. Aerosol antibiotics are tedious, time-consuming and expensive, and should probably only be used in patients requiring frequent admissions to hospital for intravenous antibiotics or in those whose condition shows a relentless decline in pulmonary function.

*Table 14.2* Aerosol antibiotics active against *Pseudomonas aeruginosa*

| Drug | Dilution |
|---|---|
| Colistin | 1 000 000 units diluted in 3-4ml normal saline |
| Gentamicin | 80mg/2ml |
| Carbenicillin | 1g in 4ml of sterile water |
| Ticarcillin | 1g in 4ml of sterile water |
| Azlocillin | 1g in 4ml of sterile water |

## Antiviral Agents

These are not of established value in respiratory infection. Influenza vaccine should be given to cystic fibrosis patients when an epidemic threatens.

## Antifungal Agents

These are rarely needed. Allergic bronchopulmonary aspergillosis should be treated with steroids and not antifungal agents. If a patient should develop invasive aspergillosis then amphotericin would be indicated.

## Mucolytic Agents

Infection increases the viscosity of sputum. Some clinicians used mucolytics such as acetylcysteine or carbocysteine for cystic fibrosis patients, but they are not of established value. Some patients find inhalations of 3ml of hypertonic (7%) saline helps expectoration of sputum.

## Bronchodilators

Many patients with cystic fibrosis have been shown to have increased bronchial lability.[42] About half the cystic fibrosis patients show an increase of 15% or more in pulmonary function after inhalation of salbutamol. Each patient should be assessed for reversibility, and if this is present should be given bronchodilator therapy before physiotherapy. Salbutamol 2.5 to 5mg, or terbutaline diluted to 3ml with saline, are suitable.

## Corticosteroids

There is a natural reluctance to use steroids in patients with chronic pulmonary infection. Prednisolone (0.5mg/kg/day) had no significant bronchodilator effect when given for three weeks in patients with severe airflow obstruction.[43] However, a recent randomised, placebo-controlled, four-year study of prednisolone (2mg/kg on alternate days) showed a significant improvement in lung function and growth in children with cystic fibrosis, suggesting the importance of inflammation in pulmonary pathology.[44] This form of treatment needs further evaluation.

Corticosteroids should be given when there is an acute deterioration in pulmonary symptoms which do not respond to intensive measures such as physiotherapy and antibiotics. They should also be given to patients who develop allergic bronchopulmonary aspergillosis. A dose of at least 30mg daily should be used initially. Steroids may also be helpful in the care of the terminal patient.

## Drugs used in the Management of Complicating Features

### Meconium Ileus

About 10% of children with cystic fibrosis present in the neonatal period with small bowel obstruction due to sticky inspissated intestinal contents. Enemas with *Gastrografin* may relieve the obstruction.[45] *Gastrografin* consists of sodium and methyl glucamine diatrizoates which are substances of high osmolality and they withdraw fluid from the circulation into the bowel and so allow the bowel contents to move along. Intravenous fluid is necessary to prevent dehydration. The enema is performed under fluoroscopic control and runs through the colon to the obstructed ileum. If this fails, surgery is necessary.

**Meconium Ileus Equivalent**

This syndrome of colicky abdominal pain, constipation and abdominal masses, is due to obstruction in the small bowel and occurs in older patients.[46] In subacute cases adjustment of the dose of pancreatic enzymes is needed, and in some cases the addition of an $H_2$-blocker, such as cimetidine 400mg given 40 minutes before food, is helpful. In acute cases rehydration using intravenous fluids is necessary. Thirty millilitres of 20% acetylcysteine diluted with 120ml of water or orange juice should be given three times daily by nasogastric tube. Thirty millilitres of 20% acetylcysteine should be added to 120 to 130ml of enema fluid, (such as *Fletchers disposable phosphate enema*) and administered three times daily.[47] The foot of the bed should be raised so that the fluid passes along the colon into the caecum. Some patients require a small maintenance dose of acetylcysteine to prevent reobstruction. *Gastrografin* is also successful in some patients.[48]

Recently it has been suggested that the subacute condition can be treated with balanced intestinal lavage solution.[49] This treatment needs further evaluation.

**Diabetes Mellitus**

The incidence of diabetes mellitus in cystic fibrosis increases with age About 10% of older patients have diabetes mellitus, and many more have impaired glucose tolerance. The majority of patients are easily controlled with oral hypoglycaemic agents or insulin. Ketoacidosis and vascular complications are rare.[50]

**Liver Disease**

Liver disease is well recognised in cystic fibrosis. That most commonly present is focal biliary cirrhosis. If the prothrombin time becomes prolonged vitamin K should be given. If varices develop and haematemesis occurs it may be treated conservatively with sedation, vitamin K, blood transfusion and vasopressin 5 to 20 units by intravenous infusion. The passage of a Sengstaken tube may be necessary. Some patients require sclerotherapy, portosystemic shunts or ligation of varices.[51]

**Salt Depletion**

In temperate climates this is rarely a problem. However, in the tropics salt supplements are necessary. For an adult, 2 to 6g daily of sodium chloride should be given. Care must be taken if the patient has cor pulmonale.

**Cardiac Failure**

This may occur in patients with severe pulmonary disease and is often present in the terminal phase of the disease. Digoxin is rarely indicated. Diuretics should be given and potassium supplements as required. Low concentrations of oxygen may be helpful.

### Sinusitis

Mucosal thickening demonstrated on the sinus X-rays is common, but requires no treatment. If acute sinusitis intervenes treatment is with antibiotics. Doxycycline is very suitable as it has good penetration into the sinuses. In a few cases lavage or antrostomy may be necessary.

### Nasal Polyps

These are more frequent in older patients.[50] Initially treatment should be with betamethasone and neomycin drops in the nose-down position.[52] In some cases surgery is needed.

### Arthritis

Hypertrophic pulmonary osteoarthropathy and other arthropathies affecting mainly the large joints of the lower limb occur in cystic fibrosis.[53,54] Treatment is with anti-inflammatory agents such as naproxen, ibuprofen, or indomethacin. Rarely in an acute episode a short course of systemic corticosteroids is indicated.

### Psychological Problems

Most adolescents and young adults are remarkably well adjusted to their disease. Sometimes a patient experiences depression which can be improved by the use of tricyclic antidepressants. Most psychological problems are treated by an experienced cystic fibrosis clinician without the use of drugs.[55] Frequently the family also requires counselling.

### Terminal Care

In the terminal phases of this disease, morphine and prochlorperazine can be helpful in relieving dyspnoea and anxiety. They should be given regularly four hourly. Steroids (15mg prednisolone daily) are also helpful in causing an elevation of mood.[55]

## Contraceptives

Females with cystic fibrosis are fertile, but many of them are not fit enough for pregnancy or to care for a toddler.[55] I have prescribed a combined oral contraceptive pill with 50$\mu$g of oestrogen to cystic fibrosis patients for many years and there have been no failures of contraception and no serious problems. A high-dose oestrogen pill was chosen because the patients have malabsorption and take frequent courses of antibiotics. However, recent work[56] suggests that the bioavailability of the Pill in cystic fibrosis patients may be as good as in normal females, so a low-dose oestrogen pill may be satisfactory. Barrier methods are less reliable, but are indicated in patients with established liver disease in whom the contraceptive pill would not be advisable.

## Drugs and Patients Who Travel

Patients who travel should take with them a good supply of their regular medications. They should also carry a letter with them for the Customs officer listing their medications, and if they are using an air compressor the letter should contain details of this, also syringes and needles necessary for measuring medications. This may save much aggravation and delay.

## References


1. Hodson ME. Cystic fibrosis. *Postgrad Med J* 1984; 60: 225-233.
2. Goodchild MC, Dodge JA. In: *Cystic fibrosis — manual of diagnosis and management*. London: Bailliere Tindall, 1985.
3. Lloyd Still D. *Textbook of cystic fibrosis*. Bristol: John Wright & Sons, 1983.
4. Hodson ME, Norman AP, Batten JC, eds. *Cystic fibrosis*. London: Bailliere Tindall, 1983.
5. Andersen DH. Cystic fibrosis of the pancreas and its relation to celiac disease. A clinical and pathological study. *Am J Dis Child* 1938; 56: 344-399.
6. Corey ML. Longitudinal studies in cystic fibrosis. In: Sturgess JM, ed. *Perspectives in cystic fibrosis*. Proceedings of the 8th International CF Congress, Toronto, Canada. Canadian CF Foundation, 1980: 246-255.
7. Phelan PD, Allan JL, Landau LI, et al. Improved survival of patients with cystic fibrosis. *Med J Aust* 1979; 1: 261-263.
8. British Paediatric Association. Working Group on Cystic Fibrosis, 1985. Unpublished report.
9. Di Sant'Agnese PA, Darling RG, Perera GA, et al. Abnormal electrolyte composition of sweat in cystic fibrosis of the pancreas, clinical significance and relationship to disease. *Am J Med* 1952; 15: 777-784.
10. Gibson LE, Cooke RE. A test for concentration of electrolytes in sweat in cystic fibrosis of the pancreas utilising pilocarpine by iontophoresis. *Pediatrics* 1959; 23: 545-549.
11. Kuzemko JA, Heeley AF. Diagnostic methods and screening. In: Hodson ME, Norman AP, Batten JC, eds. *Cystic fibrosis*. London: Bailliere Tindall, 1983.
12. Hodson ME, Beldon I, Power R, et al. Sweat tests in the diagnosis of cystic fibrosis in adults. *Br Med J* 1983; 286: 1381-1383.
13. Shwachman H. Gastrointestinal manifestations of cystic fibrosis. *Pediatr Clin North Am* 1975; 22: 787-805.
14. Zentler-Munro PL, Fine DR, Batten JC, et al. Effect of cimetidine on enzyme inactivation, bile acid precipitation and lipid solubilisation in pancreatic steatorrhoea due to cystic fibrosis. *Gut* 1985; 26: 892-901.
15. Gow R, Bradbear R, Francis P, et al. Comparative study of varying regimens to improve steatorrhoea and creatorrhoea in cystic fibrosis: effectiveness of an enteric-coated preparation with and without antacids and cimetidine. *Lancet* 1981; 2: 1071-1074.
16. Underwood BA, Denning CR. Blood and liver concentrations of vitamin A and E in children with cystic fibrosis. *Pediatr Res* 1972; 6: 26-31.
17. Congden PJ, Bruce G, Rothburn MM, et al. Vitamin status in treated patients with cystic fibrosis. *Arch Dis Child* 1981; 56: 708-714.
18. Stead RJ, Muller DPR, Matthews S, et al. The effect of abnormal liver function on vitamin E status and supplementation in adults with cystic fibrosis. *Gut*, 1985 (in press).
19. Willison HJ, Muller DPR, Matthews S, et al. A study of the relationship between neurological function and serum vitamin E concentrations in patients with cystic fibrosis. *J Neurol Neurosurg Psychiatry* 1985; 48: 1097-1102.
20. Stead RJ, Redington AN, Hinks LJ, et al. Selenium deficiency and possible increased risk of carcinoma in adults with cystic fibrosis. *Lancet* 1985; 2: 862-863.
21. Neve J, Van Geffel R, Hanocq M, et al. Plasma and erythrocyte zinc, copper and selenium in cystic fibrosis. *Acta Paediatr Scand* 1983; 72: 437-440.
22. Shwachman H. Gastrointestinal manifestations of cystic fibrosis. *Pediatr Clin North Am* 1975; 22: 787-805.

23. Dodge JA. The nutritional state and nutrition. *Acta Paediatr Scand* 1985;(suppl 317):31-37.
24. Shepherd RW, Thomas BJ, Bennett D, et al. Changes in body composition and muscle protein degradation during nutritional supplementation in nutritionally growth-retarded children with cystic fibrosis. *J Paediatr Gastroenterol Nutr* 1983; 2: 439-446.
25. Shepherd RW, Cooksley WGE, Cooke WDD. Improved growth and clinical, nutritional and respiratory changes in response to nutritional therapy in cystic fibrosis. *J Pediatr* 1980; 97: 351-357.
26. Mansell AL, Anderson JC, Muttart CR, et al. Short term pulmonary effects of total parenteral nutrition in children with cystic fibrosis. *J Pediatr* 1984; 104: 700-705.
27. Di Sant'Agnese PA, Davis PB. Cystic fibrosis in the adult. *Am J Med* 1979; 66: 121-132.
28. Penketh ARL, Wise A, Mearns MB, et al. Cystic fibrosis in adolescence and adults. *Thorax* 1986 (in press).
29. Batten JC, Matthew DJ. The respiratory system. In: Hodson ME, Norman AP, Batten JC, eds. *Cystic fibrosis*. London: Bailliere Tindall, 1983.
30. Efthimiou J, Taylor P, Hodson ME, et al. The importance of viruses and *Legionella pneumophila* in the acute respiratory exacerbations of patients with cystic fibrosis. *Thorax* 1984; 39: 150-154.
31. Hodson ME, Gaskell DV. Physiotherapy. In: Hodson ME, Norman AP, Batten JC, eds. *Cystic fibrosis*. London: Bailliere Tindall, 1983.
32. Hodson ME, Smith MJ, Batten JC. Pilot study of ciprofloxacin in the treatment of *Pseudomonas aeruginosa* infection in cystic fibrosis. Proceedings of the 14th International Congress of Chemotherapy. Japan 1985: 200.
33. Szaff M, Hoiby N, Flensborg EW. Frequent antibiotic therapy improves survival of cystic fibrosis patients with chronic *Pseudomonas aeruginosa* infection. *Acta Paediatr Scand* 1983; 72: 651-657.
34. Penketh ARL, Hodson ME, Batten JC. Ticarcillin compared with carbenicillin in the treatment of exacerbations of bronchopulmonary infection due to *Pseudomonas aeruginosa* in cystic fibrosis. *Br J Dis Chest* 1983; 77: 179-184.
35. Penketh ARL, Hodson ME, Gaya H, et al. Azlocillin compared with carbenicillin in the treatment of bronchopulmonary infection due to *Pseudomonas aeruginosa* in cystic fibrosis. *Thorax* 1984; 39: 299-304.
36. Hodson ME, Wingfield HJ, Batten JC. Tobramycin and carbenicillin compared with gentamicin and carbenicillin in the treatment of infection with *Pseudomonas aeruginosa* in adult patients with cystic fibrosis. *Br J Dis Chest* 1983; 77: 71-77.
37. British Thoracic Society Research Committee. Ceftazidime compared with gentamicin and carbenicillin in patients with cystic fibrosis, pulmonary pseudomonas infection and an exacerbation of respiratory symptoms. British Thoracic Society Research Committee 1985; 40: 358-363.
38. Hodson ME, Penketh ARL, Batten JC. Aerosol carbenicillin and gentamicin treatment of *Pseudomonas aeruginosa* infection in patients with cystic fibrosis. *Lancet* 1981; 2: 1137-1139.
39. Heaf DP, Tyson S, Matthew DJ. Effect of inhaled azlocillin, mistabron and combination therapy in children with cystic fibrosis. 13th Annual Meeting of European Working Group for Cystic Fibrosis, Jerusalem, 1985: 47. Abstract.
40. Stead RJ, Hodson ME, Batten JC. Nebulised ceftazidime compared with gentamicin and carbenicillin in adults with cystic fibrosis infected with *Ps. aeruginosa. Thorax* 1985; 40: 704.
41. Newman SP, Pellow PGD, Clarke SW. Choice of nebulisers and compressors for delivery of carbenicillin aerosol. *Eur J Resp Dis* (in press).
42. Day G, Mearns MB. Bronchial liability in cystic fibrosis. *Arch Dis Child* 1973; 48: 355-359.
43. Stead RJ, Pantin CFA, Hodson ME, et al. Prednisolone in the treatment of airflow obstruction in adults with cystic fibrosis. *Thorax* 1986; 41: 34-38.
44. Auerbach HS, Williams M, Kirkpatrick JA, et al. Alternate day prednisolone reduces morbidity and improves pulmonary function in cystic fibrosis. *Lancet* 1985; 2: 686-688.
45. Noblett HR. Treatment of uncomplicated meconium ileus by gastrografin enema: a preliminary report. *J Paediatr Surg* 1969; 4: 190-197.
46. Jensen KG, Meconium ileus equivalent in a 15 year old patient with mucoviscidosis. *Acta Paediatr Scand* 1962; 51: 344-348.

47. Hodson ME, Mearns MB, Batten JC. Meconium ileus equivalent in adults with cystic fibrosis of pancreas; a report of six cases. *Br Med J* 1976; 2: 790-791.
48. Hanley JG, Fitzgerald MX. Meconium ileus equivalent in older patients with cystic fibrosis. *Br Med J* 1983; 1: 1411-1413.
49. Cleghorn GJ, Fortstner GG, Stringer DA, et al. Treatment of distal intestinal obstruction syndrome in cystic fibrosis with a balanced intestinal lavage solution. *Lancet* 1986; 1: 8-11.
50. Batten JC. The adolescent and adult. In: Hodson ME, Norman AP, Batten Jc, eds. *Cystic fibrosis.* London: Bailliere Tindall, 1983.
51. Psacharopoulos HT, Mowat AP. The liver and biliary system. In: Hodson ME, Normam AP, Batten JC, eds. *Cystic fibrosis.* London: Bailliere Tindall, 1983.
52. Chalton R, MacKay I, Wilson R, et al. Double blind, placebo controlled trial of betamethasone nasal drops for nasal polyposis. *Br Med J* 1985; 291: 788.
53. Braude S, Kennedy A, Hodson M, et al. Hypertrophic osteoarthropathy in cystic fibrosis. *Br Med J* 1984; 288: 822-823.
54. Newman AJ, Ansell BM. Episodic arthritis in children with cystic fibrosis. *J Paediatr* 1979; 94: 594-596.
55. Norman AP, Hodson ME. Emotional and social aspects of cystic fibrosis. In: Hodson ME, Norman AP, Batten JC, eds. *Cystic fibrosis.* London: Bailliere Tindall, 1983.
56. Stead RJ, Hodson ME, Batten JC, et al. Pharmacokinetics of contraceptive steroids in cystic fibrosis. In: Lawson D, ed. *Cystic fibrosis: horizons.* Proceedings of the 9th International CF Congress, Brighton 1984. Bristol: John Wiley & Sons: 401.

# Chapter 15

# The Adult Respiratory Distress Syndrome

*Timothy J.McDonnell, Norbert F. Voelkel and Thomas L. Petty*

Since its original characterisation in 1967[1] the importance of the adult respiratory distress syndrome (ARDS) has been increasingly recognized,[2-4] It has been estimated that in excess of 150 000 cases of ARDS occur in the United States annually,[5] with an overall mortality even in the best centres remaining in excess of 50%.[6-8] A large number of these cases occur in previously healthy patients, many of whom are young and in most cases require prolonged and expensive intensive care support. Consequently, the syndrome has wide medical, economic and social implications. It is therefore important that the physician looking after such cases should be aware of current concepts in management and new understanding of the pathophysiology of the condition which have opened up potential new avenues of therapeutic intervention. It is our purpose in this chapter to briefly outline the concise clinical features of ARDS, to review the current management, which is still essentially supportive in nature, and then to discuss potential pharmacological intervention.

## Definition and Diagnosis of ARDS

Criteria for the diagnosis of ARDS have been defined and are presented in Table 15.1.[7,9,10] The syndrome essentially consists of progressive respiratory distress, severe refractory hypoxaemia, alveolar infiltrates, and reduced lung compliance which develops subsequent to a direct or indirect insult to the lungs. The characteristic chest X-ray (Figure 15.1) will show, in addition to bilateral infiltrates, a normal cardiac size, and clear costophrenic and cardiophrenic angles with a normal vascular pedicle. Regardless of the route or nature of the initiating insult, the result is the development of increased alveolar capillary permeability with subsequent non-cardiogenic pulmonary oedema.[11,12] However, to characterise ARDS merely in terms of increased permeability would be an oversimplification as evidenced, for instance, by the complex derangement present on lung biopsy.[10,11]

Despite wide recognition of the condition, no specific tests or markers for ARDS exist. Various plasma abnormalities recognised include elevated fibrin, fibrinogen degradation products (including the D antigen)[13] and C5a.[14] Measured levels of serum angiotensin converting enzyme have been low,[15] though there is still no good evidence that this is an accurate marker of endothelial cell injury. Comparison of the protein content of alveolar fluid and plasma may be useful in indicating that pulmonary oedema is

*Table 15.1* Criteria for diagnosis of ARDS

| |
|---|
| *Clinical history of catastrophic event* |
| Pulmonary (aspiration, massive infection, contusion) |
| Non-pulmonary (shock, multisystem trauma) |
| but exclude |
| Chronic pulmonary disease |
| Left ventricular failure (wedge pressure $\geq$ 16mmHg (2.1kPa)) |
| *Clinical respiratory distress* |
| Tachypnoea > 20 breaths/minute |
| Laboured breathing |
| *Chest X-ray picture* |
| Diffuse pulmonary infiltrates |
| (early interstitial, later alveolar) |
| *Physiological measurements* |
| Arterial $PO_2$ < 50mmHg (6.7kPa) when $FiO_2$ > 0.6 |
| Total respiratory compliance < 50ml/cm$H_2O$ (normal > 75ml/cm$H_2O$) |
| Increased shunt fraction and dead space ventilation |

$FiO_2$ = oxygen concentration. $H_2O$ = water.

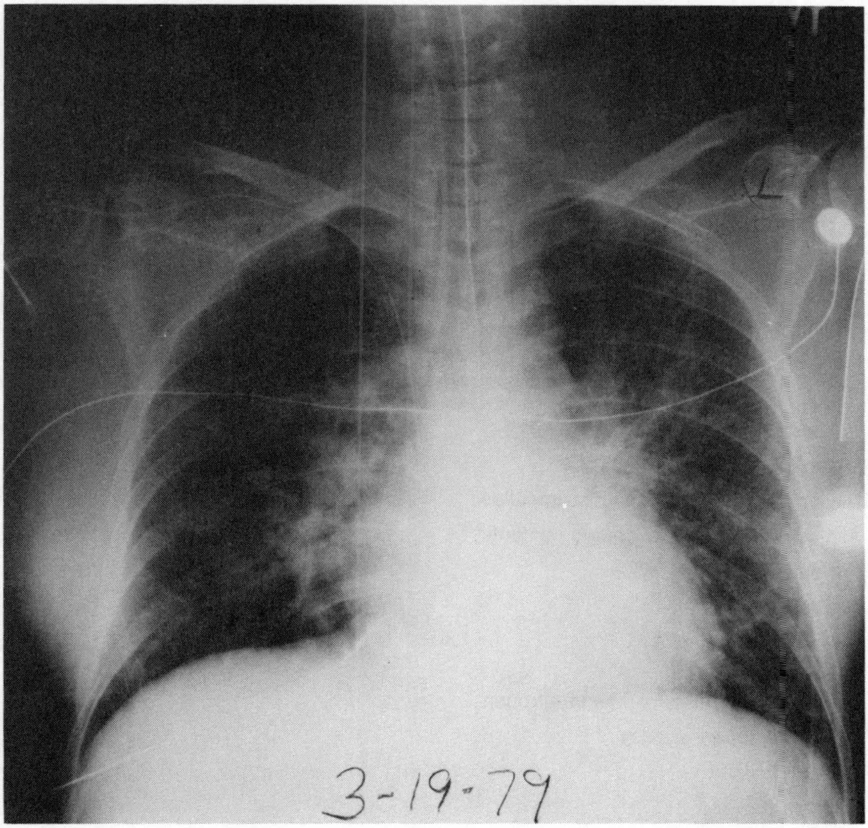


*Figure 15.1* Typical chest X-ray appearance of ARDS in an intubated patient. Note relative sparing of cardiophrenic and costophrenic angles, absence of redistribution of blood flow to upper lung zones and a normal vascular pedicle. These features should allow differentiation from cardiogenic pulmonary oedema.

cardiogenic or of permeability origin.[16] All these investigations suffer in either being non-specific or in not having gained widespread acceptance, but identification of a marker would be diagnostically useful as it would enable earlier therapeutic intervention.

## Epidemiology

Table 15.2 lists a number of conditions which are well recognised as potential causes of ARDS. A number of recent studies have investigated the influence of some of these predisposing conditions on the development and subsequent course of ARDS.[7,8,17] Fowler et al noted an incidence rate that varied from 1.7% in patients undergoing cardiopulmonary bypass to 35.6% in cases of witnessed aspiration.[7] The risk of developing the syndrome increased dramatically when more than one predisposing condition was present. A study from Seattle revealed similar findings and emphasised the high risk of ARDS in the apparently septic patient.[17]

*Table 15.2* Clinical states associated with the development of ARDS

| |
|---|
| Shock |
| Septic |
| Haemorrhagic |
| Cardiogenic |
| Anaphylactoid |
| Trauma |
| Direct pulmonary contusion |
| Non-pulmonary, multisystem trauma |
| Infection |
| Viral, bacterial and *Mycoplasma pneumoniae* |
| Miliary tuberculosis |
| Endotoxaemia |
| Multiple blood transfusions |
| Disseminated intravascular coagulation |
| Aspiration, particularly gastric contents |
| Fat emboli |
| Amniotic fluid emboli |
| Near-drowning |
| Inhaled toxins |
| Phosgene smoke, oxides of nitrogen |
| Cardiopulmonary bypass |
| Oxygen toxicity |
| Pancreatitis |
| Drug-induced |
| Salicylates, ethchlorvynol, narcotic abuse |
| Paraquat |
| Radiation lung injury |

## Mortality and Prognosis

Mortality in ARDS appears also to be related to the predisposing cause with the highest case fatalities associated with sepsis or gastric aspiration induced-ARDS.[7,17] Furthermore, sepsis or multiple organ failure (cerebral, renal, and so on), developing during ARDS are associated with a poor prognosis.[6,18] Other indicators of a poor prognosis identified recently include a tendency to acidosis, fewer than expected band forms on a blood smear, and an elevated blood urea nitrogen.[19]

In view of the severe derangement of structure and function of the lungs of patients with ARDS, it is surprising to note the excellent prognosis in survivors of the syndrome. Following weaning from mechanical ventilation patients improve symptomatically and radiographically over the following months so that over 80% are asymptomatic and have normal chest X-rays at one year.[20] Nevertheless, a minority of patients do manifest persistent abnormalities particularly on physiological testing.[21,22] The long-term progression of the pulmonary hypertension that is present in the acute stages of ARDS is not known, as follow-up haemodynamic studies have not been performed. Clinical evidence of persistent pulmonary hypertension is very rare.

## Goals of Treatment

It should be apparent that ARDS is a relatively common entity occurring in patients who were, for the most part, previously healthy and in many cases, relatively young. Those who survive have an excellent prognosis. Consequently, the potential gain in managing such patients is high. Management, however, remains essentially supportive and empirical. The main components consist of ventilatory support, fluid management, administration of nutrition and constant vigilance for the emergence of infection and other complications. Failure of other organ systems, particularly renal failure, may require additional strategies. Pharmacological interventions remain controversial and are not central to present management. Therefore, the overall goal of the clinician will be to maintain adequate oxygenation, preserve other organ systems from failure, treat if possible the underlying cause of the ARDS, and wait for the body's reparative process to heal the patient.

## Mechanical Ventilation

Ventilatory support forms the cornerstone in the management of ARDS.[9,23] It should be instituted early, following recognition of the syndrome, to prevent fatigue and respiratory arrest arising from the increased work of breathing. In ventilating the ARDS patient the physician needs to maintain adequate oxygenation without exposing the patient to unnecessarily high concentrations of oxygen. Hypoxaemia in ARDS may be severe and require a high concentration of oxygen which, in turn, may predispose to the development of pulmonary oxygen toxicity.[23-25] This may produce further inflammation, further impaired gas exchange, and in addition may increase absorption atelectasis and impair mucociliary clearance.[23] The principal features that correlate with such toxicity are the level of oxygen concentration and its duration.[24] The recognition of oxygen toxicity in the setting of ARDS is extremely difficult and, as there is no effective therapy, the clinician must strive towards its prevention by constantly attempting to reduce the oxygen concentration to the minimum that is compatible with adequate tissue oxygen delivery.

Due to decreased compliance, a volume-cycled ventilator capable of delivering high pressures will be necessary to support the ARDS patient. Tidal volumes of about 10ml/kg are useful in preventing microatelectasis.[23] Excessively high tidal volumes should be avoided as the increased pressures generated will encourage barotrauma.[23,26] There has been some controversy on the most appropriate mode of mechanical ventilation for the setting of acute respiratory failure.[23,27,28] Assist control mode (AMV) enables the awake patient to set his own minute volume on the ventilator and ensures maximum comfort. This sensitivity to patient demand is not available with the other major ventilatory mode, intermittent mandatory ventilation (IMV). Increased minute volume needs cannot be supplied by IMV without a change in ventilation settings and consequently the patient will have an increased work of breathing and resultant oxygen consumption. Only exceptionally should full sedation and controlled mechanical ventilation (CMV) be employed.

Since the initial report of its successful use,[1] positive end expiratory pressure (PEEP) has been accepted as useful in the management of ARDS, but controversy surrounds such issues as prophylactic PEEP, the optimum level of PEEP, and the degree of haemodynamic impairment produced by PEEP.[29-32] Oxygen uptake in the lungs is usually increased by PEEP producing an increase in the arterial partial pressure of oxygen ($PO_2$). In addition, PEEP will increase lung volumes and lung compliance.[23,29] PEEP may aid recruitment of new alveolar capillary units and maintain others open, but precise mechanisms underlying all these changes are unclear. PEEP may, however, increase the risk of barotrauma[23] and at higher levels will depress cardiac output, increase pulmonary artery pressure and promote oedema formation.[32-34]

Some authors have advocated the use of high levels of PEEP (30cm water or more), in an attempt to reduce the shunt fraction to a minimum.[35] This approach increases the risks substantially, and there is no good evidence that it will hasten the patient's recovery. The prophylactic use of PEEP in high-risk patients has been advocated.[36] However, a recent study by Pepe et al[37] failed to confirm earlier enthusiastic reports.

PEEP does not attack the fundamental disease process in ARDS[33] and, in view of its associated risks, it should be employed with caution. Our current approach is to use moderate levels of PEEP (between 5 and 15cm of water to aid reduction of the oxygen concentration to an acceptable level, such as 40% oxygen at sea level). Ideally, arterial $PO_2$ should be greater than 60mmHg (8kPa) and cardiac output should be maintained to ensure adequate tissue oxygen delivery.

## Non-ventilatory Aspects of Supportive Care

### Fluid Management

Due to the lack of integrity of the alveolar-capillary interface, any increase in hydrostatic pressure generated by excessive fluid administration will encourage fluid transport across the capillary endothelium and flooding of the alveoli. Consequently optimal management is to maintain the hydrostatic pressure at a minimum and keep the patient slightly dehydrated.[2,4] Appropriate monitoring of fluid status will require a pulmonary arterial catheter, at least until equilibrium is established, and usually a pulmonary arterial wedge pressure of 10mmHg (1.3kPa) or less will be the aim. Such a reduction in preload, particularly in conjunction with the use of PEEP, may lead to a reduction in cardiac output with possible hypotension and reduced tissue oxygen delivery. Cardiac performance needs to be monitored and dopamine or judicious fluid challenges may be required.[38] In the presence of anaemia, blood (preferably red cell concentrate) should be administered to improve oxygen carrying capacity and delivery to the tissues.

### Antibiotics

Sepsis is a serious problem in ARDS patients.[6,18,39] Airway colonisation occurs early in the intubated patient in an intensive care unit (ICU), putting patients at risk of developing Gram-negative pneumonia in particular.[40] Invasive monitoring also renders ARDS patients liable to become infected. Despite these risks, however, there is no place for prophylactic antibiotics. Antibiotics should be reserved until sepsis is suspected and then used in high doses intravenously, following appropriate cultures. Antibiotics should be selected by consideration of the probable site of infection and local hospital susceptibility patterns.

### Nutrition

The nutritional status of the ARDS patient must not be neglected, as these patients are usually catabolic and malnutriton with its attendant complications will rapidly ensure.[41] Supplemental feeding, preferably by the enteral route, should be introduced as soon as possible. Overfeeding may be associated with problems, particularly if high carbohydrate loads are used, as the resultant increase in carbon dioxide production may hinder eventual weaning.[42]

### Heparin

Pulmonary emboli appear to be common in respiratory intensive care units with one study reporting an incidence at autopsy of 27%.[43,44] There is some evidence that, in the absence of contraindications, subcutaneous heparin 5000 units every eight hours may be useful in the prophylaxis of thromboembolism.[45] In addition, patients should be encouraged to exercise their lower limbs.

### Prophylaxis of Gastrointestinal Bleeding

Gastrointestinal haemorrhage may be sudden and life-threatening, and occurs with an increased frequency in ventilated patients.[44,46] The administration of antacids hourly to maintain a gastric pH greater than 3.5 to 4.0 is reasonable and usually not associated with significant side effects. Cimetidine (300mg hourly) does not appear to be as effective.[47]

## Drug Treatment of ARDS

There is as yet no pharmacological agent that convincingly attacks the basic disease process in ARDS. Part of the explanation for this is that our understanding of the pathophysiology has only recently begun to expand. Early recognition that the lungs in ARDS were the site of intensive inflammation led to the empirical use of corticosteroids as anti-inflammatory agents.[1] However, with our increasing comprehension of the pathophysiological steps involved in ARDS, specific pharmacological interventions are already being postulated and some have had limited clinical use.

Our current concepts of ARDS[48,49] involve an injury to the lung producing increased vascular permeability through endothelial damage and disruption of the alveolar-capillary membrane, leading to alveolar flooding and pulmonary oedema (Figure 15.2). The intense inflammatory process destroys type 1 epithelial cells which are eventually replaced by proliferating type 2 cells. Abnormalities of surfactant have been documented which may contribute to alveolar colapse.[50,51] In addition, the airways are also involved in the inflammatory process and in conjunction with the abnormalities of the pulmonary circulation will contribute to the large ventilation-perfusion mismatch and severe hypoxaemia found in ARDS.[52,53]

How the damage is produced is not entirely clear, but a presumptive role in the progression of lung injury has been postulated for several mediators including neutrophils,[54,55] eicosanoids (active metabolites of arachidonic acid),[56,57] activated complement,[14,58] and oxygen radicals.[59] There is experimental evidence, mostly from animal work, linking these substances with various stages in the pathophysiology. For instance, activated neutrophils accumulate in the lungs of ARDS patients and are capable of releasing proteolytic enzymes and oxygen radicals, which can produce tissue injury.[60] Eicosanoids may mediate some of the pulmonary vascular and permeability responses (Figure 15.3). The precise role and inter-relationships of the agents still remain imprecise; however, other substances that appear to be less important include bradykinin, fibrinogen degradation products, platelets and histamine.[49]

### Steroids

Considering the inflammatory nature of ARDS it is not surprising that corticosteroids were used as one of the initial therapeutic manoeuvres in attacking the syndrome.[1] That steroids are not a panacea for the condition is indicated by the controversy that still surrounds their use. Steroids have a number of effects which might be considered beneficial. They are recognised

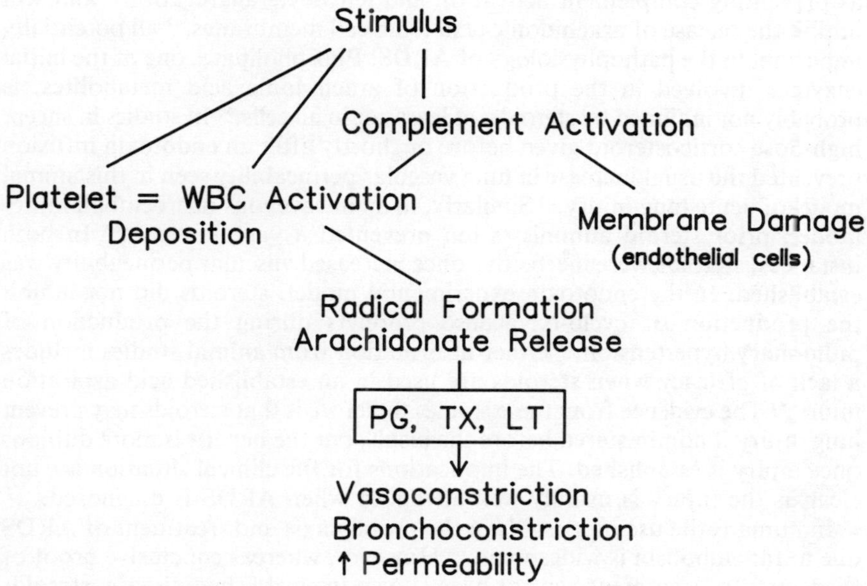


*Figure 15.2* Presumed mechanisms involved in pathophysiology of ARDS. PG = prostaglandins. TX = thromboxane. LT = leukotrienes. WBC = white blood cells.

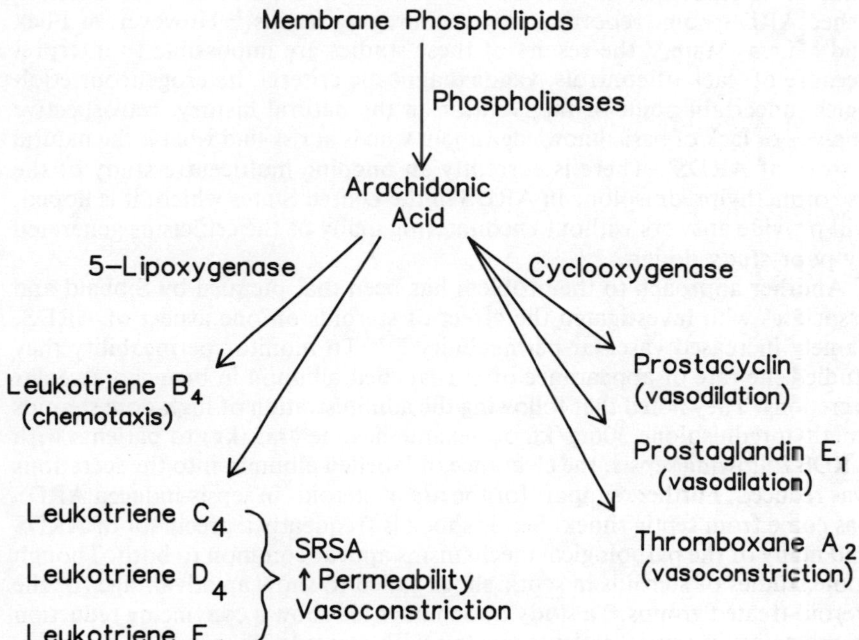


*Figure 15.3* Summary of metabolism of arachidonic acid and effects relevant to ARDS. SRSA = slow-reacting substance of anaphylaxis.

as preventing complement activation and leucocyte aggregation[61] and will inhibit the release of arachidonic acid from cell membranes,[62] all potentially important in the pathophysiology of ARDS. Phospholipase, one of the initial enzymes involved in the production of arachidonic acid metabolites, is probably not inhibited by steroids, at least not in all cells.[63] In studies in sheep, high-dose corticosteroid given before or shortly after an endotoxin infusion prevented the usual increase in lung vascular permeability seen in this animal model of acute lung injury.[64] Similarly, in an intravenous microemboli injury model, prior steroid administration prevented a vascular leak.[65] In both instances, steroids were ineffective once increased vascular permeability was established. In the endotoxin experimental model, steroids did not inhibit the production of cyclo-oxygenase products during the production of pulmonary hypertension.[66] Other information from animal studies includes a lack of efficacy when steroids are used in an established acid aspiration injury.[67] The evidence from these studies therefore is that steroids may prevent lung injury if administered before the insult, but the benefit is more dubious once injury is established. The implications for the clinical situation are not clear as the injury is usually well advanced when ARDS is diagnosed.

In humans the use of steroids in the prophylaxis and treatment of ARDS due to fat embolism is widespread.[68] However, whereas conclusive proof of the benefit of treatment has not been shown in established disease, steroids have been shown to be effective in preventing ARDS developing secondary to fat embolism.[69] Studies of prophylactic steroids in other high-risk groups, such as after gastric aspiration, have not shown any benefit.[70] There are a number of reports in the literature concerning the use of steroids in established ARDS, some reporting very encouraging results.[71] However, as Flick and Murray state,[72] the results of these studies are impossible to interpret because of 'lack of controls, vague diagnostic criteria, heterogeneous etiologies, uncertain point of intervention in the natural history, retrospective analysis or lack of basic knowledge about who is at risk and what is the natural history of ARDS'. There is currently an ongoing multicentre study of the use of methylprednisolone in ARDS in the United States which, it is hoped, will provide answers without encountering many of the criticisms generated by poor study design.

Another approach to the problem has been that pursued by Sibbald and associates who investigated the effect of steroids on one aspect of ARDS, namely increased vascular permeability.[73,74] To monitor permeability they studied the rate of appearance of $^{131}$I-labelled albumin in broncho-alveolar secretions. They noted that following the administration of high-dose steroids (methylprednisolone 30mg/kg or dexamethasone 4mg/kg) to patients with ARDS following sepsis, the clearance of labelled albumin into the secretions was reduced. Further, support for the use of steroids in sepsis-induced ARDS has come from septic shock. Septic shock is frequently a precursor of ARDS and many of the pathological mechanisms appear common to both. Though some studies of steroids in septic shock failed to show an advantage for the steroid-treated groups,[75] a study by Schumer did show a convincing reduction in mortality in septic patients treated with steroids.[76]

From our present state of knowledge, it is clear that no dogmatic guidelines can be given on the use of steroids in ARDS. It is reasonable to give 1 to 2g of methylprednisolone over a 24-hour period early in the course, but they should be discontinued subsequently. The steroids of choice would appear to be methylprednisolone because of its lack of fluid-retaining mineralocorticoid activity[77] and better penetration into the alveolar spaces.[78] It should be remembered that steroid therapy is not without risks, particularly as steroids will inhibit the bacterial defences of the lungs and predispose the patient to colonisation and sepsis.

## Eicosanoid Inhibitors

Eicosanoids have recently come under scrutiny as potential mediators of lung injury in ARDS.[56,57] Infusion of eicosanoids can produce many of the features of ARDS in experimental animals. Specifically, pulmonary hypertension,[79] loss of hypoxic pulmonary vasoconstriction,[80] leading to increased ventilation-perfusion mismatch, and increased capillary permeability[81] have all been linked to different arachidonate products (Figure 15.3). Also, in animal models of ARDS, increased production of arachidonic acid metabolites has been documented. This evidence has led to pilot studies of eicosanoid inhibitors wherever they have become available.

Most pharmacological manipulations have, to date, been directed at the presumed effects of thromboxane $A_2$, a known potent vasoconstrictor. Thromboxane is linked, in a sheep endotoxin model of lung injury, to the production of acute pulmonary hypertension.[79] Increased levels of thromboxane $B_2$, the stable inactive metabolite of thromboxane $A_2$, have been found in pulmonary lymph fluid in this situation.[57,79] Treatment of the pulmonary hypertension would have the potential benefit of increasing cardiac output and tissue oxygen delivery. Cyclo-oxygenase inhibitors such as indomethacin offer some inhibition of the hypertension,[82] but may shunt arachidonic acid metabolism down the lipoxygenase pathway with leukotriene production and potential deleterious effects.[83] Specific thromboxane synthetase inhibitors such as dazoxiben, an imidazole derivative, have been shown to inhibit the pulmonary vasoconstriction in animal studies,[84] but no beneficial effect on haemodynamics was observed in human studies.[85,86]

Other attempts to manipulate pulmonary haemodynamics in ARDS have involved the use of $PGE_1$, a vasodilator prostaglandin. Two uncontrolled studies have reported a reduction in pulmonary arterial pressure with an increase in cardiac output and oxygen transport.[87,88] A multicentre double-blind trial is now in progress to evaluate this agent further.

The agents discussed above merely attempt to adjust pulmonary haemodynamics, they do not alter increased permeability and cannot be expected to reverse the basic disease process in ARDS. Leukotrienes are linked to increased vascular permeability, and leukotriene inhibitors have been successful in attenuating lung injury induced by specific agents such as hydrogen peroxide and thiourea.[89,90] This area still requires further experimental work, but it is conceivable that leukotriene inhibitors may yet prove useful clinically in ARDS.

## Antioxidants

Neutrophils have well-recognised importance in the pathogenesis of ARDS as evidenced by their accumulation in the lung parenchyma following lung

*Table 15.3* Summary of potential drugs in ARDS and presumed mechanism of action.

| Drug | Mechanisms | Comment |
|---|---|---|
| Corticosteroids | Inhibit:<br>• Complement activation<br>• Leucocyte aggregation<br>• Release of arachidonate from cell membranes | Clinical benefit not proven.<br>Many promote sepsis including pulmonary infection |
| Eicosanoid inhibitors | | |
| • Cyclo-oxygenase inhibitors (indomethacin) | Antagonise effects of thromboxane and other prostaglandins | May increase synthesis of leukotriene. Will not affect permeability. May improve hypoxic vasoconstriction |
| • Thromboxane synthetase inhibitors (dazoxiben) | Block production of thromboxane | Will antagonise early pulmonary hypertension in animals but studies in humans negative. Will not affect permeability |
| • Leukotriene inhibitors (U60257, FPL 55712) | Will antagonise leukotriene effects | No clinical studies yet reported |
| Eicosanoid products (prostacyclin, prostaglandin $E_1$) | Will cause vasodilatation and decrease pulmonary hypertension | Limited experience in humans |
| Radical scavengers (Vitamin E, acetylcysteine) | Will neutralise oxygen radicals | No clinical studies yet reported |
| Neutrophil antagonists | May prevent neutrophil-induced injury | No studies of such agents yet reported |

injury and the attenuation of the syndrome in granulocytopenic models. One of the mechanisms by which neutrophils may produce lung damage is by generating oxygen radicals. Acetylcysteine is a recognised radical scavenger and has been used with effect in a sheep model of endotoxin lung injury.[91] However, as the authors recommend, further experimental work in animals is required before human studies should be undertaken. Interestingly, vitamin E (tocopherol), also a radical scavenger, has been used in an uncontrolled study in humans, apparently with effect.[92] Further research in this area may lead to potential useful agents for human use.

## Comment

We have displayed the potential pharmacological interventions in Table 15.3. The clarification of risk groups and predictors of outcome obtained from recent studies will enable more accurate and useful evaluation of these and other agents to be performed in patients with ARDS.[93] Multicentre studies will probably be required so that appropriate evaluation of drugs, or drug combinations, can be carried out in subgroups of patients (those with different aetiologies and severity). Regardless of whether or not a single drug or combination of drugs proves to be the 'silver bullet' it is probable that supportive care and avoidance of complications, particularly sepsis,[6] will remain paramount in the management of patients with ARDS.

## References

1. Ashbaugh DG, Bigelow DB, Petty TL, Levine BE. Acute respiratory distress in adults. *Lancet* 1967; 2: 319-23.
2. *Bernard GR, Brigham KL. The adult respiratory distress syndrome. *Ann Rev Med* 1985; 36: 195-205.
3. *Balk R, Bone RC. The adult respiratory distress syndrome. *Med Clin North Am* 1983; 67: 685-700,
4. *Petty LT, Fowler AA. The adult respiratory distress syndrome. In: Flenley DC, Petty TL, eds. *Recent advances in respiratory disease 3*. Edinburgh: Churchill Livingstone 1983: 103-114.
5. Murray JF, Staff of the Division of Lung Diseases, National Heart, Lung, and Blood Institute. Mechanisms of acute respiratory failure. *Am Rev Respir Dis* 1977; 115: 1071-1078.
6. Montgomery AB, Stager MA, Carrico CJ, Hudson LD. Causes of mortality in patients with the adult respiratory distress syndrome. *Am Rev Respir Dis* 1985; 132: 485-489.
7. Fowler AA, Hamman RF, Good JT, et al. Adult respiratory distress syndrome: risk with common predispositions. *Ann Intern Med* 1983; 98: 593-597.
8. Fein AM, Lippmann M, Holtzman H, Eliraz A, Goldberg SK. The risk factors, incidence and prognosis of adult respiratory syndrome after septicaemia. *Chest* 1983; 83: 40-42.
9. Petty TL, Ashbaugh DG. The adult respiratory distress syndrome — clinical features, factors influencing prognosis and principles of management. *Chest* 1971; 60: 233-239.
10. *Petty TL. Editor's perspective. *Semin Respir Med* 1983; 4: 321-326.
11. *Staub NC. Pathophysiology of pulmonary edema. In: Staub NC, Taylor AE, eds. *Edema.* New York: Raven Press, 1984: 719-746.
12. Dauber IM, Pluss WT, van Grondelle A, Trow RS, Weil JV. Specificity and sensitivity of noninvasive measurement of pulmonary vascular protein leak. *J Appl Physiol* 1985; 59: 564-574.

13. Haynes JB, Hyers TM, Giclas PC, Franks JJ, Petty TL. Elevated fibrin(ogen) degradation products in the adult respiratory distress syndrome. *Am Rev Respir Dis* 1980; 122: 841-847.
14. Hammerschmidt DE, Weaver LJ, Hudson LD, Craddock PR, Jacob HS. Association of complement activation and elevated plasma C5a with adult respiratory distress syndrome. *Lancet* 1980; 1: 947-949.
15. Fourrier F, Chopin C, Wallaert B, Mazurier C, Mangalaboyi J, Durocher A. Compared evolution of plasma fibronectin and angiotensin converting enzyme levels in septic ARDS. *Chest* 1985; 87: 191-195.
16. Fein A, Grossman RF, Jones JG, et al. The value of edema fluid protein measurement in patients with pulmonary edema. *Am J Med* 1979; 67: 32-38.
17. Pepe PE, Potkin RT, Reus DE, Hudson LD, Carrico CJ. Clinical predictors of the adult respiratory distress syndrome. *Am J Surg* 1982; 144: 124-130.
18. Bell RC, Coalson JJ, Smith JD, Johanson WG. Multiple organ failure and infection in adult respiratory distress syndrome. *Ann Intern Med* 1983; 99: 293-298.
19. Fowler AA, Hamman RF, Zerbe GO, Benson KN, Hyers TM. Adult respiratory distress syndrome: prognosis after onset. *Am Rev Respir Dis* 1985; 132: 472-478.
20. *Alberts WM, Priest GR, Moser KM. The outlook for survivors of ARDS. *Chest* 1983; 84: 272-274.
21. Simpson DL, Goodman M, Spector SL, Petty TL. Long term follow-up and bronchial reactivity testing in survivors of the adult respiratory distress syndrome. *Am Rev Respir Dis* 1978; 117: 449-454.
22. Buchser E, Leuenberger P, Chiolero R, Perret C, Freeman J. Reduced pulmonary capillary blood volume as a long term sequel of ARDS. *Chest* 1985; 87: 608-611.
23. *Hudson LD. Ventilatory management of patients with adult respiratory distress syndrome. *Semin Respir Med* 1981; 2: 128-139.
24. *Jenkinson SG. Pulmonary oxygen toxicity. *Clin Chest Med* 1982; 3: 109-119.
25. *Frank L, Massaro D. Oxygen toxicity. *Am J Med* 1980; 69: 117-126.
26. Cullen DJ, Caldera DL. The incidence of ventilator induced pulmonary barotrauma in critically ill patients. *Anesthesiology* 1979; 50: 185-190.
27. *Luce JM, Pierson DJ, Hudson LD. Intermittent mandatory ventilation. *Chest* 1981; 79: 678-685.
28. *Weisman IM, Rinaldo JE, Rogers RM, Saunders MH. Intermittent mandatory ventilation: state of the art. *Am Rev Respir Dis* 1983; 127: 641-647.
29. *Weisman IM, Rinaldo JE, Rogers RM. Positive end expiratory pressure in adult respiratory failure. *N Engl J Med* 1982; 307: 1381-1384.
30. *Rounds S, Brody JS. Putting PEEP in perspective. *N Engl J Med* 1984; 311: 323-325.
31. *Albert RK. Least PEEP: primum non nocere. *Chest* 1985; 87: 2-4.
32. *Luce JM. The cardiovascular effects of mechanical ventilation and positive end expiratory pressure. *JAMA* 1984; 252: 807-811.
33. *Rizk NW, Murray JF. PEEP and pulmonary edema. *Am J Med* 1982; 72: 381-383.
34. Hopewell PC. Failure of positive end expiratory pressure to decrease lung water content in alloxan-induced pulmonary edema. *Am Rev Respir Dis* 1979; 120: 813-819.
35. Kirby RR, Downs JB, Civetta JM, et al. High level positive end expiratory pressure (PEEP) in acute respiratory insufficiency. *Chest* 1975; 67: 156-163.
36. Schmidt GB, O'Neill WW, Kotb K, Hwang KK, Bennett EJ, Bombeck CT. Continuous positive airway pressure in the prophylaxis of the adult respiratory distress syndrome. *Surg Gynecol Obstet* 1976; 143: 613-618.
37. Pepe PE,. Hudson LD, Carrico CJ. Early application of positive end expiratory pressure in patients at risk for the adult respiratory distress syndrome. *N Engl J Med* 1984; 311: 281-286.
38. *Wood LDH, Prewitt RM. Cardiovascular management in acute hypoxemic respiratory failure. *Am J Cardiol* 1981; 47: 963-972.
39. Ashbaugh DG, Petty TL. Sepsis complicating the acute respiratory distress syndrome. *Surg Gynecol Obstet* 1972; 135: 865-869.
40. *Tobin MJ, Grenvik A. Nosocomial lung infection and its diagnosis. *Crit Care Med* 1984; 12: 191-199.
41. Clemmer TP, Orme JH. Nutritional support in the adult respiratory distress syndrome. *Clin Chest Med* 1982; 3: 101-108.

42. Covelli HD, Black JW, Olsen MS, Beekman JF. Respiratory failure precipated by high carbohydrate loads. *Ann Intern Med* 1981; 95: 579-581.
43. Neuhaus A, Bentz RR, Weg JC. Pulmonary embolism in respiratory failure. *Chest* 1978; 73: 460-465.
44. *Pingleton SK. Complications of acute respiratory failure. *Med Clin North Am* 1983; 67: 725-746.
45. Pingleton SK, Bone RC, Pingleton WW, Ruth WE. Prevention of pulmonary emboli in a respiratory intensive care unit. *Chest* 1981; 79: 647-650.
46. Harris SK, Bone RC, Ruth WE. Gastrointestinal haemorrhage in a respiratory intensive care unit. *Chest* 1977; 72: 301-304.
47. Priebe HJ, Skillman JJ, Bushnell LS, Long PC, Silen W. Antacid versus cimetidine in preventing acute gastrointestinal bleeding. *N Engl J Med* 1980; 302: 426-430.
48. *Rinaldo JE, Rogers RM. Adult respiratory distress syndrome: changing concepts of lung injury and repair. *N Engl J Med* 1982; 306: 900-909
49. *Niedermeyer ME, Sheller JR, Brigham KL. Pathogenesis of the adult respiratory distress syndrome. *Curr Pulmonol* 1984; 5: 229-254.
50. Petty TL, Silvers GW, Paul GW. Stanford RE. Abnormalities in lung elastic properties and surfactant function in adult respiratory distress syndrome. *Chest* 1979; 75: 571-574.
51. Hallman M, Spragg R, Harrell JH, Moser KM, Gluck L. Evidence of lung surfactant abnormality in respiratory failure. *J Clin Invest* 1982; 70: 673-683.
52. Esbenshade AM, Newman JH, Lams PM, Jolles H, Brigham KL. Respiratory failure after endotoxin infusion in sheep: lung mechanics and lung fluid balance. *J Appl Physiol* 1982; 53: 967-976.
53. Brigham KL, Karman K, Harris TR, Snapper JR, Bernard GR, Young SL. Correlation of oxygenation with vascular permeability-surface area but not with lung water in humans with acute respiratory failure and pulmonary edema. *J Clin Invest* 1983; 72: 339-349.
54. *Tate RM, Repine JE, Neutrophils and the adult respiratory distress syndrome: state of the art. *Am Rev Respir Dis* 1983; 128: 552-559.
55.*Anonymous. Neutrophils and the adult respiratory distress syndrome. *Lancet* 1984; 2: 790-791.
56. *Brigham KL, Duke SS. Prostaglandins in lung disease: adult respiratory distress syndrome. *Semin Respir Med* 1985; 7: 11-16.
57. *Brigham KL. Metabolites of arachidonic acid in experimental lung vascular injury. *Fed Proc* 1985; 44: 43-45.
58. *Hammerschmidt DE. Activation of the complement system and of granulocytes in lung injury: the adult respiratory distress syndrome. *Adv Inflamm Res* 1983; 5: 147-172.
59. Tate RM, VanBenthuysen KM, Shasby DM, McMurtry IF, Repine JE. Oxygen radical mediated permeability edema and vasoconstriction in isolated perfused rabbit lungs. *Am Rev Respir Dis* 1982; 126: 802-806.
60. Zimmerman GA, Renzetti AD, Hill HR. Functional and metabolic activity of granulocytes from patients with adult respiratory distress syndrome. Evidence for activated neutrophils in the pulmonary circulation. *Am Rev Respir Dis* 1983; 127: 290-300.
61. Hammerschmidt D, White JG, Craddock PR, Jacob HS. Corticosteroids inhibit complement-mediated granulocyte aggregation. *J Clin Invest* 1979; 63: 798-803.
62. Hong S, Levine L. Inhibition of arachidonic acid release from cells as the biochemical action of anti-inflammatory steroids. *Proc Natl Acad Sci USA* 1976; 73: 1730-1734.
63. Schleimer RP, Schulman ES, MacGloshan DW et al. Effects of dexamethasone on mediator release from human lung fragments and purified human lung mast cells. *J Clin Invest* 1983; 71: 1830-1835.
64. Brigham KL, Bowers RF, McKeen CR. Methylprednisolone prevention of increased lung vascular permeability following endotoxemia in sheep. *J Clin Invest* 1981; 67: 1103-1110.
65. Perel A, Flick M, Staub NC. Methylprednisolone partially protects against microemboli induced permeability injury in lungs of awake sheep. *Am Rev Respir Dis* 1980; 121 (part 2): 442. Abstract.
66. Begley CJ, Ogletree ML, Meyrick BO, Brigham KL. Modification of pulmonary responses to endotoxemia in awake sheep by steroidal and nonsteroidal anti-inflammatory agents. *Am Rev Respir Dis* 1984; 130: 1140-1146.

67. Glauser FL, Mitten JE, Falls R. Increased alevolar epithelial permeability with acid aspiration: the effects of high dose steroids. *Am Rev Respir Dis* 1979; 120: 1119-1123.
68. Ashbaugh D, Petty T. The use of corticosteroids in the treatment of respiratory failure associated with massive fat embolism. *Surg Gynecol Obstet* 1966; 123: 493-500.
69. Schoenfeld SA, Ploysongsang Y, Dilisio R, et al. Fat embolism prophylaxis with corticosteroids — a prospective study in high risk patients. *Ann Intern Med* 1983; 99: 438-443.
70. Wolfe JE, Bone RC, Ruth WE. Effects of corticosteroids in the treatment of patients with gastric aspiration. *Am J Med* 1977; 63: 719-722.
71. Sladen A. Methylprednisolone: pharmacologic doses in shock lung syndrome. *J Thorac Cardiovasc Surg* 1976; 71: 800-806.
72. *Flick MR, Murray JF. High dose corticosteroid therapy in the adult respiratory distress syndrome. *JAMA* 1984; 251: 1054-1056.
73. Sibbald WJ, Anderson RR, Reid B, Holliday RL, Driedger AA. Alveolo-capillary permeability in human septic ARDS: effect of high dose corticosteroid therapy. *Chest* 1981; 79: 133-142.
74. Sibbald WJ, Dredger AA, Finley RJ, et al. High dose corticosteroids in the treatment of pulmonary microvascular injury. *Ann NY Acad Sci* 1982; 384: 496-516.
75. Sprung CL, Caralis PV, Marcial EH, et al. The effects of high dose corticosteroids in patients with septic shock. *N Engl J Med* 1984; 311: 1137-1143.
76. Schumer W. Steroids in the treatment of clinical septic shock. *Ann Surg* 1976; 184: 333-341.
77. *Haynes RC, Murad F. Adrenocortrophic hormone; glucocorticoid hormones and their synthetic analogs. In: Gilman AG, Goodman LS, Rall TW, Murad F, eds. *The pharmacological basis of therapeutics.* New York: Macmillan, 1985: 1459-1484.
78. Braude AC, Rebuck AS. Prednisone and methylprednisolone disposition in the lung. *Lancet* 1983; 2: 995-997.
79. Frolich JC, Ogletree ML, Peskar BA, Brigham KL. Pulmonary hypertension correlated to pulmonary thromboxane synthesis. *Adv Prostaglandin Thromboxane Res* 1980; 7: 745-750.
80. Gerber JG, Voelkel NF, Nies AS, McMurtry IF, Reeves JT. Moderation of hypoxic vasoconstriction by infused arachidonic acid: role of $PGI_2$. *J Appl Physiol* 1980; 49: 107-112.
81. Albert R, Henderson W. Leukotriene $C_4$ increases pulmonary vascular permeability in excised rabbit lungs. *Fed Proc* 1982; 41: 1503. Abstract.
82. Ogletree ML, Brigham KL. Effect of cyclooxygenase inhibitors on pulmonary vascular responses to endotoxin in unanesthetized sheep. *Prostaglandin Leukotrienes Med* 1982; 8: 489-502.
83. Ogletree M, Brigham K. Indomethacin augments endotoxin induced lung vascular permeability in sheep. *Am Rev Respir Dis* 1979; 119: 383. Abstract.
84. Brigham KL, Ogletree ML. Effects of prostaglandin and related compounds on lung vascular permeability. *Bull Eur Physiopathol Respir* 1981; 17: 703-722.
85. Reines HD, Halushka PV, Olanoff LS, Hunt PS. Dazoxiben in human sepsis and adult respiratory distress syndrome. *Clin Pharmacol Ther* 1985; 37: 391-395.
86. Leeman M, Boeynaems JM, Degaute JP, Vincent JL, Kahn RJ. Administration of dazoxiben, a selective thromboxane synthetase inhibitor in the adult respiratory distress syndrome. *Chest* 1985; 87: 726-730.
87. Appel PL, Shoemaker WC. Haemodynamic and oxygen transport effects of prostaglandin $E_1$ in patients with adult respiratory distress syndrome. *Crit Care Med* 1984; 12: 528-529.
88. Tokioka H, Kobayashi O, Ohta Y, Wakabayashi T, Kosaku F. The acute effects of prostaglandin $E_1$ on the pulmonary circulation and oxygen delivery in patients with the adult respiratory distress syndrome. *Intensive Care Med* 1985; 11: 61-64.
89. Burghuber OC, Strife RJ, Zirrolli J, et al. Leukotriene inhibitors attenuate rat lung injury induced by hydrogen peroxide. *Am Rev Respir Dis* 1985; 131: 778-785.
90. Dauber I, Pluss W, Stenmark K, Weil J, Voelkel N. Leukotrienes in thiourea induced lung injury edema. *Am Rev Resp Dis* 1983; 127 (part 2): 304. Abstract.
91. Bernard GR, Lucht WD, Niedermeyer ME, Snapper JR, Ogletree ML, Brigham KL. Effect of n-acetylcysteine on the pulmonary response to endotoxin in the awake sheep and upon in vitro granulocyte function. *J Clin Invest* 1984; 73: 1772-1784.
92. Wolf HRD, Seeger HW. Experimental and clinical results in shock lung treatment with vitamin E. *Ann NY Acad Sci* 1982; 393: 392-409.
93. *Petty TL. Indications of risk, course and prognosis in adult respiratory distress syndrome (ARDS). *Am Rev Respir Dis* 1985; 132: 471.

*Denotes editorial or review article.

# Chapter 16

# Adult Asthma

*Richard P.G. Rothwell and J. Douglas Wilson*

Bronchial asthma is the most common chronic respiratory disease, arising at any age and persisting for years, or even for life. It is characterised by wide variations in airways resistance producing episodic symptoms of breathlessness, chest tightness, cough and wheeze.[1] For many years there has been intensive research into the pathophysiology of asthma and active pursuit of new drugs for its treatment.

Patterns of therapy have undergone many changes in recent years, in part because of new pharmacological compounds, or innovations in drug delivery systems, but also because in the United States FDA regulations delayed for many years the introduction of inhaled beta2-agonists and topically active steroids, promoting active development of alternative therapy particularly oral theophyllines. The last three or four years have seen a merging of the US and European schools of asthma treatment with exchanges of ideas and practices. As a consequence there are now available many different treatment schedules which are examined in this chapter in the light of basic and clinical data.

The clinical and therapeutic differences between childhood and adult asthma necessitate separate discussion.

## Aetiology

While the diagnosis of bronchial asthma is usually clear it remains a disorder of complex and obscure aetiology. Almost all patients, whether or not they are symptomatic, exhibit bronchial hyper-reactivity where the irritable airways react with bronchospasm to challenge by a variety of chemical, physical and pharmacological stimuli.[2] Exercise, inhalation of cold air, histamine, methacholine, sulphur dioxide or ozone can each, at certain concentrations, reliably provoke increased airways resistance in most asthmatics. Despite the consistency of the bronchial hyper-reactivity its precise nature remains unclear.

Seale in Chapter 7 reviews the contribution of chemical mediators within the lungs to the pathophysiology of asthma, showing the inter-relationships, while the reasons for differences between mediator release in asthmatics and healthy people remain unknown.

Increased activity of reflex autonomic pathways from irritant receptors beneath the tight junctions of the bronchial mucosa to the efferent limbs from the vagus to bronchial smooth muscle is a further contributing mechanism in asthma.[3] The interplay between these autonomic pathways and the production and action of the various mediators remains subject to intense investigation.

External factors which clearly exacerbate asthma, including respiratory viral infections, allergy, and inhalation of certain irritant materials, can be shown to increase the degree of bronchial hyper-reacticity for some days or weeks.[4]

Consequently a single trigger such as respiratory viral infection, by increasing bronchial hyper-reactivity, will adversely affect the patient's response to other factors such as exercise. In this fashion a vicious cycle can be built up.[5]

## Epidemiology

As wheeze can occur without bronchial asthma, as some asthmatics cough but do not wheeze, and as there remains some dispute about the exact definition and criteria for diagnosis, the prevalence of asthma in different communities cannot be accurately determined.[6] Differences in identification criteria have produced asthma prevalence figures from 2 to 30%. Woolcock et al[7] have developed a strict protocol with questionnaires, lung function tests and quantitative histamine bronchial challenge. This protocol is being applied in a number of different countries and will provide clear comparisons in asthma prevalence between countries. In most Western countries the cumulative prevalence lies approximately between 5 and 15%.

Environmental as well as racial factors influence prevalence. Waite et al[8] evaluated two groups of Tokelau Islanders, some living in New Zealand and the others in their traditional Pacific Island home. The New Zealand group exhibited a presumed or clear asthma prevalence of 25% compared with only 11% for the Pacific Island residents. As the same racial group was examined in the two countries differences must relate to environmental factors. These data also emphasise racial propensity for asthma which is more common among Polynesians than Caucasians (see Chapter 17).

## Diagnostic Features

A clear history of episodic breathlessness and wheezing, often dating back to childhood, is strong evidence of reversible airways obstruction. Associated cough, with or without prolonged cigarette smoking, may require resolution of the chronic bronchitis/asthma distinction. In some patients only a trial of anti-asthma medication will resolve the dilemma. A useful guide to reversibility of airways obstruction can be gained by contrasting the patient's symptoms at their 'best' with those at their 'worst'.

The first manifestations of bronchial asthma may occur at any age, including in the elderly, where cough may be the predominant symptom and lead to an incorrect diagnosis of chronic bronchitis.

Left ventricular heart failure occasionally can mimic bronchial asthma when wheezing is a predominant feature, but the presence of basal crackles, other evidence of ventricular failure, and radiological changes suggesting raised left atrial pressure usually allow clear differentiation.

## Examination

Between attacks no clinical abnormalities may be found on clinical examination. During attacks, and often during sleep, wheeze will be noted by auscultation and sometimes by ear. Occasionally, asthmatic symptoms are the first indication of a systemic vasculitic disorder often associated with radiological opacities, blood eosinophilia, a raised ESR and possibly evidence of multisystem involvement.

Localised wheezing due to involvement of a single main bronchus, or stridor due to upper respiratory tract narrowing, are most commonly due to intrinsic tumours, usually bronchial carcinoma, or to external compression by mediastinal masses.

### Investigation

In most instances the diagnosis of asthma is straightforward, but the following steps assist with difficult situations and also serve to measure the severity of patients' asthma, an essential part of evaluation in assessing prognosis and designing treatment schedules.

*Response to Bronchodilators*

A rapid reduction of symptoms following use of an inhaled bronchodilator provides clear evidence of reversible airways obstruction. An improvement of at least 15% in expiratory flow value with a bronchodilator is considered sufficient to diagnose asthma.

*Detailed Measurement of Expiratory Flow Rates*

The value of objective measures cannot be emphasised too strongly, for both patient and clinician can seriously underestimate the degree of obstruction. Measurement of the degree of obstruction and degree of response to treatment is essential using expiratory air flow indices, such as $FEV_1$, FVC and peak flow with various forms of spirometer or peak flow meter. Modern devices incorporate digital read-outs and can be programmed to calculate predicted values for expiratory flow levels depending on the patient's age, height and sex. Multiple airflow measurements using a portable peak flow meter are of value in patients with a convincing asthmatic history, whose measurements are normal or near-normal at the clinic visit. Some patients exhibit nocturnal airways obstruction only.[9]

Histamine, exercise, cold air, or methacholine at sufficient concentration or duration will usually provoke increased airflow obstruction in asthmatics. Various quantitative procedures have been developed using bronchial challenge to establish the degree of bronchial hyper-reactivity.[4]

*Chest X-ray Examination*

Frequently the chest X-ray is normal, but a minority of cases show evidence of overinflation with diaphragmatic flattening. Occasionally more specific changes of emphysema (bullae, or pruning of peripheral vessels) may be seen, or the non-specific inflammatory changes associated with chronic bronchitis.

Areas of atelectasis from viscid secretions or allergic aspergillosis may be found while more important causes of respiratory obstruction such as bronchial carcinoma must be excluded.

*Blood Eosinophilia*

While eosinophilia is a hallmark of atopy it also occurs in association with most forms of bronchial asthma, whether or not allergy is involved.[10]

*Tests for Potential Allergens*

Skin tests and radioallergosorbent test (RAST) assays for specific anti-allergen IgE will be of value in selected patients. At times one or two potentially avoidable allergens, such as domestic animals or occupational chemicals, can be identified. For other patients recognition of clinical allergic sensitivity can be helpful in predicting potential external triggers for asthma, while various environmental changes may assist in reducing some allergen exposure. Many asthmatics, particularly adults, have no allergy at all.

Exposure to inhaled allergens in sensitive patients is followed by an increase in bronchial hyper-reactivity. Prolonged avoidance of provocative allergens can lead to a reduction in bronchial hyper-reactivity, sometimes to normal where occupational factors are involved.[11]

*Natural History*

Older classifications into intrinsic and extrinsic asthma are not particularly helpful in determining management. Childhood asthma associated with atopy has a relatively good overall prognosis with at least 50% losing their asthma entirely and 25% showing loss for many years with some later recurrence. A significant minority has continuing problems which can be underestimated. Patients developing asthma for the first time in adult life, particularly those without atopic features, tend to have more persistent and severe disease often requiring long-term corticosteroid therapy.

The prognosis of asthma in the great majority of patients is good, with little permanent lung damage or shortened life expectancy. There remains a small but definite mortality from acute asthma which has not been reduced by the introduction of newer medication. Between 1966 and 1968 a number of countries, including the United Kingdom, Australia and New Zealand, experienced an increase in asthma mortality which in the 5 to 34 year age-group reached three times the average annual mortality of the preceding decade.[12] It was proposed that this temporary increase in asthma mortality was related to the excessive use of, or over-reliance on, pressurised bronchodilator aerosols in acute severe attacks, particularly when aerosols containing high doses of isoprenaline were used. Mortality subsequently declined, but New Zealand in the late 1970s until 1981 experienced a second epidemic of fatal asthmatic attacks.[13] A two-year national study confirmed a persistently high asthma mortality both in European and particularly in Maoris and Polynesian Islanders.[14] As with comparable British studies no single cause of this high mortality rate was identified though underuse of corticosteroids, delays in seeking medical help when self-help medication became ineffective, and inappropriate transport to hospital during acute severe episodes each appeared as contributing factors. Excessive medication did not appear to be a problem. It remains a curious phenomenon that asthma mortality has tended to increase at times when treatment patterns are changing and it seems possible that other as yet unidentified factors have contributed in part to asthma mortality.

## Treatment

### Objectives and General Principles of Treatment

Therapy in asthma is directed towards enabling patients to live a normal, active life and to prevent episodes of asthma disrupting this pattern.

Active participation of the patient in the management of his disease is essential if clinicians are to escape from merely responding to severe attacks with bronchodilator therapy then awaiting the next flare-up. Some patients with very mild, intermittent symptoms require no therapy other than reassurance. All patients must receive formal education about their disease, and its manifestations, problems and treatment. Patients must develop confidence in their capacity to maintain a full active life, to anticipate exacerbations of their disease, and to learn when and how to seek medical help. For many patients a clear understanding of their disease and its triggers is more than half the therapeutic battle.

Other forms of supportive treatment are of value in many patients. They should recognise the various external triggers for their own attacks: exercise, allergy, respiratory infection, and stress so they can respond appropriately. Physical treatment such as breathing exercises and aerobic exercise can be associated with clinical improvement.[15]

### Drug Treatment

The pharmacopoeia of drugs to treat asthma continues to increase as more is learnt of the pathophysiology of the disease and new compounds are developed to counter chemical or neural stimuli.

Respiratory obstruction is a combined effect of smooth muscle contraction, mucosal oedema and obstructed bronchial lumina with inspissated mucus and cell debris. In theory medication to relieve acute obstruction should address each of these obstructive elements, but in practice as there is no simple means of assessing the relative contribution of each in a particular asthmatic attack, medication is empirical with bronchodilator drugs used first for their effects on bronchial smooth muscle, ciliary function and oedema, and then steroids which reduce the inflammatory process.

While medication is currently empirical, advances in understanding pathophysiology, with new drugs directed against various chemical mediators involved in the asthmatic process, will in time render individual tailoring of anti-asthmatic drugs to an individual patient's disease likely. For example, anti-asthmatic medication can address: reducing bronchial hyper-reactivity; selective competition with chemical mediators such as leukotrienes; interference with reflex autonomic pathways; stimulation of beta2-receptors on bronchial smooth muscle; blockade of phosphodiesterase activity; limitation of synthesis and release of mediators; and reversal of chronic inflammatory changes in bronchial walls.

In practice, therapy is directed to the last four, but attention towards the first three is becoming clinically important: Ryan et al[16] have shown that regular therapy with inhaled steroids leads to a slow reduction in bronchial hyper-reactivity. This phenomenon is reflected in general symptomatic improvement such as growing resistance to external triggers or reduction in nocturnal asthma (Wilson JD, personal communication). While clinicians do not yet regularly monitor quantitiative changes in bronchial hyper-reactivity this practice is now emerging as a valuable indication of asthma severity and the degree of therapeutic control.

Chapter 7 reviews recent development in drugs to compete with chemical mediators.

While the original anti-asthmatic therapy was the anticholinergic stramonium it is only recently that this approach has returned with the development of the inhaled atropine-like agent ipratropium bromide (see Chapter 6). However, current practice is to administer anti-asthmatic medication empirically using trial and error to evaluate the benefits of new drugs added to a therapeutic regime.

## Details of Drug Treatment

So protean are the manifestations of asthma that therapy has to be tailored to the clinical pattern of an individual patient's disease. In general this leads to a step-wise increase in treatment according to the severity of the patient's asthma: acute and intermittent; chronic and persistent; acute, severe, and life-threatening.

Before one selects a therapeutic regime the severity of a patient's airways obstruction must be objectively established by expiratory air flow measurements. Many patients are unaware of significant persistent airways obstruction between attacks and tolerate $FEV_1$ levels at less than 50% of normal believing themselves to be quite well.[17] Obviously an acute bronchial obstructive episode on top of underlying obstruction may be more serious than bronchospasm from a state of full relaxation.

Detailed below are staged increases in treatment with a number of different protocols. The wide range of available drugs has brought a similar range of treatment options, some suiting some patients, and some suiting others. Clinicians also vary in their choice of treatment based on experience, drug availability, fashion and their particular concepts of the necessary therapeutic goals for their patients. Pharmacological details of the anti-asthmatic drugs are reviewed in Chapters 6, 7 and 8.

### *On-demand Bronchodilation*

Selective beta2-agonists by inhalation alone are the agents of choice for the rapid reversal of most acute asthmatic attacks. Non-selective drugs such as isoprenaline offer no advantage in bronchodilation while presenting unnecessary side effects. Oral medication, though suitable for some patients, is slower to act and requires higher doses with more side effects to obtain the same results.

Löfdahl and Svedmyr (Chapter 6) have reviewed the pharmacology of bronchodilators and have shown that there are no measurable differences between different bronchodilator drugs. Selection is based on dosage needed to obtain a desired clinical response, patient and clinician preference and lack of side effects. The marginal differences between the different beta2-agonists salbutamol, fenoterol, and terbutaline are of little clinical consequence for the patient. Providing that at times of stress a metered dose aerosol can be used effectively, this remains the method of choice for its effectiveness, convenience and portability. Practical problems of washing and cleaning the aerosol should be discussed.

Metered dose aerosols are of little clinical value if patients do not learn to use them correctly (Chapter 2). Clark and Newman in Chapter 2, and Asher in Chapter 17, have reviewed the place of spacer tubes which serve a valuable purpose for the very young or the poorly coordinated patient, but spacers are bulky and inconvenient to use. Inhaled powders offer a more compact alternative and salbutamol as *Rotacaps* for Rotahaler and fenoterol Inhalator offer simple convenient devices to deliver effective bronchodilators as powders which can be used by almost any patient capable of sucking through a straw. Nebulisers can effectively deliver high doses of drugs to all patients independent of their coordination, as discussed in Chapter 2.

Clinicians must be assured of patients' ability to use the metered dose aerosol effectively by understanding the doses used and the correct means of delivery (see Chapter 2).

Oral medication is necessary for some patients and preferred by others. Either beta2-agonists or theophylline preparations are satisfactory provided dosage of the latter is monitored by blood levels (Chapters 4, 17).

Therapy for more severe acute attacks often requires physician intervention and is discussed below.

### *Prophylactic Medication*

A difficult decision to make, for both clinician and patient, is when to introduce regular prophylactic medication and in what form. At present, this is a clinical judgement based on the frequency and severity of attacks. It is possible that this decision could be influenced by quantitative changes in bronchial hyper-reactivity if monitored studies establish its value as an index of disease activity, and if it can be shown that the natural history of the disease can be altered by particular patterns of therapy. Additional supportive information in decisions to commence prophylaxis include measurements of expiratory air flow to demonstrate the severity of attacks and the degree of obstruction between attacks.

The objective of prophylaxis is to decrease attack frequency and severity, and if possible to prevent attacks occurring at all, with the aim of few or no side effects from therapy. Patients' resistance to long-term regular medication, and the lack of clear long-term scientific evaluation of different treatment schedules leave a significant grey area in this decision. The importance of suppressing a persisting inflammatory reaction which may be relatively symptomless is becoming recognised.

The following treatment schedules are presented as alternatives. Different physicians for a variety of reasons favour one or more of these for different clinical situations. There is no unequivocal agreement between European and American physicians, or even among physicians in one country, on the most desirable sequence for introducing additional drugs.

### Regular Inhaled Beta2-agonist Therapy

Most European and Australasian physicians shift from bronchodilator therapy on demand to regular maintenance with inhaled beta2-agonists, using a metered dose aerosol or inhaled powder three or four times daily irrespective of symptoms. This has the advantage of a single drug regime for both prophylaxis and treatment of acute attacks.[18] While patients find this pattern easy to understand, without the confusion of two drugs, and while side effects are few, compliance remains variable.

What, if any, are the possible adverse effects of continued expoure of bronchial smooth muscle receptors to beta2-agonist drugs? As discussed in Chapter 6 there appears to be no tachyphylaxis of clinical importance, asthmatic patients remaining responsive to the drugs whether they are used regularly or intermittently. Experimentally human lymphocytes show reduction in beta-receptor density following treatment with inhaled or oral beta-agonists. This remains a laboratory observation of little clinical relevance. There is little accurate information on the impact of regular beta2-agonist therapy on bronchial hyper-reactivity.[19] Skeletal muscle tremor, a consistent beta2 effect, decreases with regular use of the drugs. Other side effects are dependent on plasma concentration and are discussed in Chapter 6.

### Maintenance Treatment with Oral Theophyllines

Groups such as those led by Weinberger and Hendeles[20] subjected theophylline medication to intensive pharmacokinetic investigation and established the desirable therapeutic plasma levels of the drug between 10 and 20mg/L (55-110micromoles/L). This has been fully reviewed in Chapters 6 and 17, but clinicians must remember the wide clinical variations in metabolism of theophylline between patients to maintain therapeutic levels. Many of the newly developed long-acting theophylline preparations will satisfactorily produce relatively constant drug levels for 10 to 12 hours. Some preparations have pH-dependent release of the drug so food intake can alter bioavailability. Newer preparations have pH-independent release so are less affected by food intake.

Patients must be told about the common side effects such as nausea, vomiting, headache, restlessness, irritability and insomnia. While these may be the early signs of toxicity occasional patients notice little amiss until more serious toxicity occurs with higher blood levels, when convulsions and cardiac irregularities supervene. For these reasons monitoring plasma concentration is mandatory in establishing patients on maintenance therapy. Details of dosage are given in Chapter 6. In practice, patients should be commenced on approximately 250mg twice daily, checking plasma levels five to six hours after drug ingestion when treatment has been stabilised for three days. The dosage can then be titrated upwards to reach maintenance levels.

In view of the predominantly hepatic clearance special care should be taken in patients with any liver dysfunction and when certain antibiotics such as erythromycin, lincomycin and triacetyloleandomycin are added to the treatment.

Clinically, where patients have no side effects at therapeutic levels regular theophylline treatment is a valuable, proven and safe therapy. The additional effects of assisting diaphragmatic contractility may also be of help during severe acute episodes (Chapter 6).

### Regular Use of Oral Beta2-agonists

As larger doses are required orally to achieve bronchodilation comparable with that from inhaled doses, side effects from oral therapy are more common and response is slower, despite which children and some adults may still prefer oral medication.

### Regular Use of Inhaled Anticholinergic Drugs

The pharmacology of ipratropium bromide has been reviewed in Chapter 6. Many patients with chronic bronchitis and some with asthma experience as much bronchodilation with ipratropium as with beta2-agonists. A few do better with the anticholinergic drug.[21] The advantage of ipratropium in responsive patients is its lack of side effects and its very wide therapeutic range so patients can increase the dosage 10 to 20 times without significant deleterious effects.[22]

In general, more asthmatics respond better to beta2-agonists that to ipratropium, but it remains a useful drug acutely or prophylactically in responsive patients. Recently combination formulation with fenoterol and ipratropium has been evaluated showing bronchodilation comparable with higher beta2-agonist doses.[21]

## *Introduction of a Second Drug*

As there are a number of bronchodilators and prophylactic agents, many different drug combinations can be developed. The treatment regimes discussed below are the most common choices.

### Addition of Inhaled Steroid

Regular use of an inhaled steroid such as beclomethasone dipropionate or budesonide is the usual practice in adult patients whose regular bronchodilator treatment proves insufficient to control symptoms. As explained in Chapter 8 modification of the steroid molecule, such as addition of the dipropionate side chain, gives drugs with potent topical activity yet ready liver detoxication. Multiple studies over 20 years have confirmed not only the major therapeutic value of these drugs but their minimal side effects, in particular their minimal effect on the adrenal-pituitary axis when used in doses of up to 1000 micrograms daily. Beclomethasone used at 400 microgram daily doses can substitute for up to 7.5mg of prednisone treatment without systemic effects.[23] Topical effects such as husky voice[24] and oral thrush can be a problem for a few patients, but are rarely an indication to discontinue treatment. Topical antifungal therapy, washing the mouth out with water immediately after inhalation, and using spacer tubes can each assist in reducing local topical effects.

Inhaled steroids, to be effective, must be used regularly two to four times daily to produce and maintain benefit. Up to three months may be needed to produce full clinical effects.[25] We believe that inhaled steroids are indicated in all adult patients not adequately controlled by regular bronchodilator therapy. Many patients who have recently developed asthma appear to benefit from inhaled steroids even if bronchodilator medication is still taken only on-demand.

By decreasing local inflammatory changes within the bronchial wall, and by decreasing mediator synthesis, steroids influence the asthmatic process by mechanisms quite different from bronchodilators. Recent evidence has clearly documented a reduction in bronchial hyper-reactivity in patients on inhaled steroids.[16] Regular use of inhaled steroids, in addition to inhibiting acute attack frequency, will effectively prevent night-time wheeze and cough, presumably a consequence of lower bronchial hyper-reactivity with reduced diurnal swings in airways calibre (Wilson et al, personal communication).

Two dosage formulations of beclomethasone are available at 50 micrograms and 250 micrograms in each puff, permitting tailoring of dosage levels up to 2000 micrograms daily if necessary in individual patients. More than 60% of patients not adequately controlled on regular bronchodilator drugs and conventional doses of beclomethasone show further improvement with high-dose medication, 1000 to 2000 micrograms.[26] The fivefold reduction in number of puffs from high-dose inhalers increases convenience and probably compliance. Surprisingly the frequency of local side effects is little increased with the high-dose formulation.

### Addition of Sodium Cromoglycate

The development of sodium cromoglycate presented an entirely new direction to anti-asthmatic medication with its capacity to inhibit release of vasoactive mediators from mast cells. While some initial clinical trials questioned its clinical value later studies of longer duration, particularly in children, clearly established its prophylactic value.[28] Recent evidence has questioned the mast cell stabilising action as having clinical relevance at doses used,[29] but the drug remains a useful and safe agent despite its uncertain mechanism of action. The wider use of inhaled steroids, and the clear lack of deleterious side effects with these agents, have limited the use of cromoglycate in adults in whom clinical responses are less predictable than in children.[30] Recent modifications to the delivery systems, originally an inhaled powder with 20mg in a capsule, have provided the more convenient metered dose aerosol with 2mg in a puff. There appears to be little difference in clinical effectiveness between the two formulations.[31] As with inhaled steroids a trial of at least four weeks is necessary to establish the degree of clinical response.

Sodium cromoglycate appears very effective in asthmatics whose prime symptom is cough and it also prevents most episodes of exercise-induced asthma, though not as effectively as inhaled beta2-agonists.[32]

### Combination of Beta2-agonists and Theophylline, both as Regular Maintenance Therapy

For a period in the early 1980s combination beta2-agonists and theophyllines were fashionable as regular prophylactic treatment. Reassessment of the various components of the obstructive process in asthma indicates that this double bronchodilator approach is likely to be less efficacious than a single bronchodilator plus an inhaled steroid.[6] But for some patients this double bronchodilator schedule has advantages and proves satisfactory.[33]

All bronchodilator drugs, at sufficient dosage, can dilate the bronchi to approximately the same extent,[34] though this may carry the price of undesirable side effects. Consequently when beta2-agonists and theophyllines are used together at submaximal bronchodilating doses greater bronchodilation will be achieved than with either drug alone with minimal side effects.[35]

Some patients maintained on regular theophylline therapy can simply add an inhaled beta2-agonist on demand.

The disadvantages of this regime are the limitations for the clinician when these patients present acutely when their maintenance bronchodilators are ineffective. They are then in need of intense bronchodilator treatment which cannot be administered as intravenous aminophylline without checking blood levels from their maintenance drugs. When these levels are within the therapeutic range all attention must be directed to intense beta2-agonist therapy, normally by nebuliser. In others low plasma theophylline levels presumably due to lack of compliance may have contributed to the acute episode.

Suggestions by one of us (JDW) that the adoption of this double bronchodilator regime to the exclusion of other prophylactic medication was in part the explanation of the increase in prevalence of fatal asthma in New Zealand in 1977 to 1981[13] have not been supported by other authorities and later evidence suggests that the lack of steroids is itself one of the predisposing factors in fatal asthma.[14]

## Oral Corticosteroid Therapy

Oral corticosteroids are used as follows: (i) as a therapeutic trial to detect reversible airways obstruction; (ii) to re-establish the patency of airways for regular inhaled therapy; (iii) as a minimum necessary supplement to regular inhaled bronchodilator and high-dose inhaled corticosteroid preventive therapy; and (iv) as treatment for acute severe asthma.

It is important that a course of systemic steroid therapy should be given if the patient has insufficient ventilatory capacity to introduce inhaled therapy such as sodium cromoglycate or beclomethasone, or during exacerbations of asthma when baseline inhaled therapy becomes temporarily ineffective.

Systemic steroid therapy should be used only as a minimum necessary supplement to optimal bronchodilator therapy, and high-dose inhaled corticosteroid therapy in those patients whose asthma is still inadequately controlled. This must be based on the patient's record of symptoms and objective ventilatory testing, balancing the interference with normal daily activities and risk of acute severe attacks on the one hand against possible long-term steroid side effects on the other. Generally speaking the severity of the asthmatic condition has tended to be under-rated and the risk of side effects from steroid therapy overestimated.

The corticosteroid drug of choice is probably either prednisone or prednisolone on the grounds of long experience with their use and the relatively short half-life compared with other steroids (Chapter 8). There is considerable evidence that a single total daily dose given in the morning has the advantage of not only minimising adrenal suppression, but also being equally effective in controlling both daytime and night-time asthmatic symptoms. The pharmacokinetics and pharmacodynamics of prednisone metabolism give no justification for giving divided or evening doses. Once the decision to use oral corticosteroid therapy has been made, either on the grounds of inadequate control of symptoms with chronic asthma or asthma initially severe enough to cause concern, it is probably best to start with a fairly high dose of 40 to 60mg of prednisone daily, giving this for long enough to get a maximal response, usually up to 7 to 10 days, and reducing thereafter fairly rapidly giving a minimum 'short' course of two to three weeks.

Whether or not a maintenance dose is required depends on the close monitoring of progress and early detection of relapse. The likelihood of significant side effects is related to both the daily dose and the duration of therapy, but in general, daily doses of less than 7.5mg are unlikely to cause significant adrenal suppression or other major side effects and should be aimed for if at all possible.[36]

Alternate-day therapy (that is, the total 48-hour dosage given as a single dose with breakfast every second day) causes significantly less adrenal suppression,[36] but in a patient whose treatment is carefully tailored to minimum requirements, it is unusual to maintain good control on twice the previous daily dosage, with likely relapse of symptoms within the 48-hour period. More comparable control is attained with approximately three times the previous daily dose given on an alternate-day basis, but the advantage of this has not been clearly proven at least in treatment for adults.

## Management of Acute Severe Asthma

Acute severe asthma has been defined as an acute episode of asthma of increased severity failing to respond to more than average treatment.[37] A patient should be given the responsibility of administering and monitoring his own therapy within certian limits. If his usual bronchodilator aerosol is failing to give adequate relief despite additional doses between the times of regular medication, and if his peak flow rate is swinging widely or falling below a predetermined level, it is important that he should urgently seek further medical advice.

Several physical signs have been found to correlate well with the severity of the underlying functional abnormality.

1. Severity of symptoms: inability to exercise, sleep, talk, swallow or inhale medication.
2. Sternomastoid retraction: this has been correlated with an $FEV_1$ of less than one litre.
3. Tachycardia greater than 110 beats per minute: in the past this has been attributed to side effects from sympathomimetic drugs, but in recent times tachycardia is virtually always related to the severity of the underlying condition.
4. Gross overinflation.
5. Pulsus paradoxus: up to 10mmHg (1.3kPa) can be regarded as normal, but anything in excess of this figure should be taken as evidence of severity.

At times the palpable pulse virtually disappears on inspiration in a severe asthmatic attack.[38]
6. Disturbances of consciousness: any disturbance of consciousness should be taken seriously as it usually indicates significant hypoxaemia and/or hypercapnia.
7. Central cyanosis: this is always indicative of severe hypoxaemia, but it should be noted that significant hypoxaemia may be present without obvious cyanosis.
8. Pneumothorax or surgical emphysema: the presence of a pneumothorax may be difficult to detect clinically due to the severe overinflation of an asthmatic attack, but reduced breath sounds may be found on the affected side. The characteristic 'crunching' sound of air in the mediastinum synchronous with the heart beat may occasionally be found with or without surgical emphysema in the neck.
9. Exhaustion: this serious symptom is still one of the commonest indications for assisted ventilation.
10. Peak flow rate: anything below 50% of the peak flow rate when 'well' should be taken seriously, and in the averate adult a peak flow rate of less than 200L/min or an $FEV_1$ of less than one litre indicates severe airflow obstruction warranting hospital admission and treatment.

Assessment of severity using a single scoring has helped distinguish patients requiring hospital admission from those likely to be able to maintain progress at home, although re-examination has suggested that this system is not completely specific or sensitive in identifying the patients most at risk.[39,40]

## Bronchodilator Therapy

More aggressive bronchodilator therapy is still the most important initial treatment in acute severe asthma despite the apparent lack of responsiveness to conventional doses by metered dose inhaler. In patients with severe airways obstruction penetration into the airways appears to be reduced as, despite high aerosol use, plasma levels remain low. In these circumstances inhaler technique is likely to be less than adequate. Despite these problems and the presence of widespread mucus plugging of small peripheral airways, the standard emergency treatment is inhaled beta2-agonists given via a nebuliser which, with equipotent doses of 5mg of salbutamol or 2.5mg of fenoterol, appears superior to other inhalation devices. The total volume of nebulised solution may be critical in minimising loss of active drug in the residual volume left after nebulisation is apparently complete. On the grounds of minimum drug wastage compatible with a reasonable nebulisation time, it appears that dilution to a volume of approximately 3ml should be optimal.[41]

Intermittent positive pressure breathing (IPPB) has been advocated for nebulisation, but a recent trial using comparable doses of inhaled salbutamol concluded that there is no advantage in using IPPB.[42] The use of oxygen rather than air as the driving gas has been advocated on the grounds that concurrent pulmonary vasodilatation may cause some increase in peripheral mismatching of ventilation and perfusion with a small additional fall in arterial oxygen tension in a patient who may already be critically hypoxaemic. Although a recent trial showed no worsening of hypoxaemia in acute severe asthma where salbutamol was nebulised by an electrically operated air compressor, it would appear prudent in this situation to use oxygen if possible.[43]

The parenteral administration of selective beta2-agonists certainly appears free of any side effects apart from a modest increase in heart rate, but despite the attractiveness of the suggestion that given in this way they may be more effective than inhaled drugs in the presence of severe airways obstruction, most studies have failed to show that intravenous salbutamol was more effective than inhaled therapy, and more tremor and tachycardia was produced.

Complications of intravenous bronchodilator therapy are seldom significant in the absence of pre-existing heart disease, but the metabolic effects of beta2-agonists, particularly in causing a fall in serum potassium concentration, should be borne in mind especially when high doses or corticosteroids are being used concurrently.

The use of a metered dose inhaler with a space chamber attachment increases airway deposition of the drug and avoids the need for critical coordination, and equal doses of drug given by nebuliser show no significant difference in the rate of onset or degree of bronchodilation between the two methods.

## Corticosteroid Treatment

The use of corticosteroids in acute severe asthma is still rather empirical, the dose being based on rather limited data with a preference for intravenous hydrocortisone hemisuccinate in a loading dose of 200 to 400mg followed by a continuous infusion of 3mg/kg over six hours for 48 hours which appears to be less likely to cause problems with hypokalaemia than repeated bolus doses.[44]

Concurrently or within a few hours, once the patient is fit enough to take oral therapy, 40 to 60mg of prednisone daily is commenced. Once some improvement has taken place intravenous corticosteroid therapy can be stopped and prednisone dosage reduced according to progress. In the initial stages any previously prescribed inhaled corticosteroid therapy is discontinued pending improvement.

It has been suggested that corticosteroid therapy is unnecessary,[45] but pending further studies it would be unwise to withhold this treatment.[46] Nevertheless, there is considerable evidence that the main value of corticosteroids is in re-establishing control in patients showing significant deterioration before the situation becomes critical. Once acute severe asthma is established, the role of steroid therapy appears to be one of hastening recovery rather than preventing death.

## Intravenous Aminophylline

There is some doubt about whether intravenous (IV) aminophylline confers additional bronchodilation once optimal doses of beta2-agonists are given, but most clinicians would still use this treatment when the initial response to maximal doses of nebulised beta2-agonists is equivocal. Aminophylline is a potentially toxic drug and particular care must be taken to first check details of any oral therapy with sustained-release preparations to ensure that the patient does not already have substantial or even fully therapeutic blood levels of theophylline before additional intravenous theophylline is given.[47] If established therapeutic drug levels are likely, a loading dose should be omitted and, if necessary, a constant infusion commenced at about the time blood levels are likely to be falling.

An approximate loading dose for a patient not on previous treatment is 5mg/kg, something of the order of 250 to 500mg in an average adult which should be given well diluted and slowly over 10 to 15 minutes if possible, to avoid nausea, vomiting and severe headache. Convulsions and serious cardiac arrhythmias have been reported virtually always in association with rapid IV 'push' doses. An initial loading dose may then be followed by an infusion of approximately 0.5mg/kg/h. Estimates of dosage are a rough guide only and must be supplemented by serum levels within 12 to 24 hours.

## Patient Instructions

Prescription of more than one drug can lead to confusion, particularly when given during a busy practice day. All patients are helped by having these instructions written down.

A crisis plan is a necessary support for all patients. They must know the circumstances which require additional medical help. As patients participate more in their own therapy the guidelines of tolerance must be defined. Delays in seeking expert help when standard medication is insufficient are an accepted contributing factor in fatal asthma.[14] An example of a crisis plan is given in Figure 16.1.

**CRISIS PLAN FOR AN ASTHMA ATTACK**

**IF**
- You are not responding as usual to your medication,
- You are waking during the night short of breath,
- You become short of breath during the day and find it difficult to do your day-to-day activities,
- Your peak flow rate is gradually falling or shows wide variations,
- Your peak flow rate is below.................

**YOUR ASTHMA IS SEVERE. Extra treatment started immediately will shorten your attack.**

Take a dose from your inhaler every 10 to 15 minutes for up to one hour.

Take prednisone if prescribed by your doctor — prednisone takes 4 to 6 hours to work.

If you haven't improved in one hour **contact your doctor or the ambulance straight away.**

IF THE ATTACK IS SUDDEN AND SEVERE, DO NOT DELAY,
CONTACT YOUR DOCTOR IMMEDIATELY OR GO TO THE
NEAREST HOSPITAL, PREFERABLY BY AMBULANCE.

Your asthma may get worse again as you decrease your prednisone or within a week or so of stopping it. If it does, **see your doctor straight away.**

**ALWAYS** report back to your doctor after a severe attack of asthma.

*Figure 16.1* Crisis plan for an asthma attack.

## Special Problems

### Nocturnal Asthma

Symptoms are often worse at night and in the early morning,[48] and many possible explanations have been considered for this including exposure to allergens in bedding and variations in autonomic responsiveness of the airways and in catecholamine levels. With greater understanding of circadian biological rhythms it appears that nocturnal asthma represents exaggeration of normal variation in bronchial tone as a manifestation of bronchial hyper-reactivity.[49]

It has been the practice to provide long-acting bronchodilator therapy taken at bed-time to control this, including slow-release oral beta2-agonists or theophylline preparations, but perhaps most effective is treatment directed towards reducing bronchial hyper-reactivity and stabilising the patient's asthma overall. A recent study by one of the authors (JD Wilson et al, personal communication) established that most patients with nocturnal asthma lost their symptoms with the introduction of inhaled steroids on a regular basis.

### Occupational Asthma

Wheezing provoked by exposure to substances at work may occur in a patient who already has asthma, or in someone who has always been well. In the latter, symptoms will usually disappear when exposure ceases, although there is always the risk that occupational exposure will trigger permanent and disabling asthma.[11]

Many organic substances have been known to provoke asthma including wood dust, especially from resinous timbers, grain dusts, various animal products and certain metals and their salts, the best known being the complex salts of platinum, nickel and chromium.[50]

Newer industries may be associated with an appreciable hazard notably the manufacture of polyurethane foam producing isocyanates, the manufacture of washing powders containing proteolytic enzymes, the use of epoxyresins, the production of new antibiotics and pharmaceuticals, and the use of solders in the manufacture of electronic circuitry.

The diagnosis is often made by the patient himself recognising the relationship between symptoms and exposure at work, although this may be obscured if the bronchial response to the provocative agent occurs several hours after exposure, or is prolonged. Confirmation of the diagnosis should be sought by monitoring ventilatory capacity using, for example, the mini-Wright Peak Flow Meter both during the working week and during holiday times.

Identification of the exact sensitising agent may be difficult and the ideal answer is to avoid exposure where possible by modifying working conditions or finding alternative employment.

## References


1. Scadding JG. Definition and clinical categories of asthma. In: Clark and Godfrey, eds. *Asthma*. London: Chapman and Hall, 1977.
2. Boushey HA, Holtzman MJ, Sheller JR, Nadel JA. State of the art: bronchial hyperreactivity. *Am Rev Respir Dis* 1980; 121: 389.
3. Nadel JA, Davies B. Autonomic regulation of mucus secretion and ion transport in airways. In: Lichtenstein and Austin, eds. *Discussion in asthma, physiology, immunopharmacology and treatment*. Second International Symposium, New York: Academic Press, 1977: 197.
4. Empey DW, Laitinen LA, Jacobs L, et al. Mechanisms of bronchial hyperreactivity in normal subjects after upper respiratory tract infection. *Am Rev Respir Dis* 1976; 113: 131.
5. Cockcroft DW. Mechanism of perennial allergic asthma. *Lancet* 1983; 2: 253.
6. Wilson JD. *Asthma and allergic diseases*. Sydney: ADIS Health Science Press, 1983.
7. Woolcock AJ, Dowse GK, Temple K, Stanley H, Alpers MP, Turner KJ. The prevalence of asthma in the South Fone people of Papua New Guinea. A method for field studies of bronchial reactivity. *Eur J Respir Dis* 1983; 64: 571.
8. Waite DA, Eyles EF, Tonkin SL, O'Donnell TV. Asthma prevalence in Tokelauan children in two environments. *Clin Allergy* 1980; 10: 71.
9. Turner-Warwick M. On observing patterns of airflow obstruction in chronic asthma. *Br J Dis Chest* 1977; 71: 73.
10. Wilson JD. Asthma: the dimension of the problem. In: Clark TJH, ed. *Steroids in asthma*. Auckland: ADIS Press, 1983.
11. Chan-Yeung M, Lam S, Koener S. Clinical features and natural history of occupational asthma due to Western red cedar (Thuja plicata). *Am J Med* 1982; 72: 411.
12. Fraser PM, Speizer FE, Waters SDM, Doll R, Mann MN. The circumstances preceding death from asthma in young people in 1968-1969. *Br J Dis Chest* 1971; 65: 71.
13. Wilson JD, Sutherland DC. Thomas AC. Has the change to beta-agonists combined with oral theophylline increased cases of fatal asthma? *Lancet* 1981; 1: 1235.
14. Sears MR, Rea HH, Beaglehole R, et al. Asthma mortality in New Zealand: a two-year national study. *NZ Med J* 1985; 98: 271.
15. Schnall RP, Landau LJ. Protective effects of repeated short sprints in exercise-induced asthma. *Thorax* 1980; 35: 828.
16. Ryan G, Latimer KM, Juniper EF, Roberts RS, Hargreave FE. Effect of beclomethasone dipropionate on bronchial responsiveness to histamine in controlled non steroid-dependent asthma. *J Allergy Clin Immunol* 1985; 75: 25.
17. Rubinfeld AR, Pain MCF. Perception of asthma. *Lancet* 1976; 1: 882.
18. Tattersfield AE. Bronchodilators in the prevention of asthma. In: Clark TJH, ed. *Bronchodilator therapy*. Auckland: ADIS Press, 1984: 76.
19. Bleeker ER. Airways reactivity and asthma: significance and treatment. *J Allergy Clin Immunol* 1985; 75: 21.
20. Weinberger M, Hendeles L. Experience with theophylline for the management of chronic asthma. *Eur J Respir Dis* 1980; 61 (suppl 109): 120.
21. Mann JS, George CF. Anticholinergic drugs in the treatment of airways disease. *Br J Dis Chest* 1985; 79: 209.
22. Allen CJ, Campbell AH. Dose-response of SCH 1000. *Thorax* 1980; 35: 137.
23. Brompton Hospital/Medical Research Council Collaborative Trial. Double blind trial comparing two dosage schedules of beclomethasone dipropionate aerosol with placebo in chronic bronchial asthma. *Br J Dis Chest* 1979; 73: 121.
24. Williams AJ, Baghat MS, Stableforth DE, Cayton RM, Skinner C. Dysphonia caused by inhaled steroids: recognition of a characteristic laryngeal abnormality. *Thorax* 1983; 38: 813.
25. Eriksson JE, Lindgren S, Lindholm B. Long term treatment of steroid dependent asthmatic patients with beclomethasone dipropionate. *Allergol Immunopathol (Madr)* 1975; 3: 77.
26. Smith ML, Hodson ME. High dose beclomethasone inhaler in the treatment of asthma. *Lancet* 1983; 1: 265.
27. Altounyan REC. Review of the clinical activity and modes of action of sodium cromoglycate. In: Pepys and Edwards, eds. *The mast cell*. East Grinstead: Pitman Medical, 1979: 199.

28. Godfrey S, Balfour-Lynn L, Konig P. The place of cromolyn sodium in the long term management of childhood asthma based on a 3 to 5 year follow-up. *J Paediatr* 1975; 87: 465.
29. Bernstein IL. Cromolyn sodium. *Chest* 1985; 87 (suppl): 685.
30. Brompton Hospital/Medical Research Council Colalborative Trial. Long-term study of disodium cromoglycate in treatment of severe extrinsic or intrinsic asthma. *Br Med J* 1972; 4: 383.
31. Paija O, Kreus KE. Clinical trial of sodium cromoglycate pressurized aerosol in the treatment of asthma. *Eur J Respir Dis* 1981; 62: 5, 168.
32. Anderson S, Seale JP, Ferris L, Schoeffel R, Lindsay DA. An evaluation of pharmacotherapy for exercise-induced asthma. *J Allergy Clin Immunol* 1979; 64: 612.
33. Svedmyr N, Löfdahl CG. Physiology and pharmacodynamics of beta-adrenergic agonist drugs. In: Jenne WK, ed. *Bronchodilating drugs.* New York: Marcel Dekker, 1986 (in press).
34. Svedmyr N. Controlled clinical trials in asthmatics. *Scand J Respir Dis* 1977; suppl 101: 35.
35. Svedmyr N, Svedmyr K. In vitro and in vivo effects of theophylline and beta 2-adreno stimulants in combination. *Eur J Respir Dis* 1980; 61 (suppl 109): 83.
36. Cochrane GM. Systemic steroids in asthma. In: Clark TJH, ed. *Steroids in asthma.* Auckland: ADIS Press, 1983; 103: 35.
37. Clark TJH. In: Clark and Godfrey, eds. *Asthma.* 2nd ed. London: Chapman and Hall, 1983: 393.
38. Knowles GK, Clark TJH. Pulsus paradoxus as a valuable sign indicating severity of asthma. *Lancet* 1973; 2: 1356.
39. Fischl MA, Pitchenik A, Gardner LB. An index predicting relapse and need for hospitalization in patients with acute bronchial asthma. *N Engl J Med* 1981; 305: 783.
40. Rose CC, Murphy JG, Swartz JS. Performance of an index predicting the response of patients with acute bronchial asthma to intensive emergency department treatment. *N Engl J Med* 1984: 310: 573.
41. Clay M. Efficiency of jet nebulizers in the production of therapeutic aerosols. *Thorax* 1982; 37: 788.
42. Fergusson RJ, Carmichael J, Rafferty P, Willey RF, Crompton GK, Grant IWB. Nebulized salbutamol in life-threatening asthma. Is I.P.P.B. necessary? *Br J Dis Chest* 1980; 74: 385.
43. Douglas JG, Rafferty P, Fergusson RJ, Prescott RJ, Crompton GK, Grant IWB. Nebulized salbutamol without oxygen in severe acute asthma. How effective, how safe? *Br J Dis Chest* 1980; 74: 385.
44. Collins JV, Clark TJH, Brown D, Townsend J. The use of corticosteroids in the treatment of acute asthma. *Q J Med* 1975; 44: 25.
45. Luksza AR. Acute severe asthma treated without steroids. *Br J Dis Chest*1982; 76: 15.
46. Grant IWB. Are corticosteroids necessary in the treatment of severe acute asthma? *Br J Dis Chest* 1982; 76: 125.
47. Anonymous. Intravenous aminophylline: a cautionary note. *Lancet* 1980; 1: 746.
48. Hetzel MR, Clark TJH, Branthwaite MA. Asthma: analysis of sudden deaths and ventilatory arrests in hospital. *Br Med J* 1977; 1: 808.
49. Clark TJH. The circadian rhythm of asthma. *Br J Dis Chest* 1985; 79: 115.
50. Pepys J, Hutchcroft BJ. Bronchial provocation tests in etiological diagnosis and analysis of asthma. *Am Rev Respir Dis* 1975; 112: 829.

## Chapter 17

# Childhood Asthma

*M. Innes Asher*

Asthma in children is a common condition which can occur even in very young children. It is characterised by episodic symptoms of wheeze, cough, and/or breathlessness which improve after the administration of bronchodilators.

## Clinical Features

Asthma can occur in children of any age, and commonly starts in young children, although it is rare under the age of six months. Although episodic wheeze is the typical feature of asthma, cough (usually dry and often nocturnal) is very common and may be the presenting or only symptom. Mild episodic symptoms are the most common pattern of asthma (75% of asthmatic children), but asthmatic children with frequent episodes (20%) or chronic asthma (5%) may have troublesome disease.[1]

The large majority of asthmatic children will suffer from exercise-induced asthma if they exercise hard enough under appropriate conditions,[2] although young children may never exercise enough to produce symptoms. There is no correlation between the severity of exercise-induced asthma and the clinical severity of asthma in an individual.[3]

## Aetiology

The three characteristic pathological features of asthma are bronchospasm, increased bronchial mucus secretion and oedema. Mucous glands and smooth muscle have been demonstrated in the bronchi of very young children,[4] indicating the potential for dysfunction even in this age-group. The mechanisms producing asthma include mediator release from mast cells.

There is an increase in asthma among parents, siblings and grandparents of asthmatic patients. While genetic factors are important for the development of asthma, non-genetic ones also contribute.

Up to half of the children who have been admitted to hospital with bronchiolitis due to respiratory syncytial virus subsequently have recurrent wheeze. Among such children there is an increased prevalence of bronchial hyper-responsiveness and decreased expiratory flow rates, but the prevalence of atopy is not increased.[5] The full relationship between asthma and respiratory syncytial virus infection will be resolved only by the completion of prospective community-based studies.

Bronchial hyper-responsiveness is present in the majority of asthmatic children, and appears to be important in the pathogenesis of asthma;

changes in bronchial hyper-responsiveness appear to reflect asthmatic symptoms and the clinical severity of asthma. Suggestions that bronchial hyper-responsiveness is potentially modifiable in the long term by drug therapy are yet to be confirmed.[6] A minority of children demonstrate bronchial hyper-responsiveness and yet are asymptomatic; a minority go on to develop clinical asthma (Sears MR et al, personal communication).

Factors which trigger asthma attacks vary between individuals and include viral infections, exercise, stress, weather changes, inhaled allergens, ingested allergens, and inhaled irritants including cigarette smoke.

## Epidemiology

Asthma is a common condition, and the estimation of its prevalence depends on the methodology used. Prevalence rates of 11% in England,[7] 6% in USA,[8] 11% in Australia[9] and 12.2% in New Zealand[10] have been found. About 70% of children with asthma have the onset of their disease under the age of three years, and about 30% between three and seven years. Asthma occurs equally commonly in children of both sexes, although more severe asthma is more common in boys.[1] Asthma has been observed in most ethnic groups, but seems to be particularly common in Western societies, especially in people who have recently moved from a non-Western community.[11] Racial differences in the prevalence of asthma have been observed between European, Pacific Island and New Zealand Maori children (Asher MI et al, unpublished observations).

## Diagnostic Features

Despite increasing awareness about asthma in children, this condition is frequently underdiagnosed and undertreated, resulting in unnecessary morbidity.[12,13]

### History

There is no difficulty recognising asthma in a child with episodic wheeze. Episodic cough, especially at night, and much less commonly episodic breathlessness alone are also characteristic. Occasionally a child will exhibit exercise-induced asthma alone and this may be manifest by any or all of the above symptoms. A careful thorough history will usually lead to the diagnosis, but other conditions which cause intrathoracic airways obstruction must be considered: cystic fibrosis, bronchiectasis, foreign body aspiration, aspiration from other causes, and heart failure.

Children with acute asthma attacks who are at particular risk of death are those with a past history of a life-threatening attack: one in which there has been impairment of consciousness and/or raised arterial $PCO_2$. Recent urgent visits to a doctor also denote high risk, as does a recent crescendo of nocturnal asthma.[14,15]

## Examination

The majority of children with asthma will have no abnormal physical features between attacks. Abnormalities that may be found in chronic asthma or during asthma attacks include audible expiratory wheeze, prolonged expiration, accessory muscle use, indrawing, hyperinflation (increased anteroposterior chest diameter, liver and spleen pushed down, hyper-resonant percussion note), reduced respiratory excursion and pulsus paradoxus. On auscultation there may be expiratory wheezes (rhonchi) and decreased air entry. Fixed chest deformity (barrel chest) indicates long-standing disease, and Harrison's sulcus indicates that chronic disease was present in the first year or two of life. Underweight indicates poor asthma control and/or inadequate food intake. Atopic children show allergic features (eczema, allergic shiners or geographic tongue). Finger clubbing is not a clinical feature of asthma.

Clinical features that indicate respiratory failure (hypoxaemia with or without hypercarbia) include central cyanosis, impaired consciousness, inability to speak, pulsus paradoxus of at least 15mmHg (2kPa), tachycardia of more than 160 beats per minute, and an unrecordable peak flow in a child who is capable of using a meter.[16]

## Investigations

The diagnostic test to confirm the presence of asthma is a test of non-specific bronchial responsiveness. This is most simply carried out by assessment of response to a bronchodilator, but in children who have normal lung function administration of a non-specific bronchial challenge will be necessary.

### *Bronchodilator Responsiveness*

A high dose of an inhaled bronchodilator is given. Lung function is measured before and 15 to 20 minutes after the dose; an increase in peak expiratory flow rate (PEFR) or forced expired volume in one second ($FEV_1$) or more than 15% is significant. Use of a nebuliser is recommended for initial testing, unless techniques of other inhaler devices have been mastered. In children who are too young to perform lung function tests, the measurement of a clinical response is satisfactory; in a positive response the respiratory rate, heart rate, and indrawing decrease, and air entry improves.

### *Non-specific Bronchial Challenge*

After initial assessment of lung function, a dose of saline is given, followed by increasing increments of histamine or methacholine until the child either has a fall in $FEV_1$ of at least 20% or until the maximum dose has been given. In children with asthma the $FEV_1$ falls before this maximum dose.[17,18]

A standardised exercise test[2] is used to make the diagnosis of exercise-induced asthma, itself diagnostic of asthma. Vigorous running exercise is followed by a fall in PEFR or $FEV_1$ from pre-exercise levels by at least 15%.

*Lung Function Testing*

Expiratory flow rates (PEFR and $FEV_1$) are commonly normal in mild infrequent asthma, but they are commonly abnormal in frequent or chronic asthma, where hyperinflation may also be evident in the lung volume measurements. These abnormalities are features of obstructive lung disease of any cause, and therefore are not diagnostic of asthma. However, lung function tests may be particularly useful to follow progress; a mini-Wright peak flow meter should be used at home by children five years old or more. Special tests have been developed for use with younger children and infants; however, it will be some years yet before such tests are widely available.

*Other Tests*

Positive tests of atopy (skin prick tests, serum IgE) support the diagnosis of allergic asthma. The chest radiograph may indicate hyperinflation and will detect complications of asthma: lobar collapse, pneumomediastinum, pneumothorax and subcutaneous emphysema. Blood gas measurement is used to detect acid-base disturbance and respiratory failure.

## Natural History and Prognosis

Fifty per cent of children with asthma have stopped wheezing by 14 years, and 60% by 21 years, but 15% are worse as adults compared with children. Of children with chronic asthma, only 5% are wheeze-free as adults, 40% have infrequent asthma and 50% have frequent or chronic asthma as adults. Factors which may increase the chance of asthma being present at 21 years of age are infantile eczema, frequent or chronic asthma at 10 to 14 years, and/or a barrel chest at 10 to 14 years.[19] The natural history of bronchial hyper-responsiveness and its relationship to clinical asthma awaits further studies. Asthma in children can result in school absences, disturbed nights and restricted physical activity if there is undertreatment.[12] Many asthmatics as young adults do not receive adequate treatment, lose time off work and restrict sporting activities; smoking of tobacco is common and is associated with troublesome asthma.

Most asthmatic children have complete reversibility of impairment of lung function; the few who do not are most likely to be children with hyperinflation, rather than airways obstruction.[20] At 21 years of age features of airways obstruction are often present during an interval phase in those with more persistent symptoms.

Asthma rarely results in death in children under the age of ten years,[15] but death is increasingly common in adolescence, with a peak for children aged 15 to 19 years.[14]

It is not known whether drug therapy is capable of improving the prognosis in children with chronic asthma and preventing the development of irreversible impairment of lung function. However, studies of mortality in New Zealand suggest that drug therapy helps to prevent death from asthma,[14] and preventive drug therapy may reduce school absences and nocturnal waking.[13]

## Goals of Treatment

The goals of treatment are to improve prognosis and optimise the quality of life, to allow the child with asthma to reach her/his potential. Therapy should aim to maintain complete reversibility of abnormalities in lung function, maximise growth potential, minimise chest deformity and eliminate mortality, while ensuring that the child is physically active and emotionally stable and participating fully in family, school and social life. These goals may be achieved by therapy which decreases symptoms, frequency and severity of attacks and by education of the child, family and teacher and any other people involved in the child's life. A child should reach adulthood with good function, appropriate knowledge of asthma and good habits in the care of her/his asthma.

### Treatment

Non-drug treatment is just as important as drug treatment and is complementary to it. Asthma and its treatment are complex and appropriate management will only be achieved by continual and thorough education of the child, parents or guardians, family, teacher and other care-givers.

The triggers for asthma in the individual child must be sought, recognised and avoided or minimised where possible. Two which are amenable to virtually complete avoidance are animals and cigarette smoke. Exercise, while a common trigger, is very important for a child's development and should be encouraged. Appropriate measures should be taken to prevent exercise-induced asthma, to enable full participation in exercise (see below).

Chest physical therapy is useful in asthma although there have been few well-designed trials of its use. Postural drainage complemented by vibration, percussion, coughing, forced expiratory technique or wing flapping may clear secretions. Thoracic mobility exercises and postural correction exercises together with relaxation techniques aim to reduce inefficient breathing movements.[21] In children aged 6 to 14 years, in a single-blind controlled study, we have seen a trend to more rapid improvement and shortened hospital stay in children with acute severe asthma receiving chest physical therapy as well as standard drug therapy (Asher MI et al, unpublished observations)

Drugs are very important in the management of acute attacks in children, and for the prevention of asthma symptoms and attacks. Unfortunately drug therapy of asthma has become increasingly complex in the last decade, with a wide range of different drugs, inhaler devices and oral routes of delivery to choose from.

### Age of Child and Choice of Delivery System

The age and capabilities of the child will determine which of the many available drug delivery systems is suitable for an individual child; a summary of guidelines is presented in Table 17.1.

*Table 17.1* Guidelines for routes of delivery by age

| Age (yr) | Inhaler device | | | | Oral preparation | | |
|---|---|---|---|---|---|---|---|
| | MDI* | Inhaled powder | Spacer | Nebuliser | Tablet | Liquid | Sprinkle |
| 0-1 | No | No | No | Yes | No | Yes | Above 6 months |
| 1-2 | No | No | No | Yes | No | Yes | Yes |
| 2-3 | No | Maybe | Maybe | Yes | No | Yes | Yes |
| 3-4 | No | Yes | Yes | \| | Maybe | Yes | Yes |
| 4-5 | No | Yes | Yes | Use | Yes | \| | |
| 5-6 | No | Yes | Yes | only | Yes | Probably | |
| 6-7 | Maybe | Yes | Yes | if | Yes | change | |
| 7-8 | Yes | Yes | Yes | specific | Yes | to | |
| >8 | Yes | Probably change to MDI | | indication | Yes | tablet | |

*MDI = metered dose inhaler.

The metered dose inhaler (MDI) is the most compact and convenient inhaler device, but it is not suitable for young children, for whom alternative devices (inhaled powder, spacer or nebuliser) are available. Children under the age of three years usually cannot take a voluntary inspiration, and for them the nebuliser is the only effective inhaler device. Children three to seven years of age can inhale voluntarily, but usually cannot achieve synchronisation of hand movement with breath for MDI usage. Inhaled powder systems are most often used in this age-group, although spacer devices may be equally effective. Children over seven years of age can usually be taught to use an MDI, but if a child is managing well on an inhaled powder system at a younger age, there is no rush to change devices. However, an MDI is more convenient for use at school.

The MDI, spacer devices and inhaled powder systems, if used correctly, are equally suitable for maintenance therapy or for use during exacerbations of mild to moderate severity. However, when airway obstruction becomes severe, the child often cannot coordinate her/his breathing pattern with actuation of the device and therefore may not obtain relief. In this situation use of a nebuliser under medical supervision is appropriate treatment and allows delivery of a larger dose of medication.

In infants and toddlers oral treatment will be used for maintenance or acute therapy unless the asthma is particularly troublesome; in that case a nebuliser may be used. Children under the age of three years are unable to swallow tablets, and therefore liquids are the oral treatment of choice in this age-group. However, the recent introduction of theophylline in the sprinkle form has made this drug more useful for very young children. In older children who are able to swallow, tablets are the preferred oral therapy for simplicity.

### *Spacers*

A large spacer confers an advantage over the MDI in young children who have difficulty coordinating a slow voluntary inspiration with actuation of the inhaler.[22] A spacer made from a coffee cup may be a useful alternative for high-dose inhaled therapy in young children where the nebuliser is either not available or not tolerated.[23]

### *Inhaled Dry Powder Systems*

Clinical trials of inhaled powder systems compared with MDIs have shown them to have equal efficacy whether used for delivery of beta2-sympathomimetic drugs,[24,25] inhaled steroids[25] or sodium cromoglycate[26] except in exercise-induced asthma where the inhaled powder showed a slight advantage.[27] Because inhaled powder systems are breath-activated, instructions for the child are very simple. The dose given is more easily checked than doses from MDIs. Dry powder systems are more compact than most spacer devices and therefore very acceptable for regular use. The sodium cromoglycate Spinhaler whistle attachment will often entice many three-year-olds and even some two-year-olds to use it satisfactorily, and this is a good learning tool for other inhaled powder devices.

### *Nebulisers*

The indications for the use of nebulisers are: (i) the inability to deliver bronchodilators or sodium cromoglycate adequately by any other inhaler device or oral route in young children; (ii) the child who is subject to life-threatening attacks, provided the parent or guardian will take further action if the nebuliser drug is ineffective; and (iii) in chronic asthma where lung function tests have shown a signficantly better response to nebulised bronchodilator inhalation compared with other methods of delivery.

Drugs should be diluted with normal saline to make up the nebuliser volume, except the sodium cromoglycate ampoule. Hypotonic solutions of water may precipitate bronchospasm;[28] however, in the home boiled water may be the only affordable diluent. Sodium cromoglycate and salbutamol may be safely mixed in a nebuliser.[29] Nebulisers, however, pose several potential problems; they are more difficult to use, are not easily portable, and deliver a large dose of drug. Overestimation of the value of nebulised treatment may lead to delays in obtaining effective therapy when there is a poor response. It is essential that the care-giver be able to use the nebuliser correctly and responsibly to ensure safe usage.

## Oxygen

Almost all asthmatic children are hypoxic during acute attacks of asthma, mainly due to ventilation/perfusion mismatch.[30] Hypoxia will be manifest clinically by tachycardia and tachypnoea, and cyanosis will appear only when hypoxia is severe (oxygen saturation less than 75%, arterial $PO_2$ approximately 40mmHg (5.3kPa). Oxygen must be given for moderate or severe hypoxia and may be safely stopped when the child has shown a marked and sustained improvement. Theoretically inhaled beta2-synpathomimetics potentiate hypoxaemia by increasing physiological shunting, but studies in adult asthmatics show this to be a rare occurrence.[31] Nevertheless it is prudent to deliver high-dose inhaled beta2-sympathomimetics with oxygen in acute severe asthma.

*Indications*

Indications for the use of oxygen include: (i) acute hypoxia during an acute attack of asthma, and (ii) delivery of inhaled high-dose beta2-sympathomimetic drugs during an attack of acute severe asthma.

*Dosage*

The dose of oxygen is 30 to 40% of inspired gas for mild to moderate attacks, and 80 to 100% for respiratory failure with carbon dioxide retention.

*Delivery Systems*

The delivery system is a mask closely applied to the face, either dry at 8L/min (which gives 30 to 40%) or humidified (for example, a Fisher and Paykel humidifier with 15L/min oxygen (40%) or 30L/min (80%)) run in.

*Side Effects*

There are none in children if oxygen is used without artificial ventilation. There is no risk of carbon dioxide retention.

**Beta2-sympathomimetic Drugs**

Agonists of the beta2-sympathomimetic adrenergic receptors are the most useful drugs in the treatment of asthma, and are especially effective when given by the inhaled route. They have surpassed the less specific adrenergic drugs such as adrenaline, isoprenaline and rimiterol, having fewer side effects.[32] There is extensive literature comparing the relative efficacy of various beta2-sympathomimetic drugs. Small advantages and disadvantages have been shown in various studies, but overall there are no major clinically relevant differences between the more selective beta2-sympathomimetics: fenoterol, hexoprenaline, orciprenaline, salbutamol, and terbutaline.[33] The drug and delivery system chosen should be determined by patient preference regarding apparent or measured efficacy, availability of an effective delivery system, patient preference regarding taste and side effects, comparative costs, and age and capabilities of the child.

Despite studies showing little benefit from the use of inhaled salbutamol in chidlren under the age of 18 months,[34] most clinicians will give a trial of inhaled beta2-sympathomimetics in a wheezy infant (unless the diagnosis is clearly bronchiolitis) and follow up with anti-asthmatic therapy if the trial is effective.[35]

*Indications*

Indications for the use of these drugs include: treatment of acute attacks, prevention of symptoms of asthma, and prevention of exercise-induced asthma.

## *Dosage*

Dosage is shown in Table 17.2. Under supervision the frequency of dosing by inhaler devices may be increased considerably above that stated in the table for up to 30 minutes without fear of overdosage. But parents or guardians must be educated to recognise worsening asthma and to seek help urgently when relief from inhaled beta2-sympathomimetics is poor. Dosage by the intravenous route is recommended only in respiratory failure (see below).

*Table 17.2* Delivery systems and doses of some long-acting beta2-sympathomimetics

| Delivery system | Drug | Dosage | Frequency | Patient's age |
|---|---|---|---|---|
| **Inhaled** | | | | |
| MDI | Fenoterol | 200μg | q 4-8h | |
| | Orciprenaline | 750μg | q 4-8h | |
| | Salbutamol | 100μg | q 4-8h | |
| | Terbutaline | 250μg | q 4-8h | |
| Inhaled powder | Fenoterol Inhalet | 200μg | q 4-8h | |
| | Salbutamol Rotacap | 200μg | q 4-8h | |
| Nebuliser | Fenoterol (5mg/ml) | 0.25-0.5ml | q 4-8h | |
| | Salbutamol (5mg/ml) | 0.5ml | q 4-8h | <6 yr |
| | | 1.0ml | q 4-8h | >6 yr |
| | Terbutaline (10mg/ml) | 0.02ml/kg | q 4-8h | |
| **Oral** | | | | |
| Liquid | Fenoterol elixir (2.5mg/5ml) | 1-2.5ml | q 6-8h | <2 yr |
| | | 2.5ml | q 6-8h | 2-4 yr |
| | | 5ml | q 6-8h | >4 yr |
| | Orciprenaline syrup (10mg/5ml) | 2mg/kg/24 h | q 6-8h | |
| | Salbutamol elixir (2mg/5ml) | 1-2.5ml | q 6-8h | <3 yr |
| | | 2.5-5ml | q 6-8h | >3 yr |
| | Terbutaline elixir (1.5mg/5ml) | 1-2.5ml | q 6-8h | <3 yr |
| | | 2.5-5ml | q 6-8h | >3 yr |
| Tablet | Orciprenaline (20mg) | 2mg/kg/24 h | q 6-8h | |
| | Salbutamol (2mg) | 2mg | q 6-8h | <12 yr |
| | | 2-4mg | q 6-8h | >12 yr |
| | 8mg Spandet | One tablet | at night | >6 yr |
| | Terbutaline (2.5mg) | 2.5mg | q 6-8h | 7-15 yr |

MDI = metered dose inhaler. q = every.

## *Delivery Systems*

Delivery systems are shown in Table 17.2. The MDI is effective in older children, but the inhaled powder[24,36] and spacer[22] are at least as potent. The inhaled powder device must be used correctly, which means high inspiratory flow rates (at least 1L/s) for the salbutamol Rotahaler[37] and variable including low flow rates for the fenoterol Inhalator. One comparison of these two inhaled powders showed no differences in bronchodilator efficacy,[38] but further studies are required to determine whether differences in design features of the devices are of clinical importance. The nebuliser delivers a large dose which is more effective than an equal dose of oral medication and a lower dose of inhaled powder.[39] An alternative to a nebuliser is a large dose of the MDI preparation given into a spacer, and even a makeshift spacer can be effective.[23] The subcutaneous route is reserved for urgent therapy in children who are intolerant of nebulised beta2-sympathomimetics and in whom an intravenous line is not available.

### *Side Effects*

These drugs are remarkably free from side effects, especially when given by the inhaled route. Tremor, tachycardia, mild increase in blood pressure[32] and anxiety are uncommon side effects, and may be dealt with by a reduction in dosage or trial of another beta2-sympathomimetic drug. In adolescents there are occasional cases of abuse reported.[40]

## Sodium Cromoglycate

This mast cell stabiliser is a very useful and safe drug for the prophylaxis of asthma in children. It compares well with theophylline for the prevention of symptoms in children with chronic asthma.[41] Some children with chronic asthma who use inhaled steroids will derive additional benefit from sodium cromoglycate, which is not surprising since the two drugs work in different ways. Sodium cromoglycate is virtually free from side effects.

### *Indications*

Indications for its use are prevention of frequent or chronic symptoms, and prevention of exercise-induced asthma.

### *Dosage*

Sodium cromoglycate should usually be given four times a day. In some individuals, a three times a day regimen may be effective. Twice a day dosage may be effective in some children in a stable phase. Standard doses are: metered dose inhaler, two puffs (2mg); inhaled powder, one Spincap (20mg); nebuliser, one ampoule (20mg).

### *Delivery Systems*

Sodium cromoglycate was first marketed as an inhaled powder and there are now two inhaled powder devices to choose from. The Spinhaler works well only at high flow rates (at least 1L/s) and allows the use of the inspiratory whistle for teaching purposes. The Halermatic works well at low flow rates, but the whistle cannot be attached. The MDI has been introduced recently and is probably as effective as the inhaled powder,[26] but the compliance advantage of the MDI is of particular importance in the adolescent. The nebuliser is used for the delivery of sodium cromoglycate in children who are too young to use the inhaled powder correctly. It is effective in children over the age of 12 months[42] and even in some younger children.[43]

## Theophylline

This bronchodilator drug also has effects on the diaphragm, central nervous system and mucociliary clearance. Theophylline is useful preventive therapy in chronic asthma[44,45] and is as effective as sodium cromoglycate in controlling asthmatic symptoms in children of all ages.[41,46] Theophylline is sometimes associated with important side effects, but sustained-release theophylline has the advantage over sodium cromoglycate of twice-daily dosage.

### *Indications*

Indications are treatment of acute attacks, and prevention of frequent or chronic symptoms.

### *Dosage*

Treatment with theophylline is more complex than treatment with other asthma drugs. The clinician needs to decide on a suitable target serum concentration, then prescribe a loading dose and maintenance therapy.

The *target serum concentration* of theophylline is decided by the need for bronchodilator efficacy balanced against the possible side effects. Although there are few studies in children which give accurate information in this matter[47-49] the following are useful guidelines.

1. Stable asthma: target concentration 10mg/L.
2. Acute severe asthma: target concentration 15mg/L.
3. Very severe acute asthma: target concentration 20mg/L.

A loading dose is given to reach the target concentration and maintenance doses maintain the target concentration. A practical guide to theophylline doses based on scientific data available[48] is given in Table 17.3.

*Table 17.3* Guidelines for theophylline dosage (if no previous theophylline)

| | Theophylline | | | | | Aminophylline | |
|---|---|---|---|---|---|---|---|
| Age | Target concentration (mg/L) | Loading dose (mg/kg) | Maintenance dose (mg/kg/h) | Clearance (L/h/kg) | Half life (h) | Loading dose (mg/kg) | Maintenance dose (mg/kg/h) |
| 3-6mth | 10 | 5 | 0.5 | 0.05 | 7 | 6 | 0.6 |
| 6-12mth | 10 | 5 | 0.6 | 0.06 | 6 | 6 | 0.75 |
| 1-9yr | 10 | 5 | 0.8 | 0.08 | 4 | 6 | 1.0 |
| 9-12yr | 10 | 5 | 0.7 | 0.07 | 5 | 6 | 0.9 |
| 12-16yr | 10 | 5 | 0.5 | 0.05 | 7 | 6 | 0.6 |

Mth = months.

The loading dose is proportional to the volume of distribution of the drug, which is dependent on the weight of the child (0.5L/kg),[48] but not the age, and is calculated as follows:

$$\text{Loading dose theophylline (mg)} = \text{volume of distribution (L)} \times \text{target serum concentration (mg/L)}$$

For example, for a child of any age, if the target serum concentration is 10mg/L, then the loading dose = 0.5L/kg × 10mg/L = 5mg/kg theophylline = 6mg/kg aminophylline.

The maintenance dose depends on the clearance of the drug from the body, which is very age-dependent; it is not dependent at all on the volume of distribution, and there is no diurnal variation. Clearance is more rapid in children aged one to nine years than at any other age, and is known to be affected by the factors listed in Table 17.4 which have a multiplicative effect.[48-55] Obesity reduces clearance and therefore if the child is more than 30% of the expected weight-for-age, clearance should be calculated based on expected body weight.

The effect of antibiotics on clearance is important, since these are commonly used in the treatment of wheezy children[13] despite lack of evidence as to their efficacy. While amoxycillin and tetracycline appear to have no effect on theophylline clearance, erythromycin and troleandomycin do. A high serum erythromycin concentration and at least three days of co-therapy seem to be necessary before an effect is seen.[54] There are conflicting reports about influenza vaccination[56,57] and until more information is available serum theophylline monitoring is recommended for a period of 48 hours after vaccination. Certainly infection with influenza may result in serious toxicity if the dose is unmodified.[51] Recently the possibility of an interaction between oral terbutaline and theophylline has been raised.[58]

| | | |
|---|---|---|
| Maintenance dose = | clearance | × target serum |
| theophylline | theophylline | concentration |
| (mg/h/kg) | (L/h/kg) | (mg/L) |

For example, in a child of four years where the clearance is 0.08L/kg/h and the target concentration is 10mg/L, the maintenance dose = 0.08L/kg/h × 10mg/L = 0.8mg/h/kg theophylline.

If there has been *previous theophylline administration* in the last 24 hours, the loading dose (but not the maintenance dose) may need to be modified, depending upon the type and timing of previous theophylline. In acute severe asthma, if the clinical condition demands immediate treatment, then half the usual loading dose should be given; for example, aminophylline 3mg/kg. A serum theophylline level measured 30 minutes after the dose will guide further therapy.

*Table 17.4* Drugs affecting theophylline clearance

| Drug | Factor | Reference |
|---|---|---|
| **Increased Clearance** | | |
| Smoking (tobacco, marijuana) | 1.6 | 48 |
| Phenytoin | 1.7 | 48 |
| Phenobarbitone | 1.3 | 48 |
| Carbamazepine | 1.9 | 50 |
| **Decreased Clearance** | | |
| Acute viral infection | 0.5 | 51 |
| Acute pulmonary oedema | 0.5 | 48 |
| Liver disease | 0.4 | 48 |
| Cimetidine | 0.7 | 48, 52 |
| Erythromycin | 0.75 | 53, 54 |
| Troleandomycin | 0.5 | 55 |

A further loading dose would be calculated as follows.

Extra loading dose (mg/kg) = 0.5L/kg × ((target − actual) serum concentration).

It will not usually be necessary to recheck the level after this extra dose. If immediate treatment is not mandatory, obtain a serum theophylline level first and give a loading dose if needed.

*Serum theophylline level* measures only theophylline, not oxtryphylline etc. These levels may be analysed from venepuncture blood, but micro-methods are available and recommended for young children. To assess the adequacy of a loading dose, obtain a level 30 minutes after the loading dose has been given. To assess the adequacy of the maintenance dose, a level should be taken after at least four half-lives have passed, regardless of the dosing frequency and route of administration. The half-life of theophylline (Table 17.4) = 0.7 × volume of distribution/clearance. In practical terms, for children of all ages this will be approximately 24 hours. In children on oral preparations therapeutic monitoring should be done using samples taken immediately before a dose, because the absorption profile is so variable that four to six hour post-dose concentrations could well be peaks or troughs.[59] The clinician should be cautious in the interpretation of a single determination, if there are problems in management or suspected toxicity.

### *Delivery Systems*

Theophylline is available for oral and intravenous use, but not for inhalation. In oral form it comes in four formulations: liquid, sprinkle (sustained-release), short-acting tablet and sustained-release tablet. Theophylline liquids have a very unpleasant bitter taste, and like the short-acting tablet must be taken six-hourly to be effective; these preparations result in major problems with compliance of the child and the parent.

Sustained-release preparations have advantages over the short-acting ones; the serum theophylline concentration during the dosing interval is more stable and the twice-daily dosage assures better patient compliance. Although dosage with sustained-release theophylline is usually 12-hourly, some patients might be treated with unequally divided doses. In some young children dosing at eight-hourly intervals may be better.[60] Sprinkles may be administered by spoon in a small amount of apple sauce, icecream or yoghurt, or tipped into a glass of liquid. Capsules of sprinkles may be split by visual estimation, with the excess discarded. In asthmatic children there is considerable interindividual variation in the time of peak and trough concentrations,[61] and there may even be considerable intraindividual variations in some children, which are related to variations in absorption from sustained release formulations. There are some important differences between the sustained-release preparations.

*Nuelin-SR (Theolair SR, Nuelin Retard)* tablet release is pH-dependent,[62] which means that food influences bioavailability.[63] In a situation where relationship to food was not controlled, *Nuelin-SR250* had unacceptably low and variable bioavailability and very large differences between day and night trough serum concentrations.[59]

*Somophylline-CRT* is completely pH-independent[62] and bioavailable, the maximum concentration occurs at about five hours, and intraindividual variation is small. Food has no effect on the extent of absorption of *Somophylline-CRT,* although it delays the average time to peak serum concentration by 1.3 hours.[59]

*Theo-Dur (Theolin-Retard)* tablet release is pH-independent, the drug is completely bioavailable and the maximum concentration occurs about six to eight hours after intake of the tablet. However, different feeding regimens produce different absorption profiles and the peak level is lower with a dry than a wet meal.[64]

Recently, a once-a-day sustained-release theophylline *(Theo-24)* has been introduced. There are wide fluctuations in serum concentrations,[65] and there is already one report of toxicity with this drug due to food-induced dumping.[66] Major concerns about this therapy have been voiced,[67] and therefore *Theo-24* cannot yet be recommended in children because of the lack of evidence of its safety.

Intravenous (IV) theophylline is currently available only as aminophylline (80% theophylline). Compatibility of aminophylline with other IV drugs is summarised in Table 17.5. IV aminophylline should be given by continuous infusion using a pump as this will sustain steady serum theophylline levels. Theophylline does not adsorb on to plastics and so it can remain in the pump for some time. Since theophylline is nearly 100% absorbed from the gastrointestinal tract, a six-hourly IV regimen would confer no advantage over a six-hourly oral regimen, except if the child were vomiting. Oral theophylline may be started as soon as the IV infusion stops; no delay is required.

*Table 17.5* Compatability of intravenous drugs

| Drug | Incompatible | Incompatible after 4 hours | Compatible |
|---|---|---|---|
| Salbutamol | Aminophylline<br>Hydrocortisone<br>Sodium bicarbonate | | |
| Aminophylline | Salbutamol<br>Cephalothin | Hydrocortisone<br>Penicillins<br>Cephradine<br>Cephazolin | Sodium bicarbonate |

## *Side Effects*

These can be a major problem with this drug in some children. Side effects are rare with theophylline serum concentrations under 15mg/L and more frequent with concentrations greater than 20mg/L. Recognised symptoms are headache, nausea, vomiting and agitation; serious cardiovascular toxicity and convulsions may occur with very high serum concentrations.[48] A small proportion of children may show significant disturbance of behaviour evidenced by an increase in restless activity, excitability, impairment of concentration or insomnia. The possibility that theophylline may have long-term deleterious effects on learning and school performance has been raised,[68] and certainly merits further investigation. Any untoward effects on behaviour, the cardiovascular, gastrointestinal or central nervous systems are indications to reduce the dose or stop the drug, except where urgent bronchodilator action is required and not available by other means.

## Anticholinergic Drugs

The new bronchodilator, ipratropium bromide, has become available more recently, and although it is effective in some patients,[69] its role in the treatment of childhood asthma is still not clear. Studies have shown an additive effect with salbutamol.[70] In some infants ipratropium has been shown to have a bronchodilator effect,[71,43] although it has not gained much use in that age-group. There do not appear to be side effects of this drug in its inhaled form.[72]

### *Indications*

Ipratropium bromide is indicated in children with severe attacks where its addition to a high dose beta2-sympathomimetic has been shown to result in a greater functional improvement than the beta2-sympathomimetic alone; and in children who are intolerant of theophylline who have chronic asthma or frequent or severe attacks.

### *Dosage*

Ipratropium is available only by the inhaled route and should be given in six to eight hourly doses, by MDI 40μg,[73] or by nebuliser 250μg.[72]

## Steroids

Use of prolonged high-dose oral steroids gave these drugs a bad name in the treatment of childhood asthma. Fortunately, the need for this approach to management has passed completely with the advent of inhaled steroids, and regular oral steroid therapy is now seldom required in children with asthma.

### *Indications*

Steroids are indicated in the following situations.
1. Preventive treatment in children with chronic asthma in whom symptoms are not adequately controlled by the use of regular beta2-sympathomimetics, and sodium cromoglycate and/or theophylline; inhaled steroids should be used in these children. Only rarely, in children with severe chronic asthma, will regular oral steroids be needed as well.
2. Treatment of acute asthma where there has been a poor response to high doses of beta2-sympathomimetics and theophylline, or where there is respiratory failure, or where the child uses regular inhaled or oral steroids. Systemic steroids are used in this situation.

### *Inhaled Steroids*

There are two drugs in this form: beclomethasone dipropionate and budesonide, which appear equally effective.[74]

Both drugs are available as MDIs, and beclomethasone is also available as an inhaled powder. Inhaled steroids for use in a nebuliser may become available in the near future.

The usual dosage of beclomethasone is 400ug/day although larger or smaller doses may be required. Twice-a-day dosage is as effective as four times a day.[75]

*Side effects:* in doses under 800ug, there are no systemic side effects, but over this dose the likelihood of these increases with increasing dose. In daily doses over 1500ug adrenal suppression is likely. Patients on more than 1500ug per day may require systemic steroids during prolonged stress. Local side effects are rare. Long-term studies have shown no effect on the respiratory mucosa.[75] However, effects of long-term inhaled steroids used in infants and young children have not been studied. The first years of life are the period of most rapid lung growth, in particular growth in alveolar number.[76] It is important to establish that lung growth is not adversely affected by the use of inhaled steroids in young children. Until this is done inhaled steroids should be used only when absolutely necessary in this age group; maximal therapy with beta2-sympathomimetics, sodium cromoglycate, theophylline and ipratropium bromide should be used first.

### *Systemic Steroids*

Intravenous steroids have been recommended for treatment of acute severe asthma[77] although another study did not confirm any benefit in children.[78] In children under the age of 18 months one study has shown no benefit from oral prednisolone 2mg/kg/day,[79] whereas there is one report of possible benefit from intramuscular dexamethasone (in combination with salbutamol) in this age group.[80] Despite the lack of conclusive evidence of their efficacy, most clinicians give systemic steroids for acute asthma as indicated above.[75]

Dosage: in the acute attack either IV hydrocortisone 5mg/kg every four hours or oral prednisone 2 to 3mg/kg statim, followed by a reducing course over 5 or 10 days in doses once a day. The progress should be monitored by PEFR where possible to determine the appropriate duration of treatment. For regular oral therapy daily doses should be avoided if possible. Alternate-day therapy (a single oral dose on the morning of each alternate day) is usually effective and is free of any effect on growth.

## Antihistamines

The effectiveness of this group of drugs in the treatment of asthma is far from certain. The new drug in this category is ketotifen, which has shown some promise in the prevention of asthma.

### *Ketotifen*

This antihistamine has additional unique anaphylactic properties. Although there has been great interest in this new drug, its efficacy as a prophylactic drug in childhood asthma is yet to be firmly established.[81,82] Of the double-blind controlled studies there are those showing some positive effects in children,[83,84] although less than theophylline,[44] while no useful prophylaxis against bronchoconstriction has been documented by others.[85] It is not effective in exercise-induced asthma.[86]

Indications: to be considered as a prophylactic or preventive drug, if sodium cromoglycate, theophylline and inhaled steroids are unsuitable or ineffective, in older children with chronic asthma or frequent or severe attacks.

Dosage: a higher dose for body weight may be given in children than in adults according to pharmacokinetic studies,[87] and it appears that a dose of 1mg twice daily is suitable for all children over the age of three years. Below that age the dosage has not been adequately studied.

Sedation, exanthemata, intestinal troubles,[83] dry mouth, and thrombocytopenia[88] are the reported side effects.

## Other Drugs

Immunotherapy has been widely used in the treatment of childhood asthma but its efficacy has not been established. Prospective double-blind trials need to be done to evaluate this therapy properly.[89]

Antibiotics are not effective in the treatment of asthma in children,[90] despite their wide usage in children with recurrent wheeze.[13]

Since the discovery of the role of leukotrienes in the pathogenesis of asthma,[91] there has been great interest in chemicals which may modify this process, such as dihomogammalinoleic acid and eicosapentanoic acid. Their efficacy has yet to be established.

## Drug Treatment for Patterns of Asthma

A framework of practical guidelines for asthma drug therapy for the three main patterns of asthma is presented in Table 17.6.

*Table 17.6* Guidelines for drug therapy for patterns of asthma

| Pattern of asthma | Drug therapy |
|---|---|
| Mild infrequent asthma | Intermittent beta2-sympathomimetic ± intermittent theophylline |
| Frequent episodic asthma | Intermittent or regular beta2-sympathomimetic and prophylactic sodium cromoglycate or preventive regular theophylline |
| Chronic asthma | Regular beta2-sympathomimetic and inhaled steroids ± sodium cromoglycate and/or regular theophylline |

## Drug Treatment of Acute Asthma

### *Acute Attacks*

The dose of beta2-sympathomimetic should be increased immediately. Very high doses may be used for a short period of time providing the response to treatment is adequately monitored (Table 17.7). Any one of the following is suitable, depending on the therapy the child uses. The MDI may be increased to four puffs every 10 minutes up to a total of 12 puffs in 20 minutes. The inhaled powder may be increased to two capsules every 10

*Table 17.7* Example of a written crisis plan for acute asthma attacks

Judith Smith dob 13 Dec 1976 No. QED6666
45 Thomas Rd, Devonport, Auckland
Doctor: John Stevens phone 666777
phone 999888 (after hours)

Fortunately asthma attacks usually respond very well to treatment.
Follow these instructions **exactly** if there is an asthma attack, or if the peak flow falls below 180 litres per minute.

1. Give *Ventolin rotacaps:* 2 every 10 minutes until Judith is improving and the peak flow is more than 180 litres per minute.
2. Then given *Ventolin rotacaps:* 2 every 2 hours until Judith is completely better. Continue regular treatment.

**If the above does not result in obvious improvement in 30 minutes**

3. Give 2 more *Ventolin rotacaps.*
4. Contact your doctor straight away for advice.

**If you cannot find your doctor within minutes**

5. Travel straight away to the nearest hospital.

**Emergencies**
If at any time Judith is so breathless she cannot speak,
or there is any **blueness,**
Dial 111 for an ambulance.
Judith should be transported with oxygen to the nearest hospital.

minutes, up to a total of four capsules in 20 minutes; or one dose may be given by nebuliser. If there has not been sufficient improvement in 30 minutes, then medical help should be sought urgently and extra therapy promptly given under medical supervision. Usually theophylline will be added (or continued if the child already takes this) and consideration should be given to starting systemic steroids.

## *Acute Severe Asthma*

This may be defined as an acute asthma attack which is poorly responsive to inhaled beta2-sympathomimetics. Therapy will need to be comprehensive and progress of the patient needs to be continually reassessed. Oxygen should be given in a concentration of 30 to 40%. A beta2-sympathomimetic should be given by nebuliser in one dose every one to four hours depending on the child's progress, although doses of 0.15mg/kg every 20 minutes may be more effective.[93] Theophylline should be given to achieve a serum concentration of 15 to 20mg/L, provided this is tolerated without serious side effects. If the patient does not rapidly improve with this approach then systemic steroids should be added. In patients who are intolerant of theophylline, or in whom an added advantage of ipratropium bromide has been shown, this drug may be added by nebuliser. Intravenous fluids need to be given to rehydrate and maintain hydration, and a deficit volume of 2.5% can be assumed on admission to hospital.

*Respiratory Failure*

Intensive emergency treatment is required. High-dose oxygen must be given. In addition to inhaled beta2-sympathomimetic, intravenous beta2-sympathomimetics may be added. Although lower doses have been recommended,[93] doses of IV salbutamol as high as 10ug/kg as a loading dose (over 15 minutes) followed by a continuous infusion of 10 to 20ug/kg/min are usually free from troublesome side effects. Aminophylline should be given intravenously to a target theophylline serum concentration of 20mg/L. Hydrocortisone should be given in a dose initially of 5mg/kg every two hours. If there is severe acidosis (pH below 7.1), then intravenous sodium bicarbonate should be added in a dose of 1mmol/kg. Patients must be under intensive observation and cardiovascular or ventilatory support may be necessary.

## Drug Treatment of Exercise-induced Asthma

Selective beta2-sympathomimetics such as fenoterol and salbutamol by inhalation are the most potent means of preventing exercise-induced asthma;[94] beta2-sympathomimetics by the oral route do not appear to be as effective.[95] For reasons that are not understood there may be no relationship between the efficacy of a drug in exercise-induced asthma and its efficacy in clinical asthma. Sodium cromoglycate protects against exercise-induced asthma,[94] although not to the same magnitude as the beta2-sympathomimetics. Theophylline inhibits exercise-induced asthma in a graded manner dependent on the serum theophylline level at the time of the exercise.[96] A direct comparison between sodium cromoglycate and theophylline suggested that greater improvement is seen in some children with theophylline.[96] The anticholinergic drugs probably have some effect on exercise-induced asthma although the extent of this is uncertain.[94,97] Corticosteroids by any route of administration have little or no effect on exercise-induced asthma, although there is one study showing diminution of exercise-induced asthma after inhalation of the newer inhaled steroid budesonide.[98] In children with chronic asthma in whom inhaled steroids are useful to control their general condition, additional medication will be necessary especially to prevent the problem of exercise-induced asthma. Ketotifen has no inhibitory effect on exercise-induced asthma.[86] A calcium blocking agent, nifedipine, has been shown in one study in adults to modify exercise-induced asthma,[99] but further studies are required to establish any usefulness of this drug.

For older children who are active, exercise-induced asthma can be a major problem and effective preventive drug therapy will be essential, although this is frequently underused.[100] Exercise-induced asthma may be lessened by physical training using inhaled beta2-sympathomimetic preventively,[101] and this is to be recommended. For most children exercise-induced asthma is prevented by the inhalation of two puffs of a beta2-sympathomimetic MDI five minutes before exercise, although one inhaled powder capsule will do equally well.

## Drug Treatment of Nocturnal Asthma

Deterioration of lung function during the night is a common problem in asthmatic children, particularly if the asthma is poorly controlled. The reduced PEFR may be associated with symptoms which usually wake the child and family (because cough is noisy) and can lead to important loss of sleep for all involved. Treatment should aim at improving the overall control of the asthma and with this will follow improved nocturnal lung function. Identification and avoidance of specific nocturnal triggers is important. The role of gastro-oesophageal reflux in the potentiation of nocturnal asthma is debated,[102] but if it is a probable contributor to an individual's problems then treatment with elevation of the head of the bed, antacids and only modest theophylline doses is recommended.

## Patient Education

Education of the child and parent is a major part of the management of asthma. The multiplicity of drugs and devices easily causes confusion among patients (and doctors!) and prescription of drugs is useless, if not dangerous, without education of all involved. Deaths from asthma, while rare in children, are contributed to by inadequate long-term care, underassessment of severity by the family doctor, failure of the family to call for help when required, and inadequate responses of medical services. Most childhood deaths should be prevented by increased family awareness, better assessment of severity, improved long-term treatment and rapid access to emergency medical care.[15]

From the time the diagnosis is made the child and parent need to learn and continue to learn about asthma. The method and extent of education of the child depend on her/his capabilities and cultural background and must be continually reviewed. Even toddlers using asthma therapy need to have some understanding about it. By the age of about ten years most children should be able to take responsibility for their own treatment although with supervision.

Knowledge about asthma in young adults is poor,[19] and might be rectified by better education of the adolescent. Adolescents need a completely different approach from the younger child, and as they become independent from their parents the education process needs to start afresh. Adolescents are subject to strong peer group pressure to start smoking, to hand around their inhaler, or to avoid usage of drugs. Adolescents in particular may suppress signs of asthma or delay seeking help.

Education of the child cannot be done in isolation, but must involve the whole family and any other care-givers. Educational tools which may be helpful are pamphlets, videos, and group sessions. Although these educational tools have not been extensively studied, teaching of self-management skills to asthmatic children and their parents in an ambulatory setting has been effective.[103] The child must understand the basic mechanisms of the disease and know her/his own trigger factors and how to avoid or minimise them. The child must know how to use the drugs and their delivery systems and any side effects to watch for. The child and care-giver must know how to monitor her/his disease by use of a peak flow meter and a written crisis plan (an example of this is given in Table 17.7). If asthma is poorly controlled, then a reassessment of the child's and family's knowledge and compliance with therapy is essential. Improvement in asthma control often results from attention to this area alone.

## References

1. Williams H, McNicol KN. Prevalence, natural history, and relationship of wheezy bronchitis and asthma in children. An epidemiological study. *Br Med J* 1969; 4: 321-325.
2. Anderson SD, Silverman M, Konig P, Godfrey S. Exercise-induced asthma. *Br J Dis Chest* 1975; 69: 1-31.
3. Balfour-Lynn L, Tooley M, Godfrey S. Relationship of exercise induced asthma to clinical asthma in childhood. *Arch Dis Child* 1981; 56: 450-454.
4. Matsuba K, Thurlbeck WM. A morphometric study of bronchial and bronchiolar walls in children. *Am Rev Respir Dis* 1972; 105: 908-913.
5. Pullan CR, Hey EN. Wheezing, asthma, and pulmonary dysfunction 10 years after infection with respiratory syncytial virus in infancy. *Br Med J* 1982; 284: 1665-1669.
6. Bleeker ER. Airways reactivity and asthma: significance and treatment. *J Allergy Clin Immunol* 1985; 75: 21-24.
7. Lee DA, Winslow NR, Speight ANP, Hey EN. Prevalence and spectrum of asthma in childhood. *Br Med J* 1983; 286: 1256-1258.
8. Dodge RR, Burrows B. The prevalence and incidence of asthma and asthma-like symptoms in a general population sample. *Am Rev Respir Dis* 1980; 122: 567-575.
9. McNicol KN, Williams HE, Gillam GL. Chest deformity, residual airways obstruction and hyperinflation, and growth in children with asthma. I: Prevalence findings from an epidemiological study. *Arch Dis Child* 1970; 45: 783-788.
10. Sears MR, Jones DT, Silva PA, Simpson A, Williams S. Asthma in seven year old children: a report from the Dunedin Multidisciplinary Child Development Study. *NZ Med J* 1982; 95: 533-536.
11. Waite DA, Eyles EF, Tonkin SL, O'Donnell TV. Asthma prevalence in Tokelauan children in two environments. *Clin Allergy* 1980; 10: 71-75.
12. Anderson HR, Bailey PA, Cooper JS, Palmer JC. Influence of morbidity, illness label, and social, family, and health service factors on drug treatment of childhood asthma. *Lancet* 1981; 1: 1030-1032.
13. Speight ANP, Lee DA, Hey EN. Underdiagnosis and undertreatment of asthma in childhood. *Br Med J* 1983; 286: 1253-1256.
14. Sears MR, Rea HH, Beaglehole R, et al. Asthma mortality in New Zealand: a two year national study. *NZ Med J* 1985; 98: 271-275.
15. Sears MR, Rea HH, Fenwick J, et al. Deaths from asthma in New Zealand. *Arch Dis Child* 1986; 61: 6-10.
16. Edmunds AT, Godfrey S. Cardiovascular response during acute severe asthma and its treatment in children. *Thorax* 1981; 36: 534-540.
17. Eisen NM, Kerrebijn KF, Quanjer PH. Guidelines for standardization of bronchial challenges with (nonspecific) bronchoconstricting agents. *Bull Europ Physiopath Respir* 1983; 19: 495-514.
18. Yan K, Salome C, Woolcock AJ. Rapid method for measurement of bronchial responsiveness. *Thorax* 1983; 38: 760-765.
19. Martin AJ, Landau LI, Phelan PD. Asthma from childhood at age 21: the patient and his disease. *Br Med J* 1982; 284: 380-382.
20. Kraemer R, Meister B, Schaad UB, Rossi E. Reversibility of lung function abnormalities in children with perennial asthma. *J Pediatr* 1983; 102: 347-350.
21. Bolton JH, Gandevia B, Ross M. The rationale and results of breathing exercises in asthma. *Med J Aust* 1956; 2: 675-679.
22. Levison H, Reilly PA, Worsley GH. Spacing devices and metered-dose inhalers in childhood asthma. *J Pediatr* 1985; 107: 662-668.
23. Henry RL, Milner AD, Davies JG. Simple drug delivery system for use by young asthmatics. *Br Med J* 1983; 286: 2021.
24. Lenney W, Milner AD, Hiller EJ. Use of salbutamol powder in childhood asthma. *Arch Dis Child* 1978; 53: 958-961.
25. Svedmyr N, Löfdahl CG, Svedmyr K. The effect of powder aerosol compared to pressurized aerosol. *Eur J Respir Dis* 1982; 63 (suppl 119): 81-88.

26. Paija O, Kreus K-E. Clinical trial of sodium cromoglycate pressurised aerosol in the treatment of asthma. *Eur J Respir Dis* 1981; 62 (suppl): 168-169.
27. Bar-Yishay E, Gur I, Levy M, Volozni D, Godfrey S., Duration of action of sodium cromoglycate on exercise-induced asthma: comparison of 2 formulations. *Arch Dis Child* 1983; 58: 624-627.
28. Allegra L, Bianco S. Non-specific broncho-reactivity obtained with an ultrasonic aerosol of distilled water. *Eur J Respir Dis* 1980; 61 (suppl): 41-49.
29. Lenney W. Nebulised salbutamol in treatment of acute asthma in children. *Lancet* 1978; 1: 440-441.
30. McFadden ER, Lyons HA. Arterial-blood gas tensions in asthma. *N Engl J Med* 1968; 278: 1027-1032.
31. Douglas JG, Rafferty P, Fergusson RJ, Prescott RJ, Crompton GK, Grant IWB. Nebulised salbutamol without oxygen in severe acute asthma: how effective and how safe? *Thorax* 1985; 40: 180-183.
32. Milner AD, Ingram D. Bronchodilator and cardiac effects of isoprenaline, orciprenaline, and salbutamol aerosols in asthma. *Arch Dis Child* 1971; 46: 502-507.
33. Paterson JW, Woolcock AJ, Shenfield GM. Bronchodilator drugs. *Am Rev Respir Dis* 1979; 120: 1149-1179.
34. Lenney W, Milner AD. At what age do bronchodilator drugs work? *Arch Dis Child* 1978; 53: 532-535.
35. Silverman M. Bronchodilators for wheezy infants? *Arch Dis Child* 1984; 59: 84-87.
36. Chambers S, Dunbar J, Taylor B. Inhaled powder compared with aerosol administration of fenoterol in asthmatic children. *Arch Dis Child* 1980; 55: 73-74.
37. Pedersen S. How to use a rotahaler. *Arch Dis Child* 1986; 61: 11-14.
38. Asher MI, Dunn C. A comparison of inhaled powders of fenoterol and salbutamol in asthma. *Aust Paed J* 1985; 21: 119-121.
39. Grimwood K, Johnson-Barrett JJ, Taylor B. Salbutamol: tablets, inhalational powder, or nebuliser? *Br Med J* 1981; 282: 105-106.
40. Brennan PO. Addiction to aerosol treatment. *Br Med J* 1983; 287: 1877.
41. Hambleton G, Weinberger M, Taylor J, et al. Comparison of cromoglycate (cromolyn) and theophylline in controlling symptoms of chronic asthma. A collaborative study. *Lancet* 1977; 1: 381-385.
42. Geller-Bernstein C, Levin S. Nebulised sodium cromoglycate in the treatment of wheezy bronchitis in infants and young children. *Respiration* 1982; 43: 294-298.
43. Henry RL, Hiller EJ, Milner AD, Hodges IGC, Stokes GM. Nebulised ipratropium bromide and sodium cromoglycate in the first two years of life. *Arch Dis Child* 1984; 59: 54-57.
44. Stratton D, Carswell F, Hughes AO, Fysh WJ, Robinson P. Double-blind comparisons of slow-release theophylline, ketotifen and placebo for prophylaxis of asthma in young children. *Br J Dis Chest* 1984; 78: 163-167.
45. Pedersen S, Nathan E. Long-term treatment of children with sustained-release theophylline. *Eur J Resp Dis* 1983; 64: 564-570.
46. Newth CJL, Newth CV, Turner JAP. Comparison of nebulized sodium cromoglycate and oral theophylline in controlling symptoms of chronic asthma in pre-school children: a double blind study. *Aust NZ J Med* 1982; 12: 232-238.
47. Levy G, Koysooko R. Pharmacokinetic analysis of the effect of theophylline on pulmonary function in asthmatic children. *J Pediatr* 1975; 86: 789-793.
48. Hendeles L, Weinberger M. Theophylline. A 'state of the art' review. *Pharmacother* 1983; 3: 2-44.
49. Simons FER, Simons KJ, Biggs CJ. Therapeutic range of serum theophylline concentrations in adolescents with asthma. *J Allergy Clin Immunol* 1979; 63: 157.
50. Rosenberry KR, Defusco CJ, Mansmann HC, McGeady SJ. Reduced theophylline half-life induced by carbamazepine therapy. *J Pediatr* 1983; 102: 472-474.
51. Kraemer MJ, Furukawa CT, Koup JR, Shapiro GG, Pierson WE, Bierman CW. Altered theophylline clearance during an influenza B outbreak. *Pediatrics* 1982; 69: 476-480.
52. Fenje PC, Isles AF, Baltodano A, MacLeod SM, Soldin S. Interaction of cimetidine and theophylline in two infants. *Can Med Ass J* 1982; 126: 1178.
53. Cummins LH, Kozak PP, Gillman SA. Erythromycin's effect on theophylline blood level. *Pediatrics* 1977; 59: 144-145.

54. Jonkman JHG, Hendeles L. The theophylline-erythromycin interaction. *Chest* 1983; 84: 309-310.
55. Weinberger M, Hudgel D, Spector S, Chidsey C. Inhibition of theophylline clearance by troleandomycin. *J Allergy Clin Immunol* 1977; 59: 228-231.
56. Renton KW, Gray JD, Hall RI. Decreased elimination of theophylline after influenza vaccination. *Can Med Ass J* 1980; 123: 288-290.
57. San Joaquin VH, Reyes S, Marks MI. Influenza vaccination in asthmatic children on maintenance theophylline therapy. *Clin Pediatr* 1982; 21: 724-726.
58. Danzinger Y, Garty M, Volwitz B, Ilfeld D, Varsano I, Rosenfeld JB. Reduction of serum theophylline levels by terbutaline in children with asthma. *Clin Pharmacol Ther* 1985; 37: 469-471.
59. Birkett DJ, Coulthard KP, Lines D, Grgurinovich N. Circadian variation in the absorption of three sustained release theophylline products in asthmatic children and the effect of food on absorption of Somophylline-CRT. *Br J Clin Pract* 1984; 38 (suppl): 17-23.
60. Newth CJL, Isles AF. Use of sustained release Somophylline-12 capsules in young asthmatic children. *Br J Clin Pract* 1984; 38 (suppl): 64-67.
61. Kelly HW, Murphy S. Serum theophylline levels in asthmatic children receiving sustained-release theophylline tablets. *Am J Hosp Pharm* 1979; 36: 1698-1701.
62. Jonkman JHG. In vitro modelling and relation to in vivo absorption. *Br J Clin Pract* 1984; 38 (suppl): 5-9.
63. Pedersen S, Moeller-Petersen J. Influence of food on the absorption rate and bioavailability of a sustained release theophylline preparation. *Allergy* 1982; 37: 531-534.
64. Pedersen S. Food and fasting intake of sustained release theophylline preparations. *Br J Clin Pract* 1984; 38 (suppl): 37-39.
65. Nerminathan V, McKenzie SA. Once a day theophylline; serum concentrations. *Arch Dis Child* 1984; 59: 762-765.
66. Hendeles L, Wubbena P, Weinberger M. Food-induced dose dumping of once-a-day theophylline. *Lancet* 1984; 2: 1471.
67. Weinberger MM. Theophylline QID, TID, BID and now QD? A report on 24-hour dosing with slow-release theophylline formulations with emphasis on analyses of data used to obtain Food and Drug Administration approval for Theo-24. *Pharmacother* 1984; 4: 181-198.
68. Furukawa CT, Shapiro GG, DuHamel T, Weimer L, Pierson WE, Beirman CW. Learning and behaviour problems associated with theophylline therapy. *Lancet* 1984; 1: 621.
69. Groggins RC, Milner AD, Stokes GM. Bronchodilator effects of clemastine, ipratropium bromide, and salbutamol in preschool children with asthma. *Arch Dis Child* 1981; 56: 342-344.
70. Beck R, Robertson C, Galdes-Sebalt M, Levison H. Combined salbutamol and ipratropium bromide by inhalation in the treatment of acute severe asthma. *J Pediatr* 1985; 107: 605-608.
71. Hodges IGC, Groggins RC, Milner AD, Stokes GM. Bronchodilator effect of inhaled ipratropium bromide in wheezy toddlers. *Arch Dis Child* 1981; 56: 729-732.
72. Davis A, Vickerson F, Worsley G, Mindorff C, Kazim F, Levison H. Determination of dose-response relationship for nebulized ipratropium bromide in asthmatic children. *J Pediatr* 1984; 105: 1002-1005.
73. Mann NP, Hiller EJ. Ipratropium bromide in children with asthma. *Thorax* 1982; 37: 72-74.
74. Field HV, Jenkinson PMA, Frame MH, Warner JO. Asthma treatment with a new corticosteroid aerosol, budesonide, administered twice daily by spacer inhaler. *Arch Dis Child* 1982; 57: 864-866.
75. Clark TJH. *Steroids in asthma. A reappraisal in the light of inhalation therapy.* Auckland: ADIS Press, 1983.
76. Thurlbeck WM. Postnatal human lung growth. *Thorax* 1982; 37: 564-571.
77. Pierson WE, Bierman CW, Kelley VC. A double-blind trial of corticosteroid therapy in status asthmaticus. *Pediatrics* 1974; 54: 282-288.
78. Kattan M, Gurwitz D, Levison H. Corticosteroids in status asthmaticus. *J Pediatr* 1980; 96: 596-599.
79. Webb MSC, Henry RL, Milner AD. Oral corticosteroids for wheezing attacks under 18 months. *Arch Dis Child* 1986; 61: 15-19.
80. Tal A, Bavilski C, Yohai D., Bearman JE, Gorodischer R, Moses SW. Dexamethasone and salbutamol in the treatment of acute wheezing in infants. *Pediatrics* 1983; 71: 13-18.

81. MacDonald GF. An overview of ketotifen. *Chest* 1982; 82 (suppl): 30-32.
82. Sutherland DC, Ketotifen. Still some unanswered questions. *New Ethicals* 1985; 22: 13-14.
83. Spicak V. The prophylactic treatment of bronchial asthma in children with ketotifen: a double blind comparison with placebo. *J Int Med Res* 1983; 11: 173-178.
84. Simons FER, Luciuk, Becker AB, Gillespie CA. Ketotifen: a new drug for prophylaxis of asthma in children. *Ann Allergy* 1982; 48: 145-150.
85. Groggins RC, Hiller EJ, Milner AD, Stokes GM. Ketotifen in the prophylaxis of childhood asthma. *Arch Dis Child* 1981; 56: 304-305.
86. Kennedy JD, Hasham F, Clay MJD, Jones RS. Comparison of actions of disodium cromoglycate and ketotifen on exercise-induced bronchoconstriction in childhood asthma. *Br Med J* 1980; 281: 1458.
87. Kennedy GR. Metabolism and pharmacokinetics of ketotifen in children. *Res Clin Forums* 1982; 4: 17-20.
88. Leupold VW, Generlich H, Kloditz E, et al. Erfahrungen mit Ketotifen beim kindlichen Asthma bronchiale. *Dtsch Gesundh-Wes* 1984; 39: 430-434.
89. Lichtenstein LM, Valentine MD, Norman PS. A reevaluation of immunotherapy for asthma. *Am Rev Respir Dis* 1984; 129: 657-659.
90. Shapiro GG, Eggleston PA, Pierson WE, Ray CG, Bierman CW. Double-blind study of the effectiveness of a broad spectrum antibiotic in status asthmaticus. *Pediatrics* 1974; 53: 867-872.
91. Weissmann G. The eicosanoids of asthma. *N Engl J Med* 1983; 308: 454-455.
92. Robertson CF, Smith F, Beck R, Levison H., Response to frequent low doses of nebulized salbutamol in acute asthma. *J Pediatr* 1985; 106: 672-674.
93. Bohn D, Kalloghlian A, Jenkins J, Edmonds J, Barker G. Intravenous salbutamol in the treatment of status asthmaticus in children. *Crit Care Med* 1984; 12: 892-896.
94. Godfrey S, Konig P. Suppression of exercise-induced asthma by salbutamol, theophylline, atropine, cromolyn, and placebo in a group of asthmatic children. *Pediatrics* 1975; 56 (suppl): 930-934.
95. Anderson SD, Searle JP, Rozea P, Bandler L, Theobald G, Lindsay DA. Inhaled and oral salbutamol in exercise-induced asthma. *Am Rev Respir Dis* 1976; 114: 493-500.
96. Pollock J, Kiechel F, Cooper D, Weinberger M. Relationship of serum theophylline concentration to inhibition of exercise-induced bronchospasm and comparison with cromolyn. *Pediatrics* 1977; 60: 840-844.
97. Borut TC, Tashkin DP, Fischer TJ, et al. Comparison of aerosolized atropine sulphate and SCH 1000 on exercise-induced bronchospasm in children. *J Allergy Clin Immunol* 1977; 60: 127-133.
98. Henricksen JM. Effect of inhalation of corticosteroids on exercise induced asthma: randomised double blind crossover study of budesonide in asthmatic children. *Br Med J* 1985; 291: 248-249.
99. Barnes PJ, Wilson NM, Brown MJ. A calcium antagonist, nifedipine, modifies exercise-induced asthma. *Thorax* 1981; 36: 726-730.
100. Crawford MKC, Asher MI. Exercise-induced asthma in children. *NZ Fam Physician* 1985; 12: 54-56.
101. Svenonius E, Kautto R, Arborelius M. Improvement after training of children with exercise-induced asthma. *Acta Pediatr Scand* 1983; 72: 23-30.
102. MacFarlane P, Miller V, Couriel J. Gastro-oesophageal reflux and childhood asthma: the acid test. *Thorax* 1986; 41: 160.
103. Fireman P, Friday GA, Gira C, Vierthaler WA, Michaels L. Teaching self-management skills to asthmatic children and their parents in an ambulatory care setting. *Pediatrics* 1981; 68: 341-347.

# Chapter 18

# Non-infective Parenchymal Diseases of the Lung

*Bruce Davidson*

Under the rubric of non-infective parenchymal diseases of the lung are at least 140 different entities. Aetiological agents have been described with certainty in perhaps one-third (primarily the inhalational pneumoconioses and hypersensitivity pneumonitides) and pathogenic mechanisms in a far smaller number. While the splitting of these syndromes is likely to be important in eventually discerning their causes, some degree of lumping is necessary for their practical discussion.

A host of non-infective disorders diffusely affecting the lungs in both confluent and patchy radiological and anatomical patterns has been termed the interstitial lung diseases. Although that label will be used for some of the conditions described in this chapter, it is a misnomer because nearly all of these conditions show airspace as well as interstitial involvement when examined histopathologically, and inflammatory cell traffic in the alveoli invariably involves the pulmonary interstices in diffuse processes. Some of these diseases appear localised to the respiratory tract, while others are multisystemic with prominent pulmonary manifestations. An exhaustive listing of therapeutic options for each of the disorders is beyond the scope of this chapter; instead, the major diseases listed in Table 18.1 and their therapies will be discussed. Sarcoidosis will be separately considered in Chapter 19, and drug-induced pneumonitis in Chapter 20.

## General Diagnostic Features

### History and Physical Examination

Interstitial lung disease is usually an indolent disorder, although patients may present with acute complaints precipitated by decompensation due to a new superimposed condition (infection, cardiac failure, pulmonary embolism) which either temporarily obscures the underlying disease or reveals its presence. Characteristic symptoms include cough (often non-productive), progressive dyspnoea on exertion, and chest pain not clearly characteristic of angina pectoris. The patient may attribute these to a respiratory infection that never fully cleared despite multiple courses of antibiotic therapy, or to progressive effects of cigarettes, if a smoker. Physical examination may reveal tachycardia, tachypnoea, 'dry' crackles (especially in the bases), a loud pulmonary component of the second heart sound, and clubbing of the fingers and toes. If the disease is advanced, cyanosis and stigmata of right ventricular failure may be apparent. Any or all of these signs may be absent.

*Table 18.1* Major non-infective parenchymal lung diseases

| |
|---|
| Sarcoidosis* |
| Idiopathic pulmonary fibrosis (cryptogenic fibrosing alveolitis) |
| Vasculitis and granulomatosis |
| Wegener's granulomatosis |
| Lymphomatoid granulomatosis |
| Benign lymphocytic angiitis and granulomatosis |
| Churg-Strauss syndrome (allergic granulomatosis and angiitis) |
| Polyarteritis nodosa (periarteritis nodosa) |
| Eosinophilic pneumonias |
| Simple (reactive) pulmonary eosinophilia (Loeffler's syndrome) |
| Tropical pulmonary eosinophilia |
| Chronic eosinophilic pneumonia |
| Pulmonary histiocytosis X (eosinophilic granuloma of the lung) |
| Hypersensitivity pneumonitis (extrinsic allergic alveolitis) |
| Inhalation of toxic gases |
| Pulmonary haemorrhage syndromes |
| Goodpasture's syndrome (pulmonary haemorrhage and nephritis with anti-glomerular basement membrane (anti-GBM) antibodies) |
| Pulmonary haemorrhage and nephritis without anti-GBM antibodies |
| Idiopathic pulmonary haemosiderosis |
| Pulmonary haemorrhage secondary to vasculitis or connective tissue disease |
| Drug-induced pneumonitis† |
| Pulmonary manifestations of connective tissue diseases |
| Systemic lupus erythematosus |
| Progressive systemic sclerosis (scleroderma) |
| Rheumatoid arthritis |
| Mixed connective tissue disease |
| Polymyositis and dermatomyositis |
| Lymphangiomyomatosis (lymphangioleiomyomatosis) |

*Discussed in Chapter 19.
†Discussed in Chapter 20.
Vasculitis, granulomatosis and pulmonary histiocytosis X will not be discussed in this chapter.

The importance of careful elicitation of the history in the patient with interstitial lung disease cannot be overemphasised. Most of the truly idiopathic disorders have guarded prognoses and vigorous diagnostic and therapeutic intervention are warranted and undertaken. On the other hand, patients with nearly identical clinical presentations with regard to physical examination, radiological and laboratory evaluation can be distinguished only by history-taking that reveals seemingly innocuous medication (such as a thiazide diuretic), occupational (organic dust), or other personal exposure (haispray aerosol). The alert physician can sometimes facilitate disease resolution in these patients simply by advising avoidance of the noxious agent, saving the morbidity of prolonged and aggressive work-up and therapy.

## Radiological Studies

While the plain chest radiograph may be normal in the presence of significant interstitial lung disease,[1] not uncommonly it is the primary clue to the presence of disease. Usually the pleura and heart are uninvolved, although radiographic densities due to fibrosis or inflammation may partially obscure the cardiac borders. Infiltrates are usually bilateral although they may be more prominent on one side, and may be upper or lower, central or peripheral in location. Densities are usually reticular, nodular, or a combination of both, and occasionally confluent. When cystic airspaces 5 to 10mm in diameter are apparent and are surrounded by thick walls, this is called 'honeycombing'. A diagnosis of fibrosis based on the radiograph should be made with caution, since inflammation and oedema may show an identical picture that disappears, unlike our current views of the permanence of lung collagen scar. Different interstitial lung diseases sometimes show characteristic radiological patterns, assisting in diagnosis.[2]

Computed tomography (CT) of the thorax may provide useful information regarding three-dimensional location of diseased parts of the lungs, and is most helpful when thin sections of 1 to 2mm are obtained. This thin-section CT allows more precise visualisation of lung architecture in diffuse non-airspace processes than conventional 10mm sections, which result in more superimposition of densities at different anatomical levels. Even so, such scans apparently cannot reliably distinguish fibrosis from interstitial or alveolar pneumonitis.[3] Consequently unless the plain chest radiograph is normal, or better definition, extent, or localisation of a density seen on the plain chest radiograph is required, routine CT scanning of the thorax does not appear warranted currently for diagnosis or management of interstitial lung diseases.

### Expectorated Sputum

In non-infective pulmonary parenchymal disease, examination of expectorated sputum is usually of no diagnostic benefit, except in rare circumstances (such as the profusion of haemosiderin-laden macrophages in Goodpasture's syndrome or idiopathic pulmonary haemosiderosis). However, since patients with interstitial lung disease are at risk of pulmonary infection, and since diffuse lung infection with certain organisms (*Pneumocystis carinii*, cytomegalovirus, *Mycobacterium tuberculosis*) may present a radiographic picture indistinguishable from non-infective disease, sputum culture and smears, stained for a variety of different organisms, may be of use in early diagnosis and subsequent management. In addition, pulmonary fibrosis may be associated with late development of lung adenocarcinoma, the latter sometimes detectable by cytological examination of sputum.

### Physiological Testing

Physiological testing in the pulmonary function laboratory usually reveals reduced lung volumes and diffusing capacity, often with normal or supranormal expiratory airflow, characteristic of restrictive lung disease. A prominent exception is pulmonary histiocytosis X (eosinophilic granuloma of the lung) in which lung destruction often produces pronounced obstructive impairment. Careful tests of small airway function may show airflow obstruction in many of these disorders. Arterial blood gas determinations usually reveal relative hypoxaemia of varying magnitude at rest that becomes more pronounced with exercise. Hypocapnia and respiratory alkalosis may be present early, and hypercapnia and acidosis late in the disease course.[4]

### The Role of Lung Biopsy in Diagnosis and Treatment

Accumulated experience with management of the interstitial lung diseases has proven that the history, physical examination and relatively non-invasive tests such as plain X-ray films, computed tomography, radionuclide scans, pulmonary function testing, and tests of sputum and venous and arterial blood will often not suffice to make a specific diagnosis. In recent years powerful anti-inflammatory and immunosuppressive drugs with their attendant deleterious side effects and complications have been used with success in the treatment of certain of these disorders, provoking enthusiasm generally for aggressive medical management of previously progressively disabling conditions. For these reasons, and because certain stages of disease are believed to be more drug-responsive, it is nearly always essential to promptly secure a firm histopathological diagnosis from an adequate sample of lung tissue.

Prospective and retrospective studies have confirmed a positive role for open lung biopsy by limited thoracotomy,[5] when less invasive tests have failed to yield a definitive diagnosis. In one study of 502 patients, a diagnosis was made in 92.2% of patients after an open biopsy procedure. One current surgical procedure of choice is an anterior second intercostal incision of 4 to 7cm begun medially about 2cm from the sternal border. In certain circumstances a submammary incision somewhat more laterally in the fourth intercostal space may be preferable. The biopsy site ought ideally to involve a 'transitional' area containing both grossly normal and abnormal tissue, since surgical experience suggests that the most abnormal tissue may reveal only end-stage fibrosis and not give a specific diagnosis. Moreover, a recent study[6] confirms several prior impressions that the lingula ought to be avoided as a biopsy site, since it often over-represents the extent of fibrosis and vasculopathy in comparison with the remainder of the pulmonary parenchyma. The open biopsy procedure is remarkably complication-free, the thoracostomy tube is usually removed within 24 hours, and patients are usually able to return home or to the medical service within three to five days after operation.[7,8]

Other less invasive biopsy procedures may be preferred for first attempts to obtain definitive histopathology. Transbronchial biopsy under fluoroscopic guidance and broncho-alveolar lavage through the fibreoptic bronchoscope may obviate the need for open biopsy in a significant number of cases,[5] and the minimal risk, discomfort, and time delay this technique involves makes it the first procedure of choice in nearly all circumstances where the expertise for its performance is available and tissue is required. Trephine drill and transthoracic needle biopsies have been enthusiastically proposed as alternatives,[9,10] but their complication rates and disappointingly low yields on occasion have prevented their widespread acceptance.[7] Whichever closed procedure is employed, the lack of a definitive diagnosis should properly lead to open biopsy in nearly every circumstance in which therapeutic response is a possibility. As always, clinical factors such as the general health of the patient, and the patient's and physician's shared views regarding disease management, should be the final determinants of what course is taken in individual cases.

## Specific Non-infective Parenchymal Lung Diseases

Differences in clinical presentation, histopathological appearance, and therapeutic response characterise a number of these diseases, and they will be discussed individually in this section.

## Idiopathic Pulmonary Fibrosis (Cryptogenic Fibrosing Alveolitis)

Idiopathic pulmonary fibrosis (IPF), also known as cryptogenic fibrosing alveolitis, refers to a syndrome in which the normal lung's delicate alveolar and interstitial structure is disturbed by collagen deposition that eventuates in thickening of the alveolar interstices and destruction of the geometrical relationship between alveoli and pulmonary capillaries that is critical for successful oxygenation of arterial blood. This collagen deposition leads to predictable physiological consequences: patients become progressively hypoxaemic as shunting of pulmonary arterial blood worsens, and ventilation becomes more difficult as the normally elastic lungs become progressively stiffer. When unchecked or complicated by superimposed ventilatory burdens such as metabolic acidosis, or hypoxaemic stresses like lung infection, death ensues from hypoxaemia and respiratory acidosis.

### *Classification of Idiopathic Pulmonary Fibrosis*

Semantic and nosological differences characterise attempts at classification of this disease and its histopathology. Generally agreed is the notion that only those cases in which there is no association with any known aetiology or coexistent disorder will be included in this category, hence the modifiers idiopathic and cryptogenic. Drug-associated pulmonary fibrosis and fibrosis associated with various connective tissue diseases are thus excluded. Categories of IPF based on biopsy histopathological findings have been proposed as a means of classification,[11] yielding the subtypes listed in Table 18.2. Desquamative interstitial pneumonia (DIP) is histologically characterised by intra-alveolar collections of alveolar macrophages and type 2 pneumocytes and only mild inflammatory changes in the alveolar walls. When present, this pattern is often uniform throughout the specimen. The histology of usual interstitial pneumonitis (UIP) shows more oedema, inflammation, fibrinous exudate, and destruction of alveolar walls without prominence of intra-alveolar cells. Lymphoid interstitial pneumonitis (LIP) displays diffuse lymphocytic infiltration of alveolar walls and spaces, bronchi and vessels, without destruction or granuloma formation. The histology of the infiltrating cells allows the pathologist to distinguish this disorder from lymphoma. Other patterns described include bronchiolitis obliterans interstitial pneumonitis (BIP) with organising pneumonia (now termed BOOP), and giant cell interstitial pneumonia (GIP).[12,13]

*Table 18.2* Histopathological classification of pulmonary fibrosis

| |
|---|
| Desquamative interstitial pneumonitis (DIP) |
| Usual interstitial pneumonitis (UIP) |
| Lymphoid interstitial pneumonitis (LIP) |
| Other patterns: |
| Bronchiolitis obliterans interstitial pneumonitis (BIP) |
| Giant cell interstitial pneumonitis (GIP) |

This schema of histological classification is not trouble-free: coexistence of DIP and UIP on the same biopsy specimen is not unusual. Moreover, these histological patterns are found not only in IPF, but in other fibrosing pneumonitis syndromes as well. Other authorities regard DIP and UIP as points on a continuous pathological and clinical spectrum, with other patterns a variant.[14]

*Natural History, Prognosis, and Goals of Treatment*

An early description of IPF by Hamman and Rich told of progressive unremitting dyspnoea leading to death within six months. More commonly, chronic cases are seen which remain stable or progress over a few years. With this variety of outcomes and no clear way to prospectively identify what category of progression an individual patient will display, crisp and convincing proof of the efficacy of therapy in IPF has been elusive. None the less, several studies suggest evidence of therapeutic benefit in certain patients.

The goal of therapy is alleviation of symptoms insofar as possible. Reversal of pulmonary fibrosis is not deemed realistic, and arresting disease progression while maximising patient comfort are twin aims in treating patients with IPF. Since the drugs used have significant risk and toxicity, it is essential that a histopathological diagnosis be made and that therapeutic effect be monitored.

*Treatment*

Successful treatment of IPF has been reported with several drug regimens. Unfortunately, only about 50% of patients will have subjective, and 20% objective, improvement. Factors that correlate with improvement after drug therapy include disease in younger patients; in women; in patients with shorter disease duration and more severe reduction in forced vital capacity (to less than 66% of predicted); in those with less radiographic abnormality; more cellular and less fibrotic biopsies; more lymphocytes together with fewer neutrophils and eosinophils in broncho-alveolar lavage (BAL) fluid; and more type 3 collagen in the biopsy specimen.[15-19] It is common to find patients who will fail to respond as these correlations would predict; hence it is practical to consider therapy in all patients.

One widely practised therapeutic regimen is oral prednisone therapy in once-daily doses of 60mg or its equivalent.[15,19] This is begun after biopsy (one to three weeks after open biopsy) and physiological testing. The latter would include spirometry and rest and exercise arterial blood gas determinations as a minimum, and diffusion capacity and lung volumes if possible. Treatment at this dose is continued for one to two months and thorough symptomatic, physiological, and radiological evaluation is again undertaken. If there is improvement the corticosteroid dosage is very gradually tapered off at 5mg decrements to a maintenance dose of 20mg, which is continued for approximately one year from the time of onset of therapy. If further reduction of dosage can be achieved without flaring of disease this is desirable, but rare patients may require low-dose (5 to 20mg) prednisone for life. If a patient's disease should flare during tapering of therapy, a higher dose is promptly instituted that will again suppress disease activity. Corticosteroid therapy need be given only once daily. An alternate-day regimen is not infrequently associated with flaring of the disease. Thus, there is some risk in adopting this alternate-day dosage approach; in patients requiring substantial (30mg of prednisone or greater) daily doses for protracted periods the risk may be worth taking if the benefits of alternate-day dosage (amelioration of adverse effects) can be realised.[20]

When two months of 60mg of daily prednisone therapy fails to significantly improve objective measurements of lung function, alternative treatment should be attempted. One approach added azathioprine at a single daily dose of 3mg/kg to 20mg of daily prednisone, maintaining this two-drug regimen for nearly a year. Eight patients of 20 studied seemed to have selective beneficial effects from azathioprine in this prospective study.[18]

Another approach to the patient who fails to improve with oral prednisone treatment employs cyclophosphamide at single daily doses of 2mg/kg. Treatment and evaluation are continued for up to six months before disease progression is regarded as treatment failure.[15] Another anecdotal report of successful therapy in patients who failed to improve on high-dose oral prednisone told of using oral cyclophosphamide at 150mg/day with prednisone 50mg/day in one patient and 200mg azathioprine orally once daily in two others.[21]

In other patients (who had associated connective tissue diseases) intramuscular methotrexate at doses of 20 to 30mg once weekly was administered to corticosteroid and azathioprine therapy failures. The drug is initially given intramuscularly at a 5mg test dose and blood count and liver function tests are checked before the higher doses are used.[22] These blood tests must be checked bi-weekly in patients who receive this drug, since hepatitis and fulminant hepatic failure as well as marked leucocytopenia and thrombocytopenia can result from methotrexate use. Methotrexate pneumonitis can also occur.

High-dose 'pulse' corticosteroid therapy has been compared with low-dose therapy in another study.[23] Weekly intravenous pulses of 2g of methylprednisolone were given to one group for six months, and both study groups received daily oral prednisone doses of 0.25mg/kg. At six months the group of five patients which received high-dose pulse therapy had diminished 'neutrophil alveolitis' as assessed by broncho-alveolar lavage and gallium radionuclide scanning, but there was no significant improvement in chest radiograph appearance or pulmonary function when this group was compared to the other. In the absence of demonstrated clinical benefit, longer-term studies of more patients would be desirable before pulse therapy is widely applied.

Of the anti-inflammatory and immunosuppressive drugs used to treat IPF, all except corticosteroids may themselves be toxic to the lungs, and all (including corticosteroids) entail the risk of significant impairment of host defence as well as other adverse effects. Such risks warrant placing the evidence for therapeutic benefit under close scrutiny. In a disease like IPF, in which the clinical course and outcome are highly variable, prospective studies involving randomisation of large numbers of comparable patients to different treatment or placebo groups would be required to rigorously prove benefit or no effect. No such trials have been performed. However, a carefully analysed retrospective study of 220 patients was undertaken and seemed to suggest that some patients will improve with steroid therapy.[16] In that report 77 patients received no treatment and 143 received corticosteroids. Of those receiving corticosteroid therapy only 22 showed objective improvement, but 72 reported substantial improvement of breathlessness. The survival of the untreated group lay between that of the steroid responders and non-responders, suggesting that steroid responsiveness identifies patients with an inherently better prognosis. Perhaps the latter group has earlier disease. In any case, since the patients with a better prognosis cannot be prospectively identified, most pulmonary physicians believe a carefully monitored attempt at therapy is warranted.

Other treatment of IPF is important, but purely palliative. Supplemental oxygen therapy, usually delivered by nasal cannulae and not requiring humidification, should be prescribed for patients whose arterial $PO_2$ drops below 55mmHg (7.3kPa). Since many patients with IPF may have this degree of hypoxaemia only with exercise, rest and exercise arterial blood gas determinations should guide application of this therapy. If pulmonary arterial hypertension and right ventricular failure supervene, additional and judicious treatment with bed rest, diuretics, vasodilators, theophylline, and cardiac glycosides may be of benefit. Episodes of respiratory infection may promote a premature demise in these patients, so it is important to provide influenza and pneumococcal vaccinations, have them avoid others with respiratory infection, and aggressively treat their own infections with supportive care and antimicrobial agents when appropriate. Bronchodilator drugs (despite the absence of reactive airflow obstruction) and chest physiotherapy are often used to help clear bronchial secretions. When patients are hospitalised, extraordinary vigilance is required to avoid nosocomial avenues of infection (such as contaminated humidified nebulisers) which may lead to intractable respiratory failure. For patients with end-stage fibrosis and a precipitating cause for superimposed acute respiratory failure, intubation and assisted ventilatory support often seems a pointless extension of the patient's and family's misery as well as a waste of medical resources. This issue ought to be resolved in advance of the event by the physician in consultation with the patient and family, as appropriate. When patients are in the terminal stages, sedation with morphine sulfate or minor tranquilisers is an important treatment to diminish the sense of unremitting dyspnoea which otherwise results in desperate distress.[24]

### *Patient Education*

General aspects of patient understanding of this disease and its treatment have already been alluded to above. Side effects of corticosteroids and immunosuppressive drugs, such as oral ulceration, thrush and abnormal bleeding, as well as early signs of infection must all be appreciated. The importance of frequent follow-up visits and laboratory studies cannot be overstated. Signs of hepatitis in patients receiving methotrexate, or bladder pain and haematuria in those receiving cyclophosphamide, merit special mention. Patients receiving the latter drug often need repeated reminders to maintain fluid intake as close to three litres a day as possible and to empty their bladders as frequently as possible to lessen the risk of haemorrhagic cystitis.

Careful home use of oxygen (Chapter 3) must be understood, as well as scrupulous cleaning of home respiratory apparatus to avoid unwitting inhalation of aerosols of pathogenic bacteria. Finally, both patient and physician will benefit from frank and sensitive discussion of treatment goals in the terminal stages of IPF.

## Vasculitis and Granulomatosis

The grouping of these disorders for discussion purposes is appropriate since both lesions may coexist in certain diseases. The most prevalent and well-known granulomatous disorder of the lungs, sarcoidosis, is considered separately in Chapter 19. The vasculitic and granulomatous disorders to be considered here are listed in Table 18.1.

## Wegener's Granulomatosis

### *Diagnostic Features*

Wegener's granulomatosis is a systemic disorder, usually of insidious onset, that involves the lungs, the upper respiratory tract (including paranasal sinuses), and the kidneys. When localised to the upper respiratory tract and airways alone it has been called 'lethal midline granuloma'. When the kidneys have appeared spared it has been called 'limited Wegener's granulomatosis'. Cutaneous, and sometimes ocular and neurological, involvement may occur. Cough and fever are common complaints, and nasal erosions and skin papules and ulcers common findings. The chest radiographic features are variable and typically bilateral: there may be nodules, sometimes cavitating, or simply hazy infiltrates. Sinus destruction and inflammation, particularly of the maxillary sinus, is frequently seen on sinus radiographs. Like chest radiographs, these should be obtained whenever the disease is suspected to assess its extent. Urinary tract involvement is signalled by microscopic haematuria; occasionally one may be fortunate enough to confirm nephritis by the detection of red blood cell casts in a carefully processed urinary sediment.[25,26]

The disease is confirmed by biopsy of an involved organ, usually from somewhere in the respiratory tract. Diagnostic histopathological findings are the coexistence of necrotising granulomas and leucocytoclastic vasculitis in involved tissues from the same patient. The latter finding, a criterion sometimes overlooked, is crucial to the diagnosis. The presence of granulocytes or lymphocytes in a vessel wall on a tissue section is not sufficient; there must be both vessel wall and neutrophil destruction in addition to the granulomas. If these findings are confirmed from a single punch biopsy of the skin in the proper clinical setting, this will be sufficient to make a diagnosis. More typically, however, such lesions as well as intranasal ulcers will not allow a microscopic diagnosis of Wegener's granulomatosis due to the extent of non-specific inflammatory change. If the disease progress is relatively indolent, repeated relatively non-invasive biopsy of the nasal ulcers and/or skin lesions is justified. However, if renal failure or respiratory tract involvement is progressive, open lung biopsy of radiologically involved areas becomes an urgent matter, since renal failure in particular can rapidly progress before treatment becomes effective. Renal biopsy usually shows only glomerulonephritis, without granulomas. Since drug treatment can be very effective and very toxic, and is usually prolonged, and since relapse is not uncommon, it is crucial to make a secure histopathological diagnosis early in the course of Wegener's granulomatosis.

*Treatment*

The superiority of cyclophosphamide over other therapy is now widely acknowledged for the acute treatment of Wegener's granulomatosis.[25-27] It is given orally at 2mg/kg once daily, although severely ill patients should receive it by intravenous infusion. Simultaneous administration of corticosteroids is not required unless the patient is not responding to cyclophosphamide; under these circumstances oral prednisone is given in single daily doses of 60mg, and cyclophosphamide is continued. Objective response to therapy is usually seen within two weeks as an improvement in the chest radiograph or nasal mucosa and symptoms. Intravenous cyclophosphamide and methylprednisolone therapy may reverse a rising serum creatinine level within days, and is probably the treatment combination of first choice when fulminant renal failure (often irreversible) is the prominent manifestation.[26] Cyclophosphamide therapy at 1 to 2mg/kg daily has usually been continued for a full year after clinical remission is achieved, in the belief that this may prevent both late relapse and progressive renal disease. For patients who are dialysis-dependent as a result of this disease such therapy is continued none the less. A year after remission has been achieved, cyclophosphamide therapy can be gradually tapered and ceased over three months, but frequent (every two to three months for several years) chest radiographs, urinalyses, and serum creatinine levels or creatinine clearance determinations ought to be obtained due to the high rate of recurrence of this disease. Renal transplantation should probably be delayed until the disease has been in remission without cytotoxic and corticosteroid therapy for at least a year. While early assessments of long-term results of therapy were extremely favourable, several series now seem to show about a 30 to 50% relapse rate, with death the most common outcome of relapse. There is a clinical sense, without firm proof, that close monitoring of patients and early reinstitution of full-dose cyclophosphamide in the face of disease recurrence will favourably affect long-term prognosis.

Long-term cyclophosphamide therapy is not without significant morbidity and mortality of its own, from haemorrhagic cystitis, 'cytoxan lung', opportunistic infection, and haematological malignancy probably due to its effect as an alkylating agent. The incidence of haemorrhagic cystitis is probably lowered by dilution in the bladder with large (three litre) daily oral fluid intake. Bone marrow suppression is a constant concern; the absolute white blood cell count ought to be kept above $3000/mm^3$ and the platelet count above $50\,000/mm^3$. Suppression of ovogenesis and spermatogenesis is common and may be long-lasting, persisting well after therapy is discontinued.

Other drugs have been used for treating Wegener's granulomatosis, all with somewhat less favourable results than cyclophosphamide. Chlorambucil has been used in daily oral doses of 0.2mg/kg with eventual tapering after several months to maintenance doses of 2 to 4mg daily.[28] Azathioprine has also been used at 2mg/kg daily.[25] The place of these therapies is in patients who are undergoing pauses or termination of cyclophosphamide therapy due to bladder pain and bleeding or pneumonitis or, uncommonly, hepatitis. Corticosteroids at starting daily oral doses of 40 to 60mg prednisone are usually given with these immunosuppressive agents, and both are tapered in tandem once remission is achieved.

Recently a series of serendipitous clinical observations suggested that the antimicrobial combination of trimethoprim-sulphamethoxazole is effective in maintaining remission of Wegener's granulomatosis achieved by standard cyclophosphamide therapy with or without a corticosteroid.[29] We and others are finding similarly promising, though not uniformly successful, results. The combination drug is given orally as one double-strength tablet twice daily to patients in whom remission has been achieved, and other drugs are gradually tapered and discontinued as the chest radiograph and other laboratory parameters noted above are carefully and frequently monitored. If the disease flares, cyclophosphamide therapy is restarted. The addition of trimethoprim-sulphamethoxazole to cyclophosphamide and prednisone therapy has also improved disease control. Side effects of the antimicrobial combination include indigestion and occasionally leucopenia, as well as haemolytic anemia in glucose-6-phosphate-dehydrogenase-deficient patients. Whether it is acting as an immunosuppressant or an antimicrobial agent is unknown.

*Patient Education*

Patients and physicians ought to be encouraged about the manner in which use of cyclophosphamide has improved long-term survival in Wegener's granulomatosis to somewhat over 50%, and it ought to be stressed to the patient that close follow-up is the key to improving an individual's course. While there may not be studies to prove the point, it is logical, and the abrupt reversal of pulmonary and renal deterioration under drug therapy has been amply demonstrated. Side effects of immunosuppressive medications should be stressed, particularly for cyclophosphamide. The presumed benefit of high oral fluid intake has already been noted, and bears repeating to patients in every office visit.

## Eosinophilic Pneumonia

Eosinophilic pneumonia is one of several disorders previously classified among the pulmonary infiltrates with eosinophilia syndromes, or PIE. In this group are the Churg-Strauss syndrome, simple (reactive) pulmonary eosinophilia or Loeffler's syndrome, tropical pulmonary eosinophilia, and chronic eosinophilic pneumonia (Table 18.1). A somewhat different approach to nosology is taken by Crofton and Douglas[24] who split PIE syndromes further.

This section will focus primarily on chronic eosinophilic pneumonia, which appears to be a specific disorder of unknown aetiology. Tropical pulmonary eosinophilia is seen where microfilarial infestation is endemic, and the condition responds dramatically to antifilarial chemotherapy with diethylcarbamazine.[30] It is believed to represent a host hypersensitivity response to filarial larvae. Simple pulmonary eosinophilia (Loeffler's syndrome) is believed to represent a transient allergic reaction in the alveoli due to a host of allergens. Implicated have been infestation with worms (*Ascaris, Ancylostoma, Trichuris, Taenia, Distoma*), hypersensitivity to drugs (para-aminosalicylic acid, aspirin, nitrofurantoin, sulfonamides, penicillin, phenylbutazone), and perhaps certain pollens. Another cause of the syndrome is treatment of schistosomal infection with anti-schistosomal chemotherapy.[31] These are transient disorders and when an aetiological agent is identified and dealt with, the syndrome generally resolves with only supportive therapy. More severe disease due to one of the aetiological agents noted above may require corticosteroid therapy and care paralleling that of chronic eosinophilic pneumonia, discussed below. For a more thorough discussion of the above syndromes the reader is referred to a review.[24]

### *Diagnostic Features*

Chronic (idiopathic) eosinophilic pneumonia occurs predominantly in middle-aged women who often have no prior atopic history. Customary complaints upon presentation include a subacute history of cough (sometimes non-productive), fever, and progressively worsening dyspnoea. No cause for a hypersensitivity reaction is generally elicited, thus the syndrome appears idiopathic. Examination reveals fever and chest crepitations as well as general signs of chronic malaise. The white blood cell count is usually in excess of 10 000/mm$^3$ and eosinophilia exceeds 10%. Serum IgE levels have been normal when reported.[32] The chest radiograph may show reticulonodular densities reaching confluence in some areas that seem to hug the periphery on the posteroanterior view: this 'photographic negative of pulmonary oedema' pattern[33] has been called sufficient to make the diagnosis.[34] However, other quite different radiographic patterns have also been described. Physiological testing usually shows mild to moderate hypoxaemia on arterial blood gas testing and restriction to airflow.[35]

Under certain circumstances, notably when the clinical, laboratory, and radiographic profiles are classical, a biopsy may not be required. Under other circumstances the diagnosis may be secured by transbronchial biopsies obtained during fibreoptic bronchoscopy.[31,32] The histopathological appearance shows alveolar and interstitial infiltration with eosinophils and histiocytes, the latter often containing eosinophilic granules. There is oedema but generally minimal destruction and fibrosis. Bronchiolitis obliterans, granuloma formation, and peribronchial fibrosis have all been reported, but the disease is believed to heal by resolution rather than organisation.[32,36]

### *Natural History and Prognosis*

The course of chronic eosinophilic pneumonia has a favourable prognosis. There is usually a protracted history including antimicrobial therapy prior to diagnosis, with spontaneous resolution seen in less than 10% of patients. Oral corticosteroid therapy results in rapid clinical and radiological improvement, but treatment may have to be continued for years at reduced doses. Discontinuation of treatment results in relapse in about one-third of patients (including eight relapses in a single patient), but remission is again readily achieved with steroid therapy. If the disease is recognised, it should seldom be lethal.[24,32,33,37]

### *Treatment*

After diagnosis is made by biopsy or chest radiograph in the appropriate clinical setting, treatment with oral prednisone should begin. In most reports 30 to 40mg is given once daily, with clinical improvement apparent in virtually all cases within 48 hours. Fever responds quickly as does peripheral eosinophilia. Radiographic infiltrates begin clearing within one week and the chest radiograph returns to baseline after one month. Prednisone is tapered slowly after several months as the blood and differential cell counts are followed, and sustained remission can usually be achieved by daily doses of 10mg or less. In one case report the drug was discontinued over two years;[36] in a larger follow-up series oral corticosteroids were discontinued after a mean of four years in eight patients. Two of the eight still required low-dose prednisone (5 to 20mg daily) at five-and-a-half and eight years after diagnosis. In others the drug had been stopped at 16 months, 18 months, 8 years and 12 years. In the patient requiring prednisone for 12 years an attempt at discontinuation of therapy six years after diagnosis resulted in disease recurrence.

The primary long-term consequence of chronic eosinophilic pneumonia is asthma which requires sustained bronchodilator therapy in half the patients, none of whom were atopic or complained of bronchospastic syndromes before onset. Pulmonary function otherwise returns to normal, and progression to more malignant pulmonary eosinophilic syndromes has not been reported.[37]

Finally, identification of an inciting agent requires careful probing of the patient's history in multiple visits. In patients taking other medications, such as thiazide diuretics for hypertension, a short-term trial without the possibly offending medication before corticosteroid therapy is begun may identify the cause of the eosinophilic pneumonia, if such a trial is safe. Rechallenge may then confirm eosinophilic pneumonia due to a drug reaction and an alternative treatment may be tried, sparing a patient the sustained prednisone therapy required to suppress a drug reaction.

### *Patient Education*

Patients should be alerted to the side effects of steroid therapy and the likely need for long-term treatment and follow-up.

## Hypersensitivity Pneumonitis

When repeated inhalation of antigen(s) results in parenchymal lung disease, it is termed hypersensitivity pneumonitis or extrinsic allergic alveolitis. Implicit in the definition are two features: first, that the triggering mechanism be immunological, that is, that the host reaction involve specificity for and memory of the antigen; and second, that the resulting inflammatory disease primarily involve the alveoli rather than the larger conducting airways. Hypersensitivity involving larger conducting airways is termed extrinsic or allergic asthma and its treatment is described in Chapter 16. In some diseases, notably allergic bronchopulmonary aspergillosis (ABPA), there is both asthma and hypersensitivity pneumonitis.

There is an ever-lengthening list of agents, most of them organic antigens from living sources, which have been identified as precipitating hypersensitivity pneumonitis in humans. It is interesting that many individuals can manifest in-vitro immune reactivity to such antigens, probably acquired by inhalation sensitisation, yet they do not display overt lung disease. From this it is presumed that host susceptibility rather than purely the presence or absence of inhaled antigen is of some importance in the development of hypersensitivity pneumonitis. Among the diseases identified as associated with inhalation of thermophilic bacteria are farmer's lung, mushroom worker's lung, bagassosis (from mouldy sugar cane) and humidifier lung. Animal proteins provoke bird fancier's (pigeon breeder's) lung in susceptible patients. The chronic form of pulmonary berylliosis is probably a similar consequence of occupational beryllium exposure. ABPA represents alveolar as well as airway hypersensitivity to the ubiquitous fungus *Aspergillus.* Excellent discussions of the pathogenesis and clinical features of these syndromes are available.[24,38-44]

*Diagnostic Features*

The characteristic clinical syndrome of hypersensitivity pneumonitis includes fever, cough, dyspnoea, and muscle aches at an interval of four to eight hours after antigen exposure. Most patients endure the syndrome for some time and even identify its cause prior to visiting the physician for relief. Occasional cases have been described in which hypersensitivity pneumonitis slowly progresses in a chronic form to causing dyspnoea at rest without simultaneous cough, fever, or other features of the acute reaction.[42] Moreover, symptoms can come at quite variable intervals of exposure and re-exposure, with a documented case of occurrence of hypersensitivity pneumonitis five years after re-exposure.

The diagnosis is a clinical one suggested by remission of symptoms within days to weeks upon withdrawal from exposure, with recrudescence upon re-exposure. Optimally re-exposure is produced by controlled inhalation of the offending agent. Skin testing (intradermal) with the suspected agent produces erythema and induration at 6 to 12 hours and IgG precipitins against it are demonstrable in the serum in most cases. However, many subjects without the pneumonitis will show such systemic evidence of immune reactivity. The chest radiograph should show evidence of 'fleeting infiltrates' in most cases (shadowing that resolves quickly, or moves in location) although patients have been described with apparently normal radiographs.[42] Pulmonary function testing may show hypoxaemia, and usually shows reduced airflow due to restriction. Obstruction may also be seen as a consequence of obliterative bronchiolitis, and in the asthma accompanying ABPA. The latter disease appears unique in also showing immediate skin reactivity to *Aspergillus* antigen, blood eosinophilia, elevated serum IgE levels, and central bronchiectasis in some cases.[44]

In most cases where hypersensitivity pneumonitis is suspected lung biopsy is not required, the remission of symptoms with avoidance and recrudesence with exposure being so characteristic. Moreover, the biopsy findings are not pathognomonic: non-caseating granulomas and a mononuclear cell infiltrate, largely composed of lymphocytes, are seen with occasional foci of necrosis. Necrotising bronchocentric granulomatosis and organising bronchiolitis obliterans may be present, as well as interstitial fibrosis (the latter in what are presumed to be cases of protracted disease). Such histopathological findings may also be seen in pulmonary sarcoidosis. In any event once the histopathology is known the diseases can be readily distinguished on other clinical grounds. In circumstances where multiple transbronchial biopsies may be easily and safely obtained and other confirming modalities (serum IgG precipitin testing, specific antigen inhalation and intradermal challenging) are not available, a compatible biopsy result taken from areas of radiographic involvement may well be a useful adjunct in diagnosis.

### *Natural History and Prognosis*

As indicated above, the natural history of hypersensitivity pneumonitis is unpredictable. Patients may develop symptoms after many years of constant exposure, which will resolve spontaneously after withdrawal from the offending antigen. Subsequent re-exposure after a prolonged period may or may not precipitate an episode.

Certain long-term clinical studies suggest that permanent impairment, while rare, can occur in hypersensitivity pneumonitis.[41] This may take the form of organising pneumonia with fibrosis and bronchiolitis obliterans, giving a combined physiological picture of restriction and obstruction.

### *Treatment*

Since hypersensitivity pneumonitis is usually a self-limited disease, avoidance of the antigen often results in relief of fever, cough, dyspnoea, and myalgia within 48 hours. When symptoms persist or are severe, a two-week course of oral corticosteroid therapy is usually successful, beginning with 40mg daily of prednisone for five days, then 20mg for five days, then 10mg for four days, then abrupt discontinuation. This treatment must be coupled with strict avoidance of the antigen. Only rarely will such a treatment programme fail to improve the patient; in that case chlorambucil may be tried, as it seems the most benign of immunosuppressive agents. A daily dose of 8mg chlorambucil with 20mg prednisone may be used until disease activity appears controlled, and the chlorambucil dosage is then tapered by 2mg every two weeks, followed by tapering of the prednisone.

The primary therapy for hypersensitivity pneumonitis is to avoid inhaling the antigen. Preventive measures for farmer's lung and bagassosis involve keeping moisture levels low in stored hay and *bagasse* to prevent growth of thermophilic actinomyces. The Baxter Pneu-Seal respirator and Racal Airstream positive pressure helmet are both effective in preventing organic dust inhalation in farm workers.[24,45] These or similar devices should be tried before a patient is advised to leave an occupation or hobby, as this may be quite difficult for the patient to accomplish.

### *Patient Education*

The prior comments about corticosteroid and immunosuppressive therapy pertain here also. Counselling the patient to avoid what provokes his hypersensitivity pneumonitis, particularly if it involves a dearly-held avocation, may prove quite time-consuming.

## Inhalation of Toxic Gases

Several toxic gases may produce damage to the airways and pulmonary parenchyma. These include smoke, steam, chlorine, ammonia, phosgene, oxides of sulphur, and oxides of nitrogen. Chlorine is used in the chemical and plastic industries and in water disinfection. Ammonia is sometimes used as a commercial refrigerant. Phosgene is used in conjunction with aniline dye production. Oxides of sulphur are released in paper manufacture and smelting of iron ore. Oxides of nitrogen are produced in a variety of circumstances: from decomposing corn in silage (silo filler's disease), in chemical and manufacturing industries in which nitric acid is used, from burning nitrocellulose and plastic fires (as when X-ray film burns), in arc welding when the electrodes are covered with nitrocellulose, and during oxyacetylene welding in closed spaces where atmospheric nitrogen is oxidised.

All such inhalations may cause cough, fever, wheezing with airflow obstruction, pulmonary infiltrates, and hypoxaemia. Initial exposure and symptoms may be followed by a period of improvement only to progress to deterioration after 24 to 48 hours.

The subject's prognosis depends upon the agent inhaled and the extent of the exposure. Inhalation of ammonia, phosgene, and oxides of sulphur generally has a favourable prognosis if the initial insult is survived, although deaths have been reported. Acute accidental and chronic inhalation of chlorine gas apparently can cause airflow obstruction that resolves rapidly without appreciable physiological disorders.[46,47] Alternatively, inhalation of oxides of nitrogen can lead to progressive bronchiolitis obliterans and death.[48] Patients who inhale smoke or steam generally have a favourable prognosis if they survive the acute insult.

### *Treatment*

Primary treatment for all such inhalation injuries is supportive, with oxygenation and circulatory support paramount considerations. Over-aggressive fluid administration in the presence of the pulmonary capillary leak syndrome (the adult respiratory distress syndrome, ARDS) may worsen oxygenation, and placing of a pulmonary artery catheter with measurement of cardiac output and oxygen delivery is prudent in such cases.[49]

Of these toxic agents, only the treatment of smoke inhalation injury has been examined in a controlled albeit retrospective fashion. In that study of 225 patients (141 steroid-treated, 84 not) in which the treated group received 10mg of intravenous dexamethasone every six hours for 48 hours, there was no difference in pulmonary-related morbidity or mortality.[50] It had previously been shown that corticosteroid administration had no positive beneficial effect on pulmonary-related morbidity or mortality and was in fact detrimental in combined smoke inhalation and thermal cutaneous injury.[51] High concentrations of inspired oxygen and hyperbaric oxygen at two atmospheres if available should be administered acutely in smoke injury in which carbon monoxide inhalation (detected by measurement of carboxyhaemoglobin in arterial blood) has occurred. For a patient breathing room air, the half-life of 50% carboxyhaemoglobin in 210 minutes, but breathing 100% oxygen this is reduced to 60 minutes. One hundred per cent oxygen should be given until the measured carboxyhaemoglobin is less than 15%.[52]

Bronchodilator drugs are usually recommended in conjunction with oxygen therapy. Various authorities further advocate the use of corticosteroid drugs to treat toxic inhalation in daily doses of 60 to 100mg of prednisone for several days or until reversal of physiological and radiographic abnormalities occurs, allowing that such use has not been confirmed in controlled studies.[24,38]

The role of antibiotic therapy in the acute injury is likewise unclear. Some physicians propose prophylactic therapy. I prefer to wait for the appearance of new radiographic infiltrates, purulent sputum, and leucocytosis as evidence for nosocomial pneumonia, and obtain appropriate Gram stains and cultures before initiating usually broad-spectrum antimicrobial therapy.

As mentioned previously, the long-term prognosis after survival of the initial and acute complicating illnesses appears dependent upon the agent inhaled and the extent of exposure. Evidence of progressive loss of function is usually inapparent on the chest radiograph (except perhaps as a progressive decrease in lung volume at maximal inspiration), and other tests such as spirometry are employed. Progressively lower values for the $FEV_1$ and FVC suggest ongoing disease, and this can often be further defined as primarily obstructive or restrictive. Usually when this occurs the picture is a mixed one, corresponding histologically (when biopsied) to bronchiolitis obliterans and organising fibrosis. If obstructive physiology is present non-steroidal bronchodilator therapy is maximised. In the face of further deterioration or restriction, a course of corticosteroid therapy at 40 to 60mg of prednisone once daily is often tried. This is continued for one to two months. In one reported case, disease stability was achieved with the addition of 150mg daily azathioprine therapy; after three months prednisone dosage was changed to 40mg every other day.[53] If pulmonary function has stabilised prednisone is continued with slow tapering at monthly intervals and usually discontinued within one year. If disease appears progressive the drug is rapidly tapered and the disease is treated similarly to idiopathic pulmonary fibrosis, described earlier in this chapter. While idiopathic bronchiolitis obliterans organising pneumonia generally has a more favourable response to corticosteroid therapy,[13] there are no series available for evaluation with regard to this complication of inhalation of irritant gases.[54,55]

## Pulmonary Haemorrhage Syndromes

A multitude of airway and other diseases can result in pulmonary haemorrhage; among them are bronchiectasis, tuberculosis, mitral stenosis, bronchial cancer, aspergilloma, and others. The diagnostic management of haemoptysis has been recently considered elsewhere.[56] This section will focus upon the primary pulmonary haemorrhage syndromes.

A classification of these has been proposed.[57] For simplification they are reclassified here (Table 18.1): (i) Goodpasture's syndrome, or pulmonary haemorrhage with nephritis and detectable serum antibody to glomerular basement membrane (anti-GBM antibodies); (ii) pulmonary haemorrhage with nephritis without detectable anti-GBM antibodies; (iii) idiopathic pulmonary haemosiderosis in which there is no nephritis; and (iv) pulmonary haemorrhage secondary to vasculitis or connective tissue (collagen vascular) disease, either known or newly presenting. The lattermost syndrome may or may not include concurrent nephritis; it will not be considered further here.

*Diagnostic Features*

All three syndromes of pulmonary haemorrhage discussed herein are characterised by confluent infiltrates on the chest radiograph, iron-deficiency anaemia, and virtually always by haemoptysis. In rare cases there may be no history of gross haemoptysis, but examination of expectorated sputum will reveal haemosiderin-laden macrophages. When nephritis is suggested by the urinalysis, idiopathic pulmonary haemosiderosis is ruled out. Renal insufficiency or renal failure may be present at the time of pulmonary presentation of the other pulmonary haemorrhage syndromes, but sometimes is delayed by months or years.

Pulmonary haemorrhage syndromes are suggested by the presence of haemoptysis and radiographic infiltrates. The bleeding and clotting, as well as the prothrombin and partial thromboplastin times, should be normal. Infectious causes of pulmonary haemorrhage are usually not overly difficult to exclude because of the usual young age of patients with primary pulmonary haemorrhage, their prior good health, and the absence of radiological signs of chronic lung abnormalities. Iron deficiency and microcytic hypochromic anaemia are readily confirmed. When tested, the single-breath diffusing capacity of carbon monoxide may be increased.[58,59] Serum for anti-GBM antibody should be quickly obtained and sent for testing. If there is evidence of nephritis and/or renal insufficiency, a percutaneous renal needle biopsy should be obtained for immunofluorescent as well as histological analysis. The presence of linear immunoglobulin deposition along the glomerular basement membrane helps secure the diagnosis of Goodpasture's syndrome. Nephritis without such a pattern is non-diagnostic; this may still be Goodpasture's syndrome and final confirmation will await the anti-GBM antibody assay. When nephritis is not present a patient should proceed expeditiously to fibreoptic bronchoscopy in order to rule out an endobronchial lesion and obtain transbronchial biopsies if feasible. These should also be submitted for immunofluorescence analysis, as linear alveolar deposition of immunoglobulins has sometimes been confirmed in this way.[60,61]

If a tissue diagnosis has not been obtained and the anti-GBM antibody result is pending, at this stage the clinician is forced to either be more aggressive in obtaining tissue for diagnosis or to treat presumptively. Because the therapy for Goodpasture's syndrome is unique and involves risk, because vasculitides may present in an identical fashion, and because even extensive transbronchial biopsying may miss diagnostic lesions (as noted earlier in this chapter), I would next proceed to open lung biopsy. In the absence of linear immunoglobulin deposition along the alveoli, the final exclusion of Goodpasture's syndrome must await the serum anti-GBM study. Granular deposition of IgG in alveoli or glomeruli suggests an immune complex pathogenesis, and this is probably pulmonary haemorrhage with nephritis without anti-GBM (group ii above) if systemic lupus erythematosus has been excluded. The absence of vasculitis probably excludes this as a cause of pulmonary haemorrhage.[62] The histopathological findings of haemorrhage with normal vessels, haemosiderin in macrophages, and variable extent of interstitial thickening are common to all these syndromes.[62]

## *Natural History and Prognosis*

Modern techniques of life support, such as renal dialysis and transplantation and ventilatory support, have dramatically altered the prognosis of what was once a virtually fatal constellation of findings. Since the use of plasmapheresis (plasma exchange) for Goodpasture's syndrome, disease remission has been achieved in approximately 50% of cases, and the relapse rate is most likely less than 10%.[63] While the detection of anti-GBM antibody is important in making the diagnosis, its titre seems to be of no prognostic value in predicting pulmonary or renal outcome.[64] The course of pulmonary haemorrhage with nephritis without anti-GBM antibodies (group ii) is uncertain with very few patients reported; prognosis is probably comparable to that of Goodpasture's syndrome.[62] Patients with idiopathic pulmonary haemosiderosis may have a fulminant course or one of chronic illness over years that eventuates in pulmonary fibrosis, believed to be secondary to organisation around haemosiderin deposition. Lacking the morbidity of renal disease this is probably the most benign (that is, has the best prognosis) of the pulmonary haemorrhage syndromes.

## *Treatment*

Since pulmonary haemorrhage may suddenly cause death from asphyxia, hypoxaemia, or exsanguination, its prompt treatment is important. Unless connective tissue disease or vasculitis is discovered, I would proceed with accepted therapy for Goodpasture's syndrome until a report of a negative study for anti-GBM antibodies were obtained. This includes intravenous administration of methylprednisolone 1g daily for five days, followed by 1 to 2mg/kg of daily prednisone. This therapy alone is often quite effective within 24 to 72 hours in minimising pulmonary haemorrhage, but immunosuppressive therapy of either cyclophosphamide (2 to 3mg/kg daily) or azathioprine (1 to 2mg/kg daily) or occasionally both[64] appears necessary to prevent progressive renal failure. There are no controlled trials comparing therapies, and many physicians will combine methylprednisolone or prednisone treatment with one immunosuppressive drug or the other.

Equally critical in achieving remission in Goodpasture's syndrome, particularly in preserving renal function, is plasmapheresis. This should be instituted shortly after or presumptively before final diagnosis if renal insufficiency appears progressive. An average of five to six litres of plasma is removed in each daily three-to-five hour procedure, with 2 to 5% normal serum albumin or plasma protein fraction constituting 80% of replacement; patients may require 12 to 30 separate treatments.[64-67] The purpose of the plasmapheresis is to remove the anti-GBM antibody, but cessation of this and other aspects of therapy is dictated by clinical improvement. Generally when results are favourable (renal function stabilised, pulmonary haemorrhage stops) plasmapheresis is discontinued and immunosuppressives are stopped, or rapidly tapered and stopped. Prednisone is usually continued at 40 to 60mg for several months in the stabilised patient and then slowly reduced to 20mg daily, where it is continued for about a year from the onset of the disease before final tapering and cessation. Renal function is followed closely and evidence of renewed or smouldering activity is again treated with immunosuppressive therapy and plasmapheresis until stabilised.

Heparin 100U intravenously every eight hours has been given as adjunctive therapy in a paediatric patient;[66] it is not part of standard treatment. Both peritoneal dialysis and haemodialysis have been employed to suppport patients during periods of renal failure. Once anuria occurs recovery of renal function is quite unusual. Such patients may successfully undergo renal transplantation in the future,[64] usually after bilateral nephrectomy and absence of anti-GBM antibodies on several determinations while off therapy. Because iron as haemosiderin cannot be reused for haem synthesis after it has been taken up by alveolar macrophages, and because its continued presence in the lung may contribute to eventual pulmonary fibrosis, patients are treated first with iron for the iron-deficiency anaemia until a satisfactory haemoglobin level is obtained, and then with desferrioxamine chelation therapy if alveolar and interstitial bleeding is believed to be quite widespread.[68]

The treatment of pulmonary haemorrhage with nephritis without anti-GBM antibodies is identical to that of Goodpasture's syndrome, except that plasmapheresis is omitted. In some circumstances, with desperately ill patients, this latter therapy is also used. All information on its efficacy is anecdotal. The risk of such therapy, from the point of view of infection in particular, is considerable.

With regard to the treatment of idiopathic pulmonary haemosiderosis, there are too few patients reported to draw definitive conclusions. No immune, inflammatory, or even microstructural abnormality has been unambiguously proven. None the less, oral corticosteroid therapy is usually applied at 1mg/kg daily with subsequent tapering as for Goodpasture's syndrome. Azathioprine has also been used at daily doses of 1.5 to 2mg/kg with remissions reported after 18 to 24 months of treatment.[69,70] Another case has been reported in which combined methylprednisolone and azathioprine therapy seemed to fail, but lung haemorrhage and hypoxaemia resolved after three plasmapheresis treatments. However, there is no mention of assay for serum anti-GBM antibodies, and it is possible that this patient had Goodpasture's syndrome without early renal involvement. In other patients idiopathic pulmonary haemosiderosis remains quiescent for years without worsening infiltrates on the chest radiograph, without progressive anaemia, and without symptoms on modest (30mg prednisone every other day) maintenance corticosteroid doses. Oral and sometimes intravenous iron replacement is required (with subsequent chelation therapy, see above) to repair the profound anaemia which may further diminish pulmonary functional reserve.

### *Patient Education*

There is little to say additional about patient education in these syndromes, except to note that the onset and exacerbation of Goodpasture's syndrome have occasionally been believed to be associated with exposure to hydrocarbon fumes.[63] Other authors find this irrelevant.[64] In any event it is probably wise to advise patients with pulmonary haemorrhage syndromes to avoid all such elective exposure to paint, refinery, and gasoline fumes.

## Pulmonary Manifestations of Connective Tissue Diseases

The connective tissue diseases (CTD) are systemic disorders with pulmonary and thoracic manifestations to varying extends. Treatment is controversial and the subject of numerous reviews, studies, and ongoing therapeutic trials.[72,73] Since specific therapy is directed to the systemic disease, rather than merely to its thoracic manifestations, the reader is referred to current texts of rheumatology and immunology for detailed discussions of the many therapeutic strategies for connective tissue diseases.[74]

## References


1. Epler GR, et al. Normal chest roentgenograms in chronic diffuse infiltrative lung disease. *N Engl J Med* 1978; 298: 934.
2. Fraser RG. The radiology of interstitial lung disease. In: Fulmer JD (ed). Interstitial lung diseases. *Clin Chest Med* 1982; 3: 375.
3. Naidich DP, Zerhouni EA, Siegelman SS. *Computed tomography of the thorax.* New York: Raven Press, 1984: 226.
4. Fulmer JD, et al. Small airways in idiopathic pulmonary fibrosis: comparison of morphologic and physiologic observations. *J Clin Invest* 1977; 60: 595.
5. Wall CP, Gaensler EA, Carrington CB, Hayes JA. Comparison of transbronchial and open biopsies in chronic infiltrative lung diseases. *Am Rev Respir Dis* 1981; 123: 180.
6. Newman SL, Michel RP, Wang N-S. Lingular lung biopsy: is it representative? *Am Rev Respir Dis* 1985; 132: 1084.
7. Gaensler EA, Carrington CB. Open biopsy for chronic diffuse infiltrative lung disease: clinical, roentenographic, and physiological correlations in 502 patients. *Ann Thoracic Surg* 1980; 30: 411.
8. Venn GE, Kay PH, Midwood CJ, Goldstraw P. Open lung biopsy in patients with diffuse pulmonary shadowing. *Thorax* 1985; 40: 931.
9. Wright PH, Heard E, Steele SJ, Turner-Warwick M. Cryptogenic fibrosing alveolitis: assessment by graded trephine lung biopsy compared with clinical, radiographic, and physiological features. *Br J Dis Chest* 1981; 75: 61.
10. Zavala DC, Schoell JE. Ultrathin needle aspiration of the lung in infectious and malignant disease. *Am Rev Respir Dis* 1981; 123: 125.
11. Liebow AA, Steer A, Billingsley JG. Desquamative interstitial pneumonia. *Am J Med* 1965; 39: 369.
12. Sokolowski JW, Cordray DW, Cantow EF, et al. Giant cell interstitial pneumonia. *Am Rev Respir Dis* 1972; 105: 417.
13. Epler GR, Colby TV, McLoud TC, et al. Bronchiolitis obliterans organizing pneumonia. *N Engl J Med* 1985; 312: 152.
14. Scadding JG, Hinson KFW. Diffuse fibrosing alveolitis (diffuse interstitial fibrosing of the lungs). *Thorax* 1967; 22: 291.
15. Turner-Warwick M. Approaches to treatment of interstitial lung disease. *Postgrad Med J* 1984; 60: 183.
16. Turner-Warwick M, Burrows B, Johnson A. Cryptogenic fibrosing alveolitis: response to corticosteroid treatment and its effect on survival. *Thorax* 1980; 35: 593.
17. Rudd RM, Haslam PL, Turner-Warwick M. Cryptogenic fibrosing alveolitis. Relationships of pulmonary physiology and bronchoalveolar lavage to response to treatment and prognosis. *Am Rev Respir Dis* 1981; 124: 1.
18. Winterbauer RH, Hamman SP, Hallman KD, et al. Diffuse interstitial pneumonitis. Clinicopathologic correlations in 20 patients treated with prednisone/azathioprine. *Am J Med* 1978; 70: 542.
19. Crystal RG, Gadek JE, Ferrans VJ, et al. Interstitial lung disease: current concepts of pathogenesis, staging, and therapy. *Am J Med* 1981; 70: 542.
20. Fauci A. Alternate-day corticosteroid therapy. *Am J Med* 1978; 64: 729.
21. Weese WC, Levine BW, Lazenri H. Interstitial lung disease resistant to corticosteroid therapy. *Chest* 1975; 67: 57.
22. Scott DGI, Bacon PA. Response to methotrexate in fibrosing alveolitis associated with connective tissue disease. *Thorax* 1980; 35: 725.

23. Keough BA, Bernardo J, Hunninghake GW, et al. Effect of intermittent high dose parenteral corticosteroids on the alveolitis of pulmonary fibrosis. *Am Rev Respir Dis* 1983; 127: 18.
24. Crofton J, Douglas A. *Respiratory diseases,* 3rd ed. Oxford: Blackwell Scientific Publications, 1981: 692.
25. Fauci A, Haynes BF, Katz P, Wolff SM. Wegener's granulomatosis: prospective clinical and therapeutic experience with 85 patients for 21 years. *Ann Intern Med* 1983; 98: 76.
26. DeRemee RA, Weiland LH, McDonald TJ. Respiratory vasculitis. *Mayo Clin Proc* 1980; 55: 492.
27. Israel HL. Pulmonary angiitis and granulomatosis. In: Fishman AP, ed. *Update, Pulmonary diseases and disorders.* New York: McGraw-Hill, 1982: 243.
28. McIlvanie SK. Wegener's granulomatosis. Successful treatment with chlorambucil. *JAMA* 1966; 197: 90.
29. DeRemee RA, McDonald TJ, Weiland LH. Wegener's granulomatosis: observations on treatment with antimicrobial agents. *Mayo Clin Proc* 1985; 60: 27.
30. Baker SJ, Rajan KT, Divadatta S. Treatment of tropical eosinophilia, a controlled trial. *Lancet* 1959; 2: 144.
31. Davidson BL, El-Kassimi F, Zaman A, Pillai DK. The "lung shift" in treated schistosomiasis: bronchoalveolar lavage evidence for eosinophilic pneumonia. *Chest* 1986 (in press).
32. Fox B, Seed WA. Chronic eosinophilic pneumonia. *Thorax* 1980; 35: 570.
33. Gaensler EA, Carrington CB. Peripheral opacities in eosinophilic pneumonia. The photographic negative of pulmonary edema. *Am J Roentgenol* 1977; 128: 1.
34. Dines DE. Chronic eosinophilic pneumonia. A roentogenographic diagnosis. *Mayo Clin Proc* 1978; 53: 129.
35. Carrington CB, Addington NW, Goff AM, et al. Chronic eosinophilic pneumonia. *N Engl J Med* 1969; 180: 787.
36. Perrault JL, Jarvis M, Wolinsky H. Resolution of chronic eosinophilic pneumonia with corticoid therapy. *Ann Intern Med* 1971; 74: 951.
37. Pearson DJ, Rosenow EC. Chronic eosinophilic pneumonia (Carrington's). *Mayo Clin Proc* 1978; 53: 73.
38. Weg JG. Chronic noninfectious parenchymal diseases. In: Guenter CA, Welsh MHJ, eds. *Pulmonary Medicine,* 2nd ed. Philadelphia: JB Lippincott, 1982: 608.
39. Reynolds HY. Hypersensitivity pneumonitis. *Clin Chest Med* 1982; 3: 503.
40. Roberts RC, Moore VL. State of the art: immunopathogenesis of hypersensitivity pneumonitis. *Am Rev Respir Dis* 1977; 116: 1075.
41. Braun SR, LoPico GA, Tsiatis A, et al. Farmer's lung disease: long-term clinical and physiologic outcome. *Am Rev Respir Dis* 1979; 119: 185.
42. Fink JN, Sosman AJ, Barboriak JJ, et al. Pigeon breeders' disease: a clinical study of a hypersensitivity pneumonitis. *Ann Intern Med* 1968; 68: 1205.
43. Epstein PE, Dauber JH, Rossman MD, Daniele RP. Bronchoalveolar lavage in a patient with chronic berylliosis: evidence for hypersensitivity pneumonitis. *Ann Intern Med* 1982; 97: 213.
44. Mendelson EB, Fisher MR, Mintzer RA, Halwig JM, Greenberger PA. Roentgenographic and clinical staging of allergic bronchopulmonary aspergillosis. *Chest* 1985; 87: 334.
45. Gourley CA, Braidwood GD. The use of dust respirators in the recurrence of farmer's lung. *Trans Soc Occup Med* 1971; 21: 93.
46. Chester EG, Gillespie DG, Krause FD. The prevalence of chronic obstructive pulmonary disease in chlorine gas workers. *Am Rev Respir Dis* 1969; 99: 365.
47. Weill H, George R, Schwarz M, Ziskind M. Late evaluation of pulmonary function after acute exposure to chlorine gas. *Am Rev Respir Dis* 1969; 99: 374.
48. Lowry T, Schuman LM. Silo-filler's disease: a syndrome caused by nitrogen dioxide. *JAMA* 1956; 162: 153.
49. Pierce AK. Acute respiratory failure. In: Guenter CA, Welsh MHJ, eds. *Pulmonary medicine.* 2nd ed. Philadelphia: JB Lippincott, 1982: 237.
50. Robinson NB, Hudson LD, Piem M, et al. Steroid therapy following isolated smoke inhalation injury. *J Trauma* 1982; 22: 876.
51. Moylan JA, Alexander TG Jr. Diagnosis and treatment of inhalation injury. *World J Surg* 1978; 2: 185.

52. Crapo RD. Smoke-inhalation injuries. *JAMA* 1981; 246: 1694.
53. Seggev JW, Masson UG, Worthen S, Stanford RE, Fernandez E. Bronchiolitis obliterans: report of three cases with detailed physiologic studies. *Chest* 1983; 83: 169.
54. Epler GR, Colby TV. The spectrum of bronchiolitis obliterans. *Chest* 1983; 83: 161.
55. Gosink BB, Friedman PJ, Liebow AA. Bronchiolitis obliterans: roentgenologic-pathologic correlation. *Radiology* 1973; 117: 816.
56. Lyons HA. Differential diagnosis of hemoptysis and its treatment. Basics of respiratory disease 1976; 5, No 2.
57. Thomas HM, Irwin RS. Classification of diffuse intrapulmonary hemorrhage. *Chest* 1975; 68: 483.
58. Addleman M, Logan AS, Grossman RF. Monitoring intrapulmonary hemorrhage in Goodpasture's syndrome. *Chest* 1985; 87: 119.
59. Greening AP, Hughes JMB. Serial estimations of carbon monoxide diffusing capacity in intrapulmonary hemorrhage. *Clin Sci* 1981; 60: 507.
60. Abboud RT, Chase WH, Ballon HS, et al. Goodpasture's syndrome: diagnosis by transbronchial lung biopsy. *Ann Intern Med* 1978; 89: 635.
61. Beechler CR, Enquist RW, Hunt KK, et al. Immunofluorescence of transbronchial biopsies in Goodpasture's syndrome. *Am Rev Respir Dis* 1980; 121: 869.
62. Leatherman JW, Sibley RK, DAvies SF. Diffuse intrapulmonary hemorrhage and glomerulonephritis unrelated to anti-glomerular basement membrane antibody. *Am J Med* 1982; 72: 401.
63. Keller F, Nekarda H. Fatal relapse in Goodpasture's syndrome three years after plasma exchange. *Respiration* 1985; 48: 62.
64. Erickson SB, Kurtz SB, Donadio JV, et al. Use of combined plasmapheresis and immunosuppression in the treatment of Goodpasture's syndrome. *Mayo Clin Proc* 1979; 54: 714.
65. Keller F, Offerman G, Schultze G, et al. Membrane plasma exchange in Goodpasture's syndrome. *Am J Med Sci* 1984; 287: 32.
66. Levin M. Rigden SPA, Pincott JR, et al. Goodpasture's syndrome: treatment with plasmapheresis, immunosuppression, and anticoagulation. *Arch Dis Child* 1983; 58: 697.
67. Shumak KH, Rock GA. Therapeutic plasma exchange. *N Engl J Med* 1984; 310 762.
68. Hyatt RW, Adelstein ER, Halazun JF, Lukens JN. Ultrastructure of the lung in idiopathic pulmonary hemosiderosis. *Am J Med* 1972; 52: 822.
69. Bailey P, Groden BM. Idiopathic pulmonary haemosiderosis: report of two cases and review of the literature. *Postgrad Med J* 1979; 55: 266.
70. Yeager H Jr, Powell D, Weinberg RM, et al. Idiopathic pulmonary hemosiderosis. Ultrastructural studies and response to azathioprine. *Arch Intern Med* 1976; 136: 1145.
71. Pozo-Rodriguiez F, Freire-Rampo JM, Gutierrez-Millet V, et al. Idiopathic pulmonary haemosiderosis treated by plasmapheresis. *Thorax* 1980; 35: 399.
72. Klippel JH, Decker JL. Clinical trials in the rheumatic diseases. *Clin Rheum Dis* 1983; 9: 489.
73. Rosenbloom D, Brooks P, Bellamy N, Buchanan W. *Clinical trials in the rheumatic diseases.* New York: Praeger Scientific, 1985.
74. Kelley WN, HArris ED Jr, Ruddy S, Sledge CB. *Textbook of rheumatology.* Philadelphia: WB Saunders Company, 1981.

# Chapter 19

# Sarcoidosis

*Bruce Davidson*

Sarcoidosis is a systemic disease of unknown aetiology characterised by the presence of non-caseating granulomas in involved tissues. Because of the presence of a constellation of immunological abnormalities, sarcoidosis is generally believed to be an immunological disorder, perhaps provoked by a yet undiscovered infection or other exogenous or endogenous agent.[1] Sarcoid granulomas have been found in nearly all organ systems, but lung, skin, liver, spleen, lymph node, ocular, salivary and lacrimal gland, bone, nasal sinus, cardiac, and brain involvement comprise the great majority of cases.[2] Pulmonary involvement is probably the most common feature, but may be present and asymptomatic or absent in those patients who present with disease elsewhere. Symptoms of pulmonary sarcoidosis include cough (usually non-productive), dyspnoea, and chest pain of a sharp or vague character that is neither anginal nor pleuritic. Fever, weakness, inanition, and weight loss may be constant, intermittent, or absent features. The disease is found worldwide, but identified more frequently where chest radiographs are frequently used. The incidence is greater in men than in women worldwide, but the reverse is true in the USA. The peak age of incidence is in the third decade, although sarcoid has been found in patients from 3 months to 80 years of age.[3]

## Diagnostic Features

In addition to the symptoms noted above, several other clinical features suggest the diagnosis of sarcoidosis. Pulmonary findings may include tachypnoea, crepitations, signs of consolidation, or wheezes. These are non-specific and may be absent in patients proven to have pulmonary involvement. Splenomegaly, hepatomegaly, lymph node enlargement, lacrimal and parotid gland enlargement, and characteristic skin lesions as well as erythema nodosum may all be present.

### The Chest Radiograph

Chest radiographs are of great value in suggesting the diagnosis. By international convention a radiological staging classification (Table 19.1) has been devised.[4] This is currently used more for classification than for staging, since staging implies determination of progression, and patient course and histopathological findings are often dissociated from the radiographic appearance. Bilateral hilar (with or without right paratracheal) adenopathy is a hallmark of the chest radiograph in sarcoidosis. While one paper suggested that this finding in asymptomatic young patients with normal examinations was enough to make a diagnosis of sarcoidosis without biopsy, the point is controversial.[5,6]

*Table 19.1* Radiological 'staging' (classification) of pulmonary sarcoidosis

| Stage | Description |
|---|---|
| O | Normal |
| 1 | Hilar, with or without paratracheal, adenopathy |
| 2 | Hilar adenopathy and parenchymal infiltrates |
| 3 | Parenchylmal infiltrates alone |

## Physiological Testing

Pulmonary physiological abnormalities are important clinical features of sarcoidosis. The arterial oxygen tension (and particularly the alveolar-arterial oxygen gradient) is the most sensitive though non-specific test of respiratory impairment, particularly when determinations are made at rest and at quantified levels of exercise. Significant haemoglobin desaturation and relative hypoxaemia upon exercise are the expected findings in disabling pulmonary sarcoidosis. Such studies remain the best and most objective measures of improvement or deterioration in an individual patient's course. Ideally they ought to be repeated periodically, particularly to document response to therapy when there are questions about its benefit or risk. Other physiological tests of help in following sarcoidosis patients include the diffusion capacity, a sensitive test of impairment in gas exchange; lung volumes, which usually show restriction; and spirometry, which usually shows a decreased vital capacity and normal or even supranormal air flow rates, reflected in the ratio of forced expiratory volume in the first second to forced vital capacity ($FEV_1/FVC$). Other tests of small airway function may show obstruction to airflow.

It should be emphasised that none of these tests taken alone or together at any single point in time can distinguish between the extent of active inflammatory sarcoidosis and fibrosed inactive disease.[1]

## Gallium-67 Scanning

The radionuclide gallium-67 scan has been studied extensively in the diagnosis and management of sarcoidosis. Its advantages are that isotope uptake identifies sites of disease activity, which can be used to advantage in selecting possible biopsy locations (lung, lacrimal glands, mediastinal lymph nodes). The extent and intensity of lung radionuclide uptake have been further proposed as an index of disease activity. Disadvantages include the fact that many interstitial lung diseases and neoplasia can all exhibit positive gallium scans. Moreover, an increased gallium index has only a weak correlation with clinical signs and symptoms, radiographic stage, and physiological data.[6,7]

## Broncho-alveolar Lavage

Broncho-alveolar lavage (BAL) is yet another technique that has been studied in relation to the diagnosis and management of sarcoidosis. BAL through the fibreoptic bronchoscope samples cells and fluid from the distal airspaces, and in sarcoidosis has shown high percentages of T lymphocytes from radiographically clear lungs, leading to the current concept of lymphocyte alveolitis in the disease.[1] Lymphocyte alveolitis may also be found in hypersensitivity pneumonitis, berylliosis, and Crohn's disease. Some authors have written that patients with more than 28% T lymphocytes in their BAL fluid have a worse prognosis and will require corticosteroid therapy.[8] This has not been a uniform finding, however, and a host of variables in lavage procedure and cell analysis, as well as new discoveries regarding lack of uniformity of lung T lymphocyte surface marker expression, lead me to regard BAL as a clinically inessential research procedure in the diagnosis and management of sarcoidosis.[9-11]

## Serum Angiotensin Converting Enzyme

Serum levels of angiotensin converting enzyme (ACE) and lysozyme have been found to be elevated in sarcoidosis, particularly with pulmonary involvement. They are, however, neither sufficiently sensitive nor specific enough to serve as a diagnostic test. In certain patients ACE levels may be a valuable indication of disease activity or response to therapy, although this also is controversial.[12]

## Biopsy

In nearly all cases of sarcoidosis, and particularly in those where therapy is considered, the diagnosis should be made by histopathological demonstration of non-caseating granulomas in biopsied tissue. This finding, together with negative stains and cultures for infecting organisms which lead to granulomatous inflammation (such as mycobacterial and fungal infections), and supporting clinical features allow a secure diagnosis. While sarcoidosis is a disease of multiple organ systems, biopsy of one is usually sufficient. For cases of suspected pulmonary involvement we and others rely on fibreoptic bronchoscopy under topical anaesthesia with endobronchial and/or transbronchial biopsies. With this approach, and with at least six adequate transbronchial biopsies obtained, the diagnosis can be made in more than 90% of patients even when the chest radiograph shows adenopathy without parenchymal infiltrates.[6,13] Where cutaneous involvement is apparent a skin punch biopsy is the procedure of first choice; in certain patients lacrimal, conjunctival, and lymph node biopsies may be preferable if there is apparent involvement of these tissues. Liver biopsy, once a mainstay of tissue diagnosis, is no longer highly preferred because of the host of unrelated causes that can lead to hepatic granulomas.

## The Kveim test

The Kveim test is another means of making a tissue diagnosis of sarcoidosis. Like biopsy, only a positive result (the identification of granulomatous inflammation at the site of prior injection of Kveim suspension) is of help; up to 70% of patients with stage 0 or stage 3 radiographs have negative Kveim tests. Because of the difficulty in obtaining reliable Kveim test materials and the four to six week wait after injection to biopsy the Kveim-induced papule, the Kveim reaction is not currently in frequent usage worldwide as a diagnostic test.[14]

## Natural History and Prognosis

Recent studies have focused on the natural history of sarcoidosis.[15] Large numbers of patients must be followed for long periods of time to give useful answers to natural history questions in this chronic disease, and satisfying those criteria will inherently cause possibly significant trends in smaller patient subsets to be diluted and overlooked. Therefore this sort of data can only be a guide, and is certainly not rigorously applicable to individual patients.

Studied by radiological classification, stage 1 patients had the best prognosis with 50% showing a normal radiograph within 15 months of the diagnosis; this included between 50 and 73% of all patients diagnosed. Stage 2 sarcoidosis was present in 21 to 34% of patients at diagnosis; it was six months before 50% of these patients had normal chest radiographs. For patients with stage 3 radiographs at diagnosis, 37% would show clearing of the chest X-ray, but this could take up to seven years. Approximately 10% of all patients in all stages would progress to some degree of permanent impairment with pulmonary fibrosis. Interestingly, the overall lifetime incidence of sarcoidosis in this study from Sweden was 1.3% for women and nearly 1% for men.

## Goals of Treatment

Ideally, the goals of drug treatment in sarcoidosis are twofold: to minimise disease symptoms, and to reverse or at least arrest the abnormalities associated with disease progression. Unfortunately, no such result has been reliably obtained in the drug therapy of sarcoidosis.

Corticosteroids have been used in the treatment of sarcoidosis for their anti-inflammatory and immunosuppressive effects. Regrettably, the data from numerous retrospective, many prospective, and even some prospective controlled and randomised studies have failed to substantiate the long-term efficacy of corticosteroid therapy in patients with pulmonary sarcoidosis.[6] Most of these studies show early improvement in symptoms and signs, but variable results with regard to chest radiographs and pulmonary function; however, evaluation of such patients at six months to three years after commencement of therapy shows no significant differences in symptoms, signs, chest radiographs, or pulmonary function between those treated with corticosteroids and those not treated. Some patients will show improvement with therapy that is early and sustained; others will show progressive deterioration despite years of high-dose corticosteroid therapy. The issues of when and how long to use corticosteroid therapy with its attendant complications are thus far from clarified, and are best decided by the physician and the informed patient. I reserve corticosteroid therapy for patients with systemic symptoms and findings that are not controlled with lesser measures. For example, fever and weight loss due to the disease will usually require corticosteroid therapy for alleviation. Granulomatous skin lesions will respond to periodical local steroid injection and painful erythema nodosum and mild arthralgia and myalgia will respond to aspirin therapy.

## Treatment

Major and significant manifestations of sarcoidosis are best treated with once-daily oral administration of corticosteroids. Indications for such treatment will vary with the patient and physician. What follows is my opinion based on literature review and personal experience. A summary appears in Table 19.2.

### Systemic Symptoms

Fever and weight loss are two systemic symptoms that nearly always require and will respond to corticosteroid therapy. These manifestations are subacute

*Table 19.2* Guidelines for treatment of manifestations of sarcoidosis*

| Manifestations | Treatment |
|---|---|
| Fever, inaniton, weight loss | Prednisone 20mg/day |
| Cough, dyspnoea | Prednisone 20-60mg/day |
| Ocular disease: | |
| Anterior uveitis; conjunctivitis | 1% Prednisone eye drops, mydriatics |
| Posterior uveitis, iridocyclitis | Prednisone 20-60mg/day |
| Neurosarcoidosis | Prednisone 40-60mg/day |
| Glandular sarcoidosis | Prednisone 20mg/day |
| Cutaneous disease: | |
| Pruritus and diffuse skin granulomas | Antipruritic lotion, oral antihistamine |
| Erythema nodosum | Aspirin, non-steroidal anti-inflammatory drugs |
| Disfiguring lesions | Intralesional steroids<br>Prednisone 20-40mg/day<br>Methotrexate 20mg/week |
| Liver disease | Prednisone 20-40mg/day |
| Myocardial disease | Prednisone 20-60mg/day<br>Anti-arrhythmic therapy |
| Complete heart block | Pacemaker |
| Myosarcoidosis | Prednisone 20-40mg/day |
| Arthritis and arthralgia | Aspirin, non-steroidal anti-inflammatory drugs<br>Colchicine |
| Hypercalcaemia and hypercalciuria | Oral phosphate<br>Restrict calcium intake<br>Prednisone 20mg/day<br>Colchicine |
| Alternatives to corticosteroid therapy and steroid-sparing agents: | Chlorambucil 4-14mg/day<br>Azathioprine 100mg/day<br>Methotrexate 5-20mg/week |

*See text for details of and indications for therapy.

in onset and their gradual rather than abrupt reversal is the therapeutic goal. This can nearly always be achieved over two to four weeks with single daily oral doses of 20mg of prednisone or its equivalent, and the therapeutic response is assessed by periodic weight and temperature checks. Therapy is best continued at this dose for four to six months before bi-monthly tapering at 5mg decrements. Quite commonly 10 to 15mg daily of prednisone is required long-term to prevent re-occurrence of these symptoms, although periodic attempts to further decrease corticosteroid therapy should be undertaken.

## Pulmonary Involvement

Not all pulmonary involvement with sarcoidosis requires therapy. Hilar adenopathy or even radiographic pulmonary infiltrates may be asymptomatic and thus would not require treatment. On the other end of the disease spectrum, impairment from pulmonary fibrosis is not expected to improve with corticosteroid therapy. Between these points lie the manifestations of pulmonary sarcoidosis worthy of a trial of corticosteroid therapy. Therapy is best guided by initial and subsequent objective evaluation of pulmonary function in the form of resting and exercise arterial blood oxygen tension, spirometry, lung volumes, and diffusing capacity.[16] Sarcoidosis can occur in patients with asthma, or with chronic obstructive pulmonary disease with or without bronchospasm, and bronchodilator therapy and cessation of cigarette smoking are important facets of treatment in these cases. When breathlessness occurs in the absence of significant oxygen desaturation of haemoglobin (more than 5%), in the absence of more than 30% impairment of a corrected diffusion capacity, or in the absence of at least 20 to 30% impairment of vital capacity, corticosteroid therapy is best withheld and another cause for breathlessness should be sought. If these criteria are present, a trial of therapy is worthwhile. I begin patients on 20mg of oral prednisone once daily and re-evaluate the patient's symptoms, chest radiograph, and vital capacity at two to four weeks. Improvement, rather than resolution, is the goal. In certain patients with moderate to severe impairment 40 to 60mg of prednisone once daily is begun. While some authors will start all patients at these higher doses, two points are worthy of emphasis: doses higher than 60mg of prednisone or its equivalent are rarely justified, and once-daily therapy is sufficient. Once begun, and in the absence of troublesome side effects, therapy is continued for four to six months before attempts are made to taper it. As in treating systemic symptoms, gradual decrements in dosage is the approach, with periodical evaluation of the parameters noted above. Flaring of disease is sometimes heralded by an increase in serum ACE level, and is dealt with by increasing the corticosteroid dose to the lowest level that will gradually suppress the abnormalities. Persistent breathlessness despite therapy should prompt a search for other complications, such as fixed upper airway obstruction or undiscovered pulmonary hypertension. Cough and chest pain respond favourably to analgesics and antitussive medications. In those patients with persistently active pulmonary sarcoidosis corticosteroid therapy may be needed for many years, and thus ought to be given at the lowest possible dose which can alleviate symptoms. Of note, inhaled steroid aerosols have not been found to be effective in pulmonary sarcoidosis.[17]

There are reports of successful use of alternate-day oral administration of corticosteroids, usually employed some months after disease control is achieved with a daily administered dose.[18,19] Since alternate-day administration does often ameliorate deleterious side effects, it can be tried in patients on chronic therapy. I will double the daily dose and give this every other day, and taper the dose over time. Failure of such a regimen usually dictates a return to a daily dosage schedule.

Systemic corticosteroid administration may provoke certain side effects unacceptable to the patient or physician, such as weight gain, diabetes mellitus, hypertension, acne, psychological changes, and so on. Numerous other drugs have been tried either in its place or for steroid-sparing effect. Most successfully used has been chlorambucil, which is begun at oral doses of 4 to 6mg once daily and increased to a maximum of 12mg/day. Improvement should be noticed within two to three months or the drug is discontinued. Because of chlorambucil's suppressive effect on the bone marrow, blood counts are monitored weekly initially and then every two to four weeks once a stable dose is achieved; the total white blood cell count is kept above 3500 per $mm^3$, and the platelet count above 80 000 per $mm^3$.[20] Azathioprine has been used at an oral dosage of 100mg once daily, and methotrexate at 20mg once weekly.[21,22] Both drugs may cause significant hepatotoxicity and are of uncertain efficacy.[23] Chloroquine, phenylbutazone, levamisole, and numerous other drugs have been used with widely varying views as to their therapeutic success.[23] Cyclosporin A, an immunosuppressive agent, was found ineffective for controlling pulmonary sarcoidosis in one small as yet unpublished prospective randomised trial.

**Extrapulmonary Sarcoidosis**

*Ocular involvement,* including anterior and posterior uveitis, scleral plaques, conjunctivitis, and papilloedema must be treated when diagnosed and managed in concert with an ophthalmologist. Ideally, all patients with the diagnosis of sarcoidosis ought to have a slit-lamp examination at the time of diagnosis. Fluorescein angiography may be required. Acute anterior uveitis and conjunctivitis can usually be successfully managed by instillation of a mydriatic solution and 1% prednisone eye drops. Certain patients with anterior and those with posterior uveitis will require oral corticosteroids and chronic iridocyclitis may be poorly responsive to topical and oral use of these agents.[23]

*Neurosarcoidosis* may present as a space-occupying lesion(s), meningitis, facial or other cranial nerve palsy, polyneuropathy, diabetes insipidus, papilloedema, or epilepsy. This is an indication for sustained steroid therapy at a dosage of 40 to 60mg of prednisone daily.[24]

*Glandular* involvement of sarcoidosis, apparent in the salivary or lacrimal glands, usually responds to low-dose (20mg) daily prednisone therapy.[24]

*Cutaneous* sarcoidosis may take the form of reactive erythema nodosum, a lesion not specific to sarcoidosis but which confers a good prognosis, or sarcoidal granulomas including lupus pernio of the face. Sarcoidal lesions on the skin do not necessarily scar or require therapy, and their presence tends to parallel disease activity. If pruritus is a problem, oral antihistamines and topical lubricating lotions containing menthol and phenol are indicated. Cosmetically disfiguring facial granulomas, often occurring on the nasal alae, are best treated with injections through a 25 to 27G needle of between

0.3 to 1.0ml of a 10mg/ml triamcinolone acetate suspension diluted with equal parts of 1% lignocaine (lidocaine) or procaine, to make a 5mg/ml solution. Injections may be repeated weekly or bi-weekly, and lesions should regrees over several weeks; they may recur if therapy is discontinued. Moderately severe lupus pernio may be improved by 5mg oral methotrexate given once weekly,[23,25] but liver function tests and blood counts must be periodically checked. Once disease control is achieved, the weekly methotrexate dose is slowly decreased by 2 to 5mg decrements.

*Hepatic* involvement with sarcoidosis is common, reflected by hepatomegaly and by granulomas seen in liver biopsies. Serum alkaline phosphatase levels may be elevated, but involvement extensive enough to cause cholestasis or symptoms is unusual.[26] When hepatic sarcoidosis must be treated, prednisone therapy at 20 to 40mg daily is the preferred therapy.

*Myocardial* conduction disease and *symptomatic muscle* sarcoidosis are best treated with corticosteroids. In one study, atrioventricular block and atrial and ventricular arrhythmias were improved in 16 to 25 patients with corticosteroids alone; daily dosages of 40 to 60mg of prednisone are generally used.[27-29] Myocardial involvement has led to sudden death, and anti-arrhythmic and pacemaker treatment may be required. Skeletal muscle involvement can be treated with 20 to 40mg of daily prednisone, and serum creatine phosphokinase (CPK) and aldolase levels are followed to assess response to therapy.

Sarcoidal *arthritis* and arthralgia are not uncommon. They may respond to aspirin and other non-steroidal anti-inflammatory drugs, or be so disabling that prednisone and chlorambucil are required. Colchicine at 0.5mg two or three times daily has been used for acute bouts of arthritis.[24]

*Hypercalcaemia* and *hypercalciuria* are caused by heightened gastrointestinal calcium absorption, a consequence of elevated calcitriol (dihydroxy vitamin $D_3$). Because these may lead to nephrocalcinosis and urinary calculi, patients with these findings are wise to restrict calcium intake and take oral phosphate in the form of 1 to 2g of effervescent phosphate daily in divided doses with meals. I prefer this conservative therapy to immediate institution of corticosteroids for this indication alone; the latter also are efficacious at low dosage (20mg prednisone daily) but may need to be continued for years. Recently, the intermittent administration of 500 mg of chloroquine phosphate with low-dose prednisone was reported to be successful in difficult cases.[30] Periodic determinations of 24-hour urinary calcium excretion allow assessment of adequacy and need for therapy.

## Summary of Treatment

In summary, drug therapy of sarcoidosis is individualised for each patient and is based on the principle that this is a chronic disorder with a usually favourable prognosis. Disease manifestations may be suppressed, but the final outcome is not significantly altered by potentially toxic drug therapy. Patient understanding and acceptance of these principles make therapeutic decisions and compliance more easily attained.

## Patient Education

As in any chronic disease, the reaction of the patient to his disease determines to a significant extent what the intensity of treatment will be. The admonition that sarcoidosis is a chronic disease, that its symptoms did not arise overnight and will not regress overnight, is a pithy and helpful way to explain the issue.

Patients ought to be alerted to the germane features of disease prognosis: that only 20 to 25% of patients experience appreciable deterioration in pulmonary function, with 5 to 10% eventually dying from the disease.[31,32] Additionally, the concept that corticosteroid therapy may ameliorate symptoms without altering the outcome requires careful explanation.

The reader is referred to the detailed discussion of corticosteroid therapy in Chapter 8. A preference for low-dose chronic therapy except under unusual circumstances has already been expressed in this chapter, and the physician must be willing to stop therapy if objectionable symptoms such as weight gain, or untoward events, such as diabetes mellitus, ensue. Patients must recognise that corticosteroid therapy requires close follow-up to monitor effectiveness and side effects. Physicians can, however, take some comfort in knowing that patients who precipitously stop taking their 15 or 20mg of daily prednisone are probably in less danger than if they were taking higher doses, and that they will probably not be deleteriously affecting the course of the sarcoidosis.

Patients must be cautioned that administration of immunosuppressive agents such as chlorambucil and methotrexate requires close follow-up, and must be alerted to signs of thrombocytopenia and bone marrow suppression as well as hepatitis. It is wise for the physician to prescribe small quantities of these medications frequently for those patients, where doubt exists as to the patient's reliability in returning for regular supervision of their drug therapy.

## References

1. Crystal RG, Roberts WC, Hunninghake GW, et al. Pulmonary sarcoidosis: a disease characterized and perpetuated by activated lung T-lymphocytes. *Ann Intern Med* 1981; 94: 73.
2. Mayock RL, Bertrand P, Morrison CE, et al. Manifestations of sarcoidosis. *Am J Med* 1963; 35: 67.
3. James DG, Neville E, Siltzbach LE, et al. A worldwide survey of sarcoid. In: Siltzbach LE, ed. Seventh International Conference on Sarcoidosis. *Ann NY Acad Sci* 1976; 278: 32.
4. Siltzbach LE, James DG, Neville E, et al. Course and prognosis of sarcoidosis around the world. *Am J Med* 1974; 57: 847.
5. Winterbauer RH, Belic N, Moores KK. A clinical interpretation of bilateral hilar adenopathy. *Ann Intern Med* 1983; 78: 65.
6. Thrasher DR, Briggs DD. Pulmonary sarcoidosis. In: Fulmer JD, et. Interstitial lung diseases. *Clin Chest Med* 1982; 3: 537.
7. Line BR, Fulmer JD, Reynolds HY, et al. Gallium-67 scanning to stage the alveolitis of sarcoidosis: correlation with clinical studies, pulmonary function studies, and bronchoalveolar lavage. *Am Rev Respir Dis* 1981; 123: 440.
8. Keough BA, Hunninghake GW, Line BR, Crystal RG. The alveolitis of pulmonary sarcoidosis: evaluation of natural history and alveolitis-dependent changes in lung function. *Am Rev Respir Dis* 1983; 128: 256.

9. Davidson BL, Faust J, Pessano S, Daniele RP, Rovera G. Differentiation and activation phenotypes of lung T lymphocytes differ from those of circulating T lymphocytes. *J Clin Invest* 1985; 76: 60.
10. Lin YH, Haslam PL, Turner-Warwick M. Chronic pulmonary sarcoidosis: relationship between lung lavage cell counts, chest radiograph, and results of standard lung function tests. *Thorax* 1985; 40: 501.
11. DeRemee RA. The alveolitis of pulmonary sarcoidosis. *Am Rev Respir Dis* 1984; 129: 343.
12. Cohen RD, Bunting PS, Meindok HO, et al. Does serum angiotension converting enzyme reflect intensity of alveolitis in sarcoidosis? *Thorax* 1985; 40: 497.
13. Rothe RA, Fuller PB, Byrd BR, et al. Transbronchoscopic lung biopsy in sarcoidosis: optimal number and sites of diagnosis. *Chest* 1980; 77: 400.
14. Israel HL. Diagnostic value of the Kveim reaction. In: Fanburg BL, ed. *Sarcoidosis and other granulomatous disorders of the lung*. New York: Marcel Dekker, 1983: 273.
15. Hillerdal G, Nou E, Osterman K, Schmekel B. Sarcoidosis: epidemiology and prognosis. *Am Rev Respir Dis* 1984; 130: 29.
16. Keough BA, Lakatos E, Price D, et al. Importance of the lower respiratory tract in oxygen transfer: exercise testing in patients with interstitial and destructive lung disease. *Am Rev Respir Dis* 1984; 129 (suppl S76).
17. Williams MH. Pulmonary function in sarcoidosis. In: Fanburg BL, ed. *Sarcoidosis and other granulomatous disorders of the lung*. New York: Marcel Dekker, 1983: 77.
18. Block AJ, Light RW. Alternate day steroid therapy in diffuse pulmonary sarcoidosis. *Chest* 1973; 63: 495.
19. Selroos O, Sellergren TL. Corticosteroid therapy of pulmonary sarcoidosis. *Scand J Respir Dis* 1979; 60: 215.
20. Kataria YP. Chlorambucil in sarcoidosis. *Chest* 1980; 78: 36.
21. Sharma O, Hughes DTD, James DG, et al. Immunosuppressive therapy with azathioprine in sarcoidosis. In: Levinsky L, Macholda F, eds. Fifth International Conference on Sarcoidosis, Universita Karlova, Praha, Prague. 1971: 635.
22. Israel HL. Effects of chlorambucil and methrotrexate in sarcoidosis. In: Levinsky L, Macholda F, eds. Fifth International Conference on Sarcoidosis, Universita Karlova, Praha, Prague. 1971: 632.
23. James DG, Williams WJ. *Sarcoidosis and other granulomatous disorders*. Philadelphia: WB Saunders, 1985.
24. Sharma OP. *Sarcoidosis*. London: Butterworths, 1984: 165.
25. Veien NK, Brodthagen H. Cutaneous sarcoidosis treated with methotrexate. *Br J Dermatol* 1977; 97: 213.
26. Crofton J, Douglas A. *Respiratory diseases*. 3rd ed. Oxford: Blackwell Scientific Publications, 1981: 463.
27. Sekigudi M, Suda T, Furni T, et al. Long-term prognosis of cardiac sarcoidosis patients with permanent pacemaker implantation. In: Chretien J, Marsac J, Saltiel J, eds. Proceedings of the Ninth International Congress on Sarcoidosis, Paris: Pergammon Press, 1981: 658.
28. Ishikawa T, Kondoh H, Nakagawa S, et al. Steroid therapy in cardiac sarcoidosis: increased left ventricular contractility concomitant with electrocardiographic improvements after prednisolone. *Chest* 1984; 85: 445.
29. Stein E, Stimmel B, Siltzbach LE. Clinical course of cardiac sarcoidosis. *Ann NY Acad Sci* 1976; 278: 470.
30. O'Leary TJ, Jones G, Yip A, et al. The effects of chloroquine on serum 1,25-dihydroxyvitamin D and calcium metabolism in sarcoidosis. *N Engl J Med* 1986; 315: 727.
31. Mitchell DN, Scadding JG. State of the art: sarcoidosis. *Am Rev Respir Dis* 1974; 110: 774.
32. Israel HL. Prognosis of sarcoidosis. *Ann Intern Med* 1970; 73: 1038.

# Chapter 20

# Adverse Effects of Drugs on the Lungs

*J. Allen D. Cooper Jr and Richard A. Matthay*

Pulmonary reactions occur in response to a variety of drug treatments. Although cancer chemotherapeutic agents are most commonly associated with pulmonary injury, drugs utilised in the treatment of benign disorders also have been implicated. Currently more than 30 commonly used agents are known to affect the respiratory system directly (Table 20.1); others cause pulmonary alterations as part of a systemic reaction.

This chapter deals with direct adverse effects of these pharmacological agents on the respiratory system. Although effects on any organ system may indirectly affect the respiratory system, indirect effects are not discussed here. In addition, although a brief discussion of the effects of certain drugs on respiratory muscle function is included, effects of drugs on the respiratory control centre are not addressed. The discussion is limited to commonly used therapeutic agents; syndromes such as talc-induced pulmonary granulomatosis, and hypertension secondary to illicit drugs, or pulmonary hypertension due to formerly used agents such as aminorex are not included. These syndromes are discussed in several previous reviews.[1,2] This review outlines common pulmonary syndromes associated with administration of commonly employed pharmacological agents.

The discussion is organised by individual clinical syndromes. Three important ways that drugs may affect respiratory function are through (i) pulmonary parenchymal damage, (ii) airway alterations resulting in bronchospasm, and (iii) respiratory muscle dysfunction. The most common drug-induced alteration is pulmonary parenchymal damage. This category can be subdivided into clinical syndromes of chronic fibrosis/pneumonitis, hypersensitivity lung disease, non-cardiogenic pulmonary oedema, bronchiolitis obliterans, and a pulmonary/renal syndrome resembling Goodpasture's syndrome. We first discuss basic mechanisms of these clinical syndromes associated with drug administration, then outline potential risk factors, and finally present the clinical aspects. Because of space constraints each drug cannot be discussed in detail. The reader is referred to a recent review for further definition of the subject.[3]

## Chronic Pneumonitis/Fibrosis

### Mechanism

Drugs that cause this clinical syndrome are listed in Table 20.2. There are three basic mechanisms by which drugs may produce pulmonary fibrosis: (i) oxidant production; (ii) immunological alterations; and (iii) effects on

*Table 20.1* Pharmacological agents causing respiratory system alterations

| Cytotoxic agents | Frequency (%) | Non-cytotoxic agents | Frequency (%) |
|---|---|---|---|
| Bleomycin | 4-6 | Nitrofurantoin | <1 |
| Mitomycin | 3-12 | Amphotericin† | <1 |
| Neocarzinostatin | <1 | Other antibiotics | <1 |
| Busulphan | 4 | Sulphasalazine | <1 |
| Cyclophosphamide | <1 | Aspirin‡ | 22 |
| Chlorambucil | <1 | Heroin‡ | 33 |
| Melphalan | <1 | Dextropropoxyphene‡ | <1 |
| Carmustine | 20-30 | Methadone‡ | <1 |
| Other nitrosoureas | <1 | Ethchlorvynol‡ | <1 |
| Methotrexate | 7 | Chlordiazepoxide‡ | <1 |
| Azathioprine | <1 | Phenytoin | <1 |
| Cytarabine | NK | Carbamazepine | <1 |
| Procarbazine | NK | Hydrochlorothiazide | <1 |
| Teniposide | <1 | Haloperidol | <1 |
| Vinblastine* | NK | Amiodarone | 5 |
| Vindesine* | NK | Lignocaine (lidocaine) | <1 |
| | | Tocainide | <1 |
| | | Gold salts | <1 |
| | | Penicillamine | <1 |
| | | Colchicine‡ | <1 |

*In conjunction with mitomycin therapy.
†In conjunction with leucocyte transfusions.
‡Reported with overdose only.
NK = not known.

collagen metabolism. Oxidants such as the superoxide anion ($O_2^-\cdot$), hydrogen peroxide ($H_2O_2$), the hydroxyl radical ($OH\cdot$), singlet oxygen ($^1O_2$) and hypochlorous acid (HOCl) have been implicated in a variety of disease states including the adult respiratory distress syndrome, pulmonary oxygen toxicity and radiation-induced pulmonary damage.[4] Toxic effects appear to occur through fatty acid oxidation which may lead to membrane instability.[4] Bleomycin, cyclophosphamide and nitrofurantoin produce oxidants *in vitro*.[3] This suggests that a mechanism of pulmonary damage by certain toxic pulmonary pharmacological agents may be similar to that of oxygen and radiation, that is, oxidant-induced membrane damage.

*Table 20.2* Drugs that cause chronic pneumonitis/fibrosis

| Cytotoxic agents | Non-cytotoxic agents |
|---|---|
| Bleomycin | Nitrofurantoin |
| Mitomycin | Sulphasalazine |
| Neocarzinostatin | Amiodarone |
| Busulphan | Tocainide |
| Cyclophosphamide | Gold salts |
| Chlorambucil | Penicillamine |
| Melphalan | |
| Carmustine | |
| Other nitrosoureas | |
| Methotrexate | |

Alteration of the pulmonary immunological system by certain drugs also may be important in producing chronic pneumonitis. Resident pulmonary cells release a number of mediators that may amplify toxic reactions by attracting and activating inflammatory cells; drug administration may enhance this mediator release. For example, bleomycin administration may result in the release of factors chemotactic for polymorphonuclear leucocytes (PMN) by alveolar macrophages,[3] and cyclophosphamide has been shown to enhance delayed hypersensitivity in non-pulmonary systems.[5] In addition, non-cytotoxic drugs including nitrofurantoin[3] and gold salts[3] enhance blastogenesis of lymphocytes from patients with pneumonitis due to these agents. Finally, in humans, bronchoalveolar lavage (BAL) — a technique helpful in examining pulmonary inflammatory disorders — has shown evidence of a lymphocyte alveolitis in patients with pneumonitis due to methotrexate,[6] gold salts[7] and amiodarone.[8] All these studies suggest that influx of inflammatory cells may be important in propagating pulmonary damage due to pharmacological agents.

The balance between collagen deposition and degradation is important in the lung. An imbalance towards increased amounts of collagen, or deposition of collagen that is resistant to degradation, may result in fibrosis. Drugs that may affect this system include bleomycin, penicillamine and gold salts.[3] Bleomycin directly stimulates fibroblasts,[9] cells that are primarily responsible for deposition of collagen. Paradoxically, alveolar macrophages from bleomycin-treated animals produce soluble factors that suppress fibroblast growth. Production of these factors may be important in regulating the amount of pulmonary fibrosis produced by bleomycin.[10] Both penicillamine and gold salts affect collagen directly. Penicillamine causes a reduction in insoluble collagen and impairs wound healing in rats;[3] gold salts increase cross-linking of the collagen molecule, thus altering its structure.[3]

## Risk Factors

Risk factors are outlined in Table 20.3. Both cumulative and maintenance doses appear to be important in the drug-related development of chronic pneumonitis/fibrosis. Cumulative dosage is important in the case of chronic pneumonitis due to bleomycin[11] and carmustine.[11] In fact, carmustine shows a linear relationship between cumulative dose and toxicity.[11] In contrast, the risk of developing amiodarone-induced pneumonitis increases with increasing maintenance dose although cumulative dose does not appear to play a role.[12]

Age may be another important risk factor for pneumonitis caused by cancer chemotherapeutic agents and drugs used for benign conditions. This may be due to the decreased antioxidant defences manifested with increasing age.[3] Radiation therapy and oxygen therapy potentiate pulmonary damage due to bleomycin[13,14] and possibly mitomycin.[3] Oxygen therapy alone potentiates pulmonary injury due to cyclophosphamide[15] and nitrofurantoin[16] in animal models. This synergy between the toxicity of oxygen or radiation therapy and drug-induced pulmonary toxicity may be due to the common production of reactive oxygen species.

Use of combined cancer chemotherapeutic agents increases the likelihood of pulmonary reactions.[3] Chemotherapeutic drugs that exhibit such a relationship include carmustine, mitomycin, cyclophosphamide, bleomycin

*Table 20.3* Risk factors for drug-induced pulmonary disease

| Risk factor | Drug(s) implicated |
|---|---|
| Cumulative dose | Bleomycin, busulphan, carmustine |
| Maintenance dose | Amiodarone |
| Age | Bleomycin |
| Concurrent or previous radiotherapy | Bleomycin, busulphan, mitomycin |
| Oxygen therapy | Bleomycin, cyclophosphamide, mitomycin, nitrofurantoin |
| Other drug therapy | Carmustine, mitomycin, cyclophosphamide, bleomycin, methotrexate |
| Pre-existing pulmonary disease | Carmustine |
| Leucocyte transfusions | Amphotericin |

and methotrexate.[3] Also, although cyclophosphamide alone rarely produces chronic pneumonitis or any pulmonary toxicity, it is a common component of these multiple drug regimens which show increased pulmonary toxicity.[3]

## Clinical and Histological Features

Chronic pneumonitis/fibrosis is the most common manifestation of drug-induced pulmonary disease and has been associated with virtually all categories of pneumotoxic cancer chemotherapeutic drugs in addition to selected non-cytotoxic drugs (Table 20.2).[3] Bleomycin is the drug most commonly associated with this syndrome; approximately 4% of patients receiving this drug develop some degree of pneumonitis.[3] Typical symptoms include progressive dyspnoea on exertion, a non-productive cough, and fatigue and malaise developing over a period of several weeks or months. Physical examination commonly reveals bi-basilar end-expiratory crackles and, less commonly, muscle wasting or digital clubbing. Laboratory examination may show an elevated erythrocyte sedimentation rate (ESR) which, in the case of amiodarone-induced pulmonary toxicity, returns to normal with resolution of the disease.

The chest radiograph in drug-induced chronic pneumonitis/fibrosis commonly shows a reticulonodular infiltrate (Figure 20.1) although findings may be normal even in a setting of abnormal pulmonary function tests or histologically proven pulmonary fibrosis. Unusual chest radiographic manifestations include large nodular lesions simulating metastatic disease[17] and diffuse acinar infiltrates.[18] Diffuse pulmonary gallium uptake has also been documented.[19] Pleural effusions are rare.

Pulmonary function testing in patients with clinically significant chronic pneumonitis/fibrosis due to drug administration commonly shows a restrictive ventilatory defect and a reduced diffusing capacity. In addition, an isolated reduction in the diffusing capacity for carbon monoxide may occur in asymptomatic patients. Numerous investigators have examined the diffusing capacity for carbon monoxide as a screening procedure in patients receiving bleomycin. They have found that, although a significant reduction from the baseline value is a useful warning sign, it is not absolutely predictive of

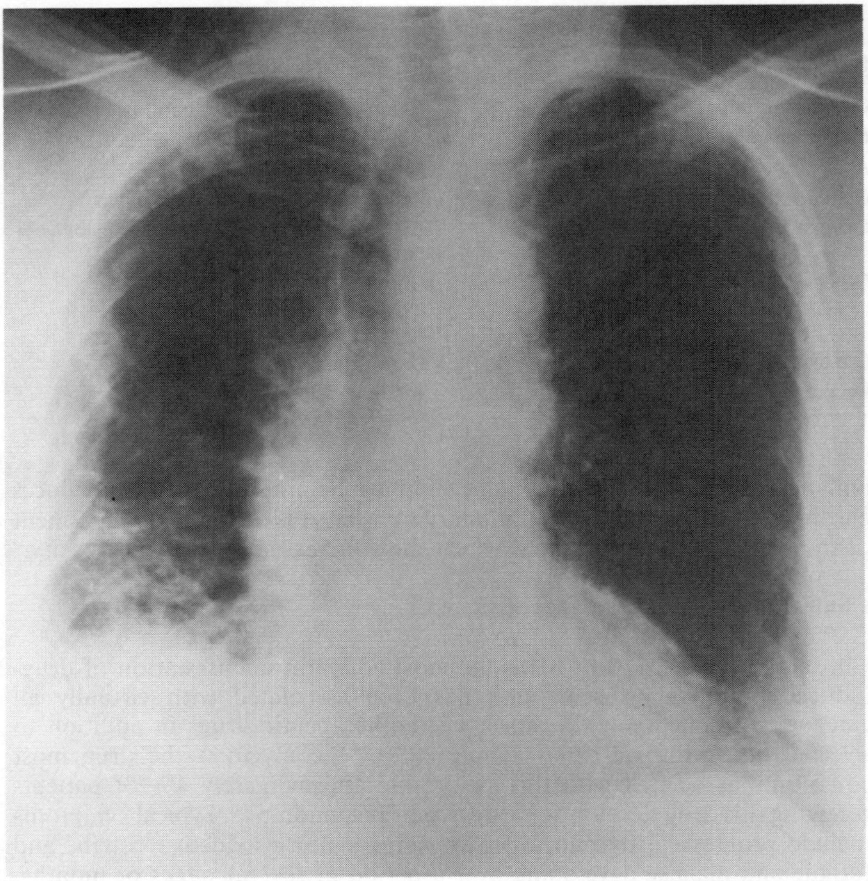

*Figure 20.1* Chest radiograph of a patient with diffuse histiocytic lymphoma who developed shortness of breath and radiographic abnormalities after therapy with a multidrug regimen containing bleomycin. Note the bi-basilar reticular infiltrates and apparent lung volume loss.

significant pulmonary disease. Recently, Van Barneveld et al[20] showed that a combination of a low creatinine clearance with decreased lung volume and vital capacity in the absence of a reduction in the pulmonary capillary blood volume is the best predictor of clinically significant bleomycin-induced pulmonary disease.

The histological picture of drug-induced chronic pneumonitis/fibrosis consists of endothelial cell damage with swelling and blebbing, epithelial abnormalities with desquamation of type 1 pneumocytes and type 2 pneumocyte dysplasia and fibroblast proliferation with fibrosis.[21] Patients developing the clinical syndrome in association with penicillamine therapy also may show some degree of bronchiolitis. In general, treatment of this syndrome is difficult. Discontinuation of the offending agent should be the first manoeuvre. Use of corticosteroids has been helpful in selected cases especially when associated with mitomycin[22] or bleomycin[18] therapy. However, even with improvement, residual symptoms may occur and radiographic or pulmonary function abnormalities often persist.

## Hypersensitivity Lung Disease

### Mechanism

Drugs causing hypersensitivity reactions are listed in Table 20.4. The overwhelming evidence suggests that these reactions are due to activation of the pulmonary immunological system. This evidence includes the reversibility of the syndrome and response to corticosteroids, the common association of peripheral eosinophilia and fever, other signs of hypersensitivity such as dermatitis or hepatitis, and the histological picture of acute inflammation. However, to date no experimental studies have established the basic mechanisms of this syndrome.

*Table 20.4* Drugs that cause hypersensitivity lung disease

| Cytotoxic drugs | Non-cytotoxic drugs | |
|---|---|---|
| Bleomycin | Nitrofurantoin | Para-aminosalicylic acid |
| Methotrexate | Sulphasalazine | Penicillin |
| Procarbazine | Sulphadimethoxine | Sodium cromoglycate |
| | Phenytoin | Dantrolene |
| | Carbamazepine | Methylphenidate |
| | Chlorpropamide | Mephenesin carbamate |
| | Imipramine | Hydrallazine |
| | Isoniazid | Mecamylamine |
| | | Ampicillin |

### Risk Factors

There are no clear-cut risk factors for development of this syndrome secondary to drug treatment. Some patients developing the syndrome have exhibited previous hypersensitivity reactions in other organ systems to the implicated drug.[33] However, the majority of patients have not shown such a history. Tapering of corticosteroids that have been part of a multidrug regimen may be a risk factor for developing the syndrome in association with methotrexate or procarbazine therapy.[3]

### Clinical and Histological Features

An acute syndrome often associated with peripheral eosinophilia has been described in association with numerous non-cytotoxic drugs and three cancer chemotherapeutic agents (Table 20.4)[24-26] The clinical presentation is similar for all drugs causing this syndrome and consists of dyspnoea, non-productive cough and fever developing rapidly over several hours to days. Development of the syndrome is unrelated to cumulative drug dosage. Laboratory examination reveals significant peripheral eosinophilia in up to 80% of cases[3] and an elevated ESR in the majority of cases.

The chest radiograph in drug-induced hypersensitivity lung disease is the same as that seen in idiopathic forms of the syndrome. Findings include peripheral acinar infiltrates (Figure 20.2) commonly associated with unilateral or bilateral pleural effusions. Diffuse reticular infiltrates are also uncommonly noted. Pulmonary function tests generally show a restrictive ventilatory defect and diffusion impairment. Chest radiographic and pulmonary function abnormalities rapidly reverse with improvement of the syndrome.

Histological findings in drug-induced hypersensitivity pulmonary syndromes are characteristic and show alveolar and interstitial cellular infiltration with significant numbers of eosinophils. There is a general lack of surrounding pulmonary fibrosis. Treatment includes withdrawal of the offending agent and institution of corticosteroids. Improvement is as rapid as the onset of the syndrome and may occur within days or, at most, a week. The minority of patients (fewer than 10%) exhibit residual pulmonary abnormalities several months after resolution of the syndrome.

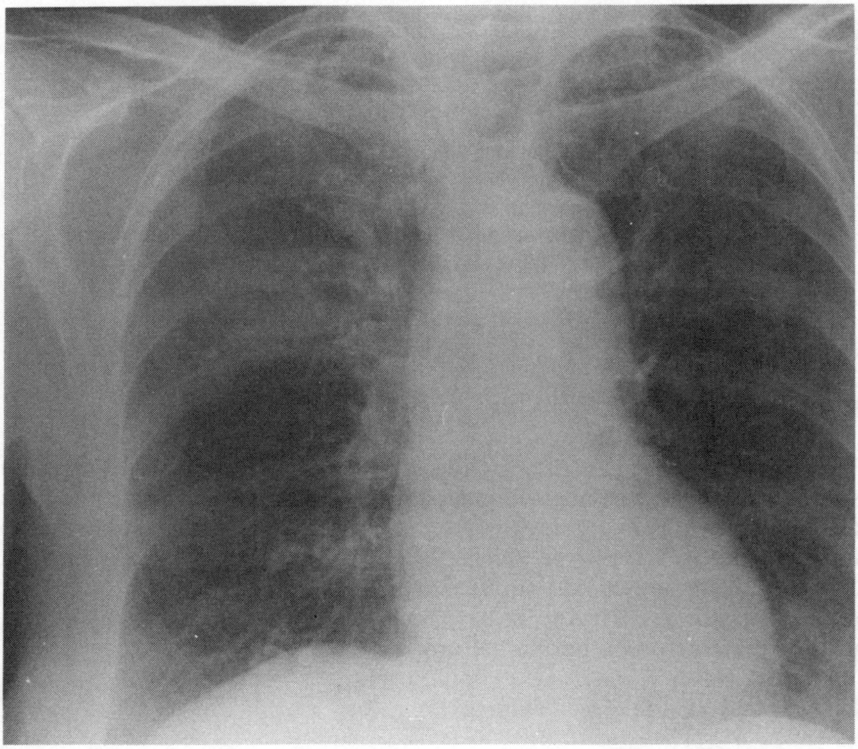

*Figure 20.2* Chest radiograph of a patient receiving imipramine therapy who developed shortness of breath in conjunction with a significant peripheral eosinophilia. Note the right upper zone acinar infiltrate. This infiltrate cleared rapidly with discontinuation of the offending drug and institution of corticosteroid therapy.

## Non-cardiogenic Pulmonary Oedema

### Mechanism

Drugs thought to cause this syndrome are listed in Table 20.5. Little work has been done concerning mechanisms of drug-induced non-cardiogenic pulmonary oedema. However, complement activation may be important; patients with this syndrome due to terbutaline[27] and heroin[28] have shown evidence of serum complement activation. In review, complement activation results in the production of multiple inflammatory components that have been implicated in causing non-cardiogenic pulmonary oedema during dialysis or in the setting of sepsis.

Direct effects of leucocytes also may be an important mechanism of drug-induced non-cardiogenic pulmonary oedema. Amphotericin, a drug thought to cause this syndrome, is directly toxic to polymorphonuclear leucocytes,[3] and non-cardiogenic pulmonary oedema due to this agent occurs in the setting of leucocyte transfusions,[29] a situation that results in abnormal circulating polymorphonuclear leucocytes.

Mechanisms of drug-induced non-cardiogenic pulmonary oedema that have been proposed, but have no supporting clinical or laboratory data, include central nervous system effects of the drugs[30] and alterations in arachidonic acid metabolism.[30] The first proposal is attractive because patients presenting with non-cardiogenic pulmonary oedema secondary to drugs such as aspirin[30] and opiates[31] often have altered sensoria. In addition, opiate receptors are present near the respiratory control centre,[3] and application of drugs in this area may result in pulmonary oedema.[3] Alterations in arachidonic acid metabolism have been proposed as a mechanism for aspirin-induced non-cardiogenic pulmonary oedema.[30] Aspirin inhibits the cyclo-oxygenase enzyme,[32] which may result in an overabundant production of permeability-inducing arachidonic acid metabolities, namely leukotrienes. However, there is no strong experimental evidence to support this theory to date.

## Risk Factors

A risk factor for this syndrome is drug overdose. In fact, non-cardiogenic pulmonary oedema due to aspirin, colchicine, sedatives and opiates[3] occurs only in the setting of overdose of these agents. In addition, leucocyte transfusions precipitate non-cardiogenic pulmonary oedema due to amphotericin therapy.[29] Amphotericin alone does not appear to cause this syndrome.

## Clinical and Histological Features

Non-cardiogenic pulmonary oedema is associated primarily with drugs used for benign conditions and usually in the setting of overdose.[27,30,31] However,

*Table 20.5* Drugs that cause non-cardiogenic pulmonary oedema

| Cytotoxic agents | Non-cytotoxic agents | |
|---|---|---|
| Cyclophosphamide | Nitrofurantoin | Ethchlorvynol |
| Methotrexate | Amphotericin | Chlordiazepoxide |
| Cytarabine | Aspirin | Hydrochlorothiazide |
| Teniposide | Heroin | Haloperidol |
| | Propoxyphene | Lignocaine |
| | Methadone | Colchicine |

certain cancer chemotherapeutic agents are associated with it as well (Table 20.5).[33,34] Methotrexate-induced non-cardiogenic pulmonary oedema has been reported after intrathecal administration of the drug,[33] a unique feature of this agent. Onset of symptoms is acute and the syndrome is fully developed within one to two days of onset. Clinical manifestations include severe dyspnoea, obtundation and hypoxaemia.

Chest radiograph abnormalities are the same as those seen in other forms of non-cardiogenic pulmonary oedema and consist of diffuse reticular or acinar infiltrates without cardiomegaly (Figure 20.3). Pulmonary function tests, performed in a few patients, have shown a reduction in total lung compliance and a restrictive ventilatory defect. Histological abnormalities include diffuse pulmonary oedema with hyaline membrane formation. Treatment is primarily supportive with oxygen administration and ventilatory assistance. The prognosis is variable. There is a high mortality with development of non-cardiogenic pulmonary oedema after methotrexate[24,33] or cytosine arabinoside[3,34] administration. However, the prognosis is better when the syndrome is due to administration of other drugs than when the cause is non-drug related, presumably because the precipitating stimulus can be removed.[3]

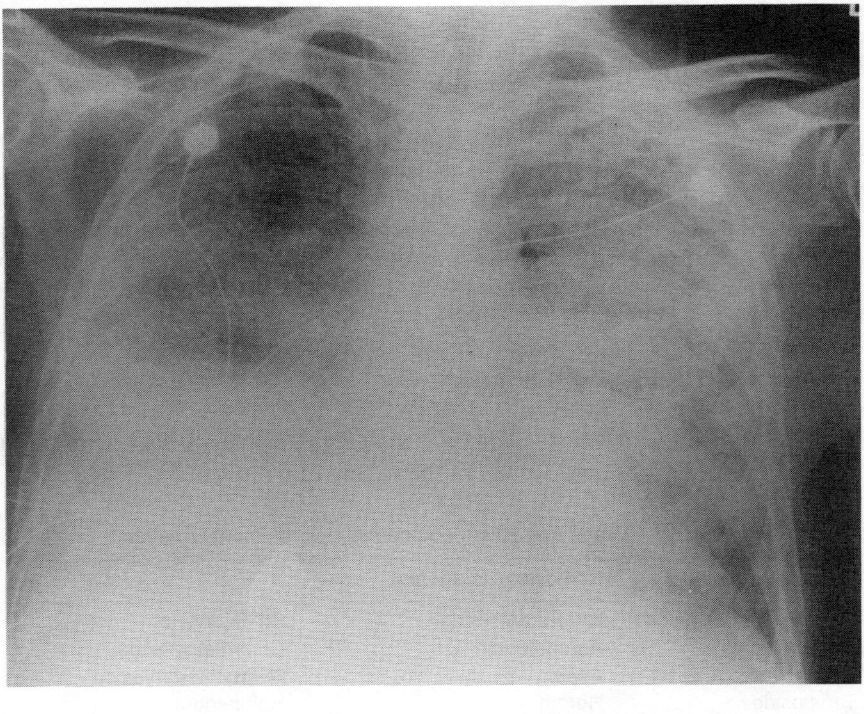

*Figure 20.3* Chest radiograph of a patient presenting with non-cardiogenic pulmonary oedema after a methadone overdose. Note the diffuse acinar infiltrates.

## Bronchiolitis Obliterans

### Mechanism

Penicillamine[35,36] and sulphasalazine[37] are the only two drugs associated with this syndrome. Although there are no studies of specific mechanisms of drug-induced bronchiolitis obliterans, penicillamine does affect collagen metabolism as previously described,[3] and this may be one way in which this drug causes bronchiolitis.

### Risk Factors

It is not known whether the underlying diseases (rheumatoid arthritis and ulcerative colitis) of the patients reported with this syndrome are important risk factors. However, rheumatoid arthritis itself has resulted in bronchiolitis obliterans;[38] an interaction between drug and disease state may be important.

### Clinical and Histological Features

Bronchiolitis obliterans is an uncommon complication of drug administration and has been reported in association with sulphasalazine[37] and penicillamine[35,36] therapy. Because eight of the nine cases reported have occurred in a setting in which the underlying disease (ulcerative colitis or rheumatoid arthritis) may involve the lungs, determination of causality is difficult. However, each case showed some evidence that the pharmacological agent was the inciting factor. Symptoms, developing insidiously, are similar to those seen with chronic pneumonitis/fibrosis including dyspnoea on exertion and a non-productive cough. The chest radiograph may be normal or may show localised acinar infiltrates. Gallium uptake in areas of radiographic abnormalities has also been documented.[3]

In contrast to the previous clinical syndromes, pulmonary function tests in patients with drug-induced bronchiolitis obliterans primarily show airway obstruction,[37] although a restrictive component may also be present, and the diffusing capacity of carbon monoxide is commonly reduced as well. Pulmonary histological abnormalities consist of characteristic obliteration of bronchioles with surrounding parenchymal inflammation.[3] Effective treatment is unclear, because few cases are available for analysis. Even with withdrawal of the agent and institution of corticosteroids, the prognosis is poor; four of the patients died and the others showed some residual pulmonary impairment.[3]

## Pulmonary Renal Syndrome

### Mechanism

Penicillamine is the only pharmacological agent associated with a disorder similar to Goodpasture's syndrome.[39] Paradoxical exacerbations of systemic autoimmune phenomena have been reported after therapy with this drug; this may be a mechanism for the syndrome. The similarity to Goodpasture's syndrome is consistent with this theory.

### Risk Factors

In the few patients reported with this syndrome, length of treatment and cumulative dose appear to be important risk factors. Penicillamine was administered for longer than one year in the four cases reported.[39]

### Clinical and Histological Features

Development of pulmonary infiltrates and haemoptysis in conjunction with haematuria and uraemia has been described in four patients treated with penicillamine.[39] The clinical presentation is indistinguishable from the idiopathic form of Goodpasture's syndrome except for the relationship to penicillamine therapy and an atypical immunofluorescence pattern on renal biopsy. Signs and symptoms, which occur one to two years after initiation of penicillamine therapy and develop rapidly, include haemoptysis, haematuria, dyspnoea and pleuritic chest pain. The chest radiograph shows diffuse reticular or acinar infiltrates with multiple large nodular lesions noted in one patient.[39] Lungs from patients with the pulmonary renal syndrome due to penicillamine therapy show evidence of alveolar haemorrhage and mild fibrosis. Prognosis is poor; three of the four patients have died. The survivor underwent plasmapheresis while receiving corticosteroids and azathioprine.[39]

## Drug-induced Bronchospasm

### Mechanism

Numerous pharmacological agents may induce bronchospasm. The majority of these reactions are in association with systemic type 1 allergic reactions, and these are not discussed here. The reader is referred to a previous review of the subject.[40] However, there are categories of drugs that induce bronchospasm primarily in asthmatics through non-allergic mechanisms (Table 20.6). These are discussed briefly in this section.

*Table 20.6* Drugs that cause bronchospasm by non-allergic mechanisms

| | |
|---|---|
| Aspirin | Isoetharine |
| Indomethacin | Terbutaline |
| Zomepirac | Propranolol |
| Ibuprofen | Timolol |
| Phenylbutazone | Pindolol |
| Methacholine | Naldolol |
| Carbachol | Sodium cromoglycate |
| Bethanechol | Ethanol |
| Pilocarpine | Penicillamine |

Although the mechanism by which non-steroidal anti-inflammatory agents induce bronchospasm is unclear, the inhibition of cyclo-oxygenase with a subsequent increase in the known bronchoconstricting arachidonic acid metabolites, 12-L-hydroxy-5,8,10,14-eicosatetraenoic acid (HETE) and leukotrienes may be important.[32] Beta-antagonists such as propranolol also induce bronchospasm, probably through inhibition of beta activity of the bronchial smooth muscle, which may be important in maintaining a degree of bronchodilatory tone.[41] However, other mechanisms may be important in the bronchoconstricting effect of these agents. At least one study has suggested that beta-antagonistic effects do not totally explain the bronchoconstriction induced by 'beta blockers'.[42] Cholinergic agents also may precipitate bronchospasm, probably through stimulation of cholinergic innervation of bronchial smooth muscle and subsequent bronchoconstriction.[43]

## Risk Factors

An overwhelming risk factor for drug-induced bronchospasm is a history of asthma.[40] Of the drugs that precipitate bronchospasm by apparent non-allergic mechanisms, only propranolol has been implicated in normal individuals without a history of asthma.[44] In the case of non-steroidal anti-inflammatory agent-induced bronchospasm, age, female gender, and the presence of nasal polyps are risk factors.[32] Removal of the polyps may transiently exacerbate the asthmatic condition.

## Clinical and Histological Features

Non-steroidal anti-inflammatory agents such as aspirin, indomethacin, ibuprofen and phenylbutazone have been shown to induce bronchospasm in 4 to 19% of adult asthmatics.[32] This analgesic intolerance increases with age and is often associated with peripheral eosinophilia (in up to 50% of the cases). Such reactions are commonly associated with nasal polyposis and rhinitis and occur more frequently in females. Onset of bronchospasm generally occurs 30 to 90 minutes after ingestion of the drug. Treatment is similar to that for other forms of bronchospasm and includes bronchodilators and corticosteroids. Progressive desensitisation with aspirin has had variable results.[32] This procedure should only be attempted under closely supervised conditions because severe bronchospasm may occur if desensitisation is not done correctly.

Cholinergic agents such as methacholine, carbachol, bethanechol and pilocarpine may cause acute airway obstruction, also primarily in asthmatics. Pilocarpine may reduce flow rates in asthmatics when administered locally to the eye.[45] Clinical features of these reactions are not well documented. However, treatment consists of withdrawal of the drug and administration of atropine parenterally or by inhalation. Other bronchodilators such as beta-sympathetic agonists and methyl xanthines may be of some use, as well.

Paradoxically, beta-sympathetic agonists such as terbutaline and isoetharine rarely induce bronchospasm in asthmatics.[46] This is ironic because these agents are commonly used to treat bronchospasm. However, there is some evidence that components of the drug preparation other than the beta-agonist are responsible for the bronchoconstricting effect. Treatment of this condition includes alternate bronchodilator therapy.

Beta-sympathetic antagonists such as propranolol, timolol, pindolol and naldolol[47] have also been shown to induce bronchospasm, primarily in asthmatics. There is some evidence that normal subjects are not totally immune from this effect.[44] The association of timolol with this syndrome is especially important because patients who react to this drug do so after ophthalmic treatment,[48] a situation that can be easily overlooked. As with aspirin-induced bronchospasm, symptoms occur one hour after use of the beta-blocker and may be severe; several patients have required mechanical ventilation. Treatment includes supportive measures, administration of bronchodilators and withdrawal of the offending beta-antagonist. Prevention by maintaining a high index of suspicion and avoiding beta-blocker therapy in high-risk patients is of utmost importance.

Other drugs that induce bronchospasm through non-allergic mechanisms include inhaled sodium cromoglycate,[49] ethanol[50] and penicillamine.[51] The reader is referred to the referenced case reports of these reactions.

## Respiratory Muscle Dysfunction

### Mechanism

The aminoglycoside antibiotics have a curare-like effect, blocking acetylcholine receptors and subsequently causing paralysis.[52] Succinylcholine causes paralysis by inducing membrane depolarisation and then a prolonged insensitivity to neuromuscular transmission and subsequent paralysis.[53]

### Risk Factors, Clinical and Histological Features

Succinylcholine may induce severe apnoea within one to two minutes after administration.[53] This effect may be extremely prolonged in patients with pseudocholinesterase deficiency. Antibiotics including aminoglycosides,[52] penicillin[52] and polymixin[54] can cause acute repiratory failure secondary to respiratory muscle dysfunction. An antihypertensive agent trimetaphan camsylate has also caused respiratory paralysis in one patient.[55] Signs and symptoms include severe dyspnoea with an orthopnoeic component, hypoxaemia and reduced motion of the diaphragm. The chest radiograph may show an elevated hemi-diaphragm and reduced lung volumes. Treatment involves supportive measures including mechanical ventilation in severe cases. Some improvement may occur with calcium or neostigmine therapy.

## Summary

The drug-induced pneumopathies are a heterogeneous group of disorders that may be caused by a variety of pharmacological agents. Damage to the respiratory system culminates in a limited number of manifestations including pulmonary parenchymal damage, airway alterations and respiratory muscle dysfunction. By recognising these syndromes and knowing risk factors for drug-induced pulmonary alterations, the physician can avoid serious pumonary reactions.

## References


1. Rosenow EC. The spectrum of drug-induced pulmonary disease. *Ann Intern Med* 1972; 77: 977-991.
2. Robertson CH Jr, Reynolds RC, Wilson JE III. Pulmonary hypertension and foreign body granulomas in intravenous drug abusers. Documentation by cardiac catheterization and lung biopsy. *Am J Med* 1976; 61: 657-664.
3. Cooper JAD Jr, White DA, Matthay RA. Drug-induced pulmonary disease. *Am Rev Respir Dis* 1986 133: 321-340, 488-505.
4. Freeman BA, Crapo JD. Biology of disease: free radicals and tissue injury. *Lab Invest* 1982; 47: 412-426.
5. Askenase PW, Hayden BJ, Gershon RK. Augmentation of delayed-type hypersensitivity by doses of cyclophosphamide which do not affect antibody responses. *J Exp Med* 1974; 141: 697-702.
6. White DA, Gellene R, Rankin JR, Gupta S, Gunningham-Rundles C, Stover DE. Methotrexate pneumonitis: bronchoalveolar lavage findings suggest an immune mediated disorder. *Am Rev Respir Dis* 1984; 129: A64. Abstract.
7. Ettensohn DB, Roberts NJ, Condemi JJ. Bronchoalveolar lavage in gold lung. *Chest* 1984; 85: 569-570.
8. Akoun GM, Gauthier-Rahman S, Milleron BJ, Perrot JY, Mayaud CM. Amiodarone-induced hypersensitivity pneumonitis. Evidence of an immunological cell-mediated mechanism. *Chest* 1984; 85: 133-135.
9. Otsuka K, Murota S, Mori Y. Stimulatory effect of bleomycin on the synthesis of acid glycosaminoglycans in cultured fibroblasts derived from rat granuloma. *Biochim Biophys Acta* 1976; 444: 359-368.
10. Clark JG, Kostal KM, Marino BA. Bleomycin-induced pulmonary fibrosis in hamsters. An alveolar macrophage product increases fibroblast prostaglandin E2 and cyclic adenosine monophosphate and suppresses fibroblast proliferation and collagen production. *J Clin Invest* 1983; 72: 2082-2091.
11. Ginsberg SJ, Comis RL. The pulmonary toxicity of antineoplastic agents. *Sem Oncol* 1982; 9: 34-51.
12. Marchlinski FE, Gansler TS, Waxman HL, Josephson ME. Amiodarone pulmonary toxicity. *Ann Intern Med* 1982; 97: 839-845.
13. Phillips TL, Fu KK. Quantification of combined radiation therapy and chemotherapy effects on critical normal tissues. *Cancer* 1976; 37: 1186-1200.
14. Goldiner PL, Carlon GC, Cvitkovic E, Schweizer O, Howland WS. Factors influencing postoperative morbidity and mortality in patients treated with bleomycin. *Br Med J* 1978; 1: 1664-1667.
15. Hakkinen PJ, Whiteley JW, Witschi HR. Hyperoxia, but not thoracic x-irradiation, potentiates bleomycin and cyclophosphamide-induced lung damage in mice. *Am Rev Respir Dis* 1982; 126: 281-285.
16. Boyd MR, Catignani GL, Sasame HA, Mitchell JR, Stiko AW. Acute pulmonary injury in rats by nitrofurantoin and modification by vitamin E, dietary fat and oxygen. *Am Rev Respir Dis* 1979; 120: 93-99.
17. Glasier CM, Siegel MJ. Multiple pulmonary nodules: usual manifestation of bleomycin toxicity. *Am J Roentgenol* 1981; 137: 155-156.
18. White DA, Stover DE. Severe bleomycin-induced pneumonitis: clinical features and response to corticosteroids. *Chest* 1984; 86: 723-728.
19. Richman SD, Levenson SM, Bunn PA, Flinn GS, Johnston GS, DeVita VT. $^{67}$Ga accumulation in pulmonary lesions associated with bleomycin therapy. *Cancer* 1975; 6: 1966-1972.
20. Van Barneveld PWC, Van Der Mark W, Sleijfer DTh, Mulder NH. Schraffordt Koop predictive factors for bleomycin-induced pneumonitis. *Am Rev Respir Dis* 1984; 130: 1078-1081.
21. Muggia FM. Pulmonary toxicity of antitumor agents. *Cancer Treat Rev* 1983; 10: 221-243.
22. Buzdar AU, Legha SS, Luna MA, Tashima CK, Hortobagyi GN, Blumenschein GR. Pulmonary toxicity of mitomycin. *Cancer* 1980; 45: 236-244.
23. Michael JR, Rudin ML. Acute pulmonary disease caused by phenytoin. *Ann Intern Med* 1981; 95: 452-454.

24. Sostman HD, Matthay RA, Puytman CE. Methotrexate-induced pneumonitis. *Medicine* 1976; 55: 371-388.
25. Holoye PY, Luna MA, MacKay B, Bedrossian CWM. Bleomycin hypersensitivity pneumonitis. *Ann Intern Med* 1978; 88: 47-49.
26. Jones SE, Moore M, Blank N, Castellino RA. Hypersensitivity to procarbazine (Matulane) manifested by fever and pleuropulmonary reaction. *Cancer* 1972; 29: 498-500.
27. Bowen RE, Dedhia HV, Beatty J, Schiebel F, Koss W, Granados J. ARDS associated with the use of sympathomimetics and glucocorticoids for the treatment of premature labor. *Crit Care Med* 1983; 11: 671-672.
28. Smith WR, Wells ID, Glauser FL, Novey HS. Immunologic abnormalities in heroin lung. *Chest* 1975; 68: 651-653.
29. Wright DG, Robichaud KJ, Pizzo PA, Deisseroth AB. Lethal pulmonary reactions associated with the combined use of amphotericin B and leukocyte transfusions. *N Engl J Med* 1981; 304: 1185-1189.
30. Heffner JE, Sahn SA. Salicylate-induced pulmonary edema: clinical features and prognosis. *Ann Intern Med* 1981; 95: 405-409.
31. Steinberg AD, Karliner JS. The clinical spectrum of heroin pulmonary edema. *Arch Intern Med* 1968; 122: 122-127.
32. Slepian IK, Mathews KP, McLean JA. Aspirin-sensitive asthma. *Chest* 1985; 87: 386-391.
33. Bernstein ML, Sobel DB, Wimmer RS. Noncardiogenic pulmonary edema following injection of methotrexate into the cerebrospinal fluid. *Cancer* 1982; 50: 866-868.
34. Haupt HM, Hutchins GM, Moore GW, Ara-C lung: noncardiogenic pulmonary edema complicating cytosine arabinoside therapy of leukemia. *Am J Med* 1981; 70: 256-261.
35. Scott DL, Bradby GVH, Altman TJ, Zaphiropoulos GC, Hawkins CF. Relationship of gold and penicillamine therapy to diffuse interstitial lung disease. *Ann Rheum Dis* 1981; 40: 136-141.
36. Epler GR, Snider GL, Gaensler EA, et al. Bronchiolitis and bronchitis in connective tissue disease. A possible relationship to the use of penicillamine. *JAMA* 1979; 242: 528-532.
37. Wang KK, Bowyer BA, Fleming CR, Schroeder K. Pulmonary infiltrates and eosinophilia associated with sulfasalazine. *Mayo Clin Proc* 1984; 59: 343-346.
38. Lyle WH. D-Penicillamine and fatal obliterative bronchiolitis. *Br Med J* 1977; 1: 105.
39. Matloff DS, Kaplan MM. D-Penicillamine-induced Goodpasture's-like syndrome in primary biliary cirrhosis. Successful treatment with plasmapheresis and immunosuppressives. *Gastroenterol* 1980; 78: 1046-1049.
40. Kounis NG. A review: drug-induced bronchospasm. *Ann Allergy* 1976; 37: 285-291.
41. Trautlein J, Allegra J, Field J, Gillin M. Paradoxic bronchospasm after inhalation of isoproterenol. *Chest* 1976; 70: 711-714.
42. Maclagan J, Ney UM. Investigation of the mechanism of propranolol-induced bronchoconstriction. *Br J Pharmacol* 1979; 66: 409-418.
43. Taytard A, Vergeret J, Auzerie J, Freour P. Ascetylcholine-induced bronchospasm in asthma patients: dose/response curves. *Eur J Respir Dis* 1983; 128 (suppl): 513-514.
44. Fraley DS, Bruns FJ, Segel DP, Adler S. Propranolol-related bronchospasm in patients without history of asthma. *South Med J* 1980; 73: 238-240.
45. Taylor P. Cholinergic agonists. In: Gilman AG, Goodman LS, Gilman A, eds. *The pharmacological basis of therapeutics.* New York: Macmillan, 1980.
46. Koepke JW, Christopher KL, Chai H, Selner JC. Dose-dependent bronchospasm from sulfites in isoetharine. *JAMA* 1984; 251: 2982-2983.
47. Mattson K, Poppius H. Controlled study of the bronchoconstriction effect of pindolol administered intravenously or orally to patients with unstable asthma. *Eur J Clin Pharmacol* 1978; 14: 87-92.
48. Charan NB, Lakshminarayan S. Pulmonary effects of topical timolol. *Arch Intern Med* 1980; 140: 843-844.
49. Serup J. Severe asthmatic reaction during long-term treatment with disodium cromoglycate powder inhalations. *Acta Med Scand* 1979; 205: 447-448.
50. Gong H Jr, Tashkin DP, Calvarese BM. Alcohol-induced bronchospasm in an asthmatic patient. Pharmacologic evaluation of the mechanism. *Chest* 1981; 80: 167-173.
51. Tanphaichitr K. D-Penicillamine-induced bronchial spasm. *South Med J* 1980; 73: 788-790.

52. Pittinger C, Adamson R. Antibiotic blockade of neuromuscular function. *Annu Rev Pharmacol* 1972; 12: 169-184.
53. Argov Z, Mastaglia FL. Disorders of neuromuscular transmission caused by drugs. *N Engl J Med* 1979; 301: 409-413.
54. Colvard MC Jr. Respiratory paralysis secondary to the use of polymixin B. *South Med J* 1971; 64: 652.
55. Dale RC, Schroeder ET. Respiratory paralysis during treatment of hypertension with trimethaphan camsylate. *Arch Intern Med* 1976; 136: 816-818.

# Index